T0226982

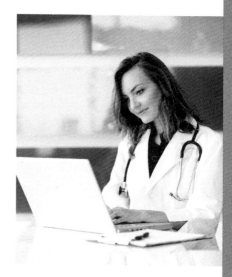

Chest Imaging

Editors

DAVID A. LYNCH
JONATHAN H. CHUNG

CLINICS IN CHEST MEDICINE

www.chestmed.theclinics.com

June 2015 • Volume 36 • Number 2

ELSEVIER

1600 John F. Kennedy Boulevard • Suite 1800 • Philadelphia, Pennsylvania, 19103-2899

http://www.theclinics.com

CLINICS IN CHEST MEDICINE Volume 36, Number 2
June 2015 ISSN 0272-5231, ISBN-13: 978-0-323-38880-1

Editor: Patrick Manley
Developmental Editor: Casey Jackson

Clinics in Chest Medicine (ISSN 0272-5231) is published quarterly by Elsevier Inc., 360 Park Avenue South, New York, NY 10010-1710. Months of issue are March, June, September, and December. Periodicals postage paid at New York, NY and additional mailing offices. Subscription prices are $345.00 per year (domestic individuals), $556.00 per year (domestic institutions), $165.00 per year (domestic students/residents), $380.00 per year (Canadian individuals), $690.00 per year (Canadian institutions), $470.00 per year (international individuals), $690.00 per year (international institutions), and $230.00 per year (international and Canadian students/residents). International air speed delivery is included in all Clinics subscription prices. All prices are subject to change without notice. **POSTMASTER:** Send address changes to Clinics in Chest Medicine, Elsevier Health Sciences Division, Subscription Customer Service, 3251 Riverport Lane, Maryland Heights, MO 63043. **Customer Service: Telephone: 1-800-654-2452** (U.S. and Canada); **1-314-447-8871** (outside U.S. and Canada). **Fax: 1-314-447-8029. E-mail: journalscustomerservice-usa@elsevier.com (for print support); journalsonlinesupport-usa@elsevier.com (for online support).**

Reprints. For copies of 100 or more of articles in this publication, please contact the Commercial Reprints Department, Elsevier Inc., 360 Park Avenue South, New York, NY 10010-1710. Tel.: 212-633-3874; Fax: 212-633-3820; E-mail: reprints@elsevier.com.

Clinics in Chest Medicine is covered in *MEDLINE/PubMed (Index Medicus), Current Contents/Clinical Medicine, EMBASE/ Excerpta Medica, Science Citation Index,* and *ISI/BIOMED.*

Contributors

EDITORS

DAVID A. LYNCH, MB
Professor, Department of Radiology, National
Jewish Health, Denver, Colorado

JONATHAN H. CHUNG, MD
Associate Professor, Department of Radiology,
National Jewish Health, Denver, Colorado

AUTHORS

JEFFREY B. ALPERT, MD
Assistant Professor of Radiology, Thoracic
Section, Department of Radiology, NYU
Langone Medical Center, New York,
New York

MATTHEW R. BENTZ, MD
Fellow, Cardiothoracic Radiology, Department
of Radiology, Oregon Health and Science
University, Portland, Oregon

SONIA L. BETANCOURT CUELLAR, MD
Assistant Professor, Section of Thoracic
Imaging, Department of Diagnostic Radiology,
The University of Texas MD Anderson Cancer
Center, Houston, Texas

SANJEEV BHALLA, MD
Professor, Cardiothoracic Imaging,
Mallinckrodt Institute of Radiology,
Washington University School of Medicine in
St Louis, St Louis, Missouri

KATRINA H. BUSBY, MD
Associate Professor of Internal Medicine,
Division of Pulmonary, Critical Care and
Sleep Medicine, University of New Mexico
Health Science Center, Albuquerque,
New Mexico

BRETT W. CARTER, MD
Assistant Professor, Section of Thoracic
Imaging, Department of Diagnostic Radiology,
The University of Texas MD Anderson Cancer
Center, Houston, Texas

CAROLINE CHILES, MD
Professor, Department of Radiology, Wake
Forest University Health Sciences Center,
Winston-Salem, North Carolina

JARED D. CHRISTENSEN, MD
Assistant Professor, Department of Radiology,
Duke University Medical Center, Durham,
North Carolina

JONATHAN H. CHUNG, MD
Associate Professor, Department of Radiology,
National Jewish Health, Denver, Colorado

KRISTOPHER W. CUMMINGS, MD
Senior Associate Consultant; Assistant
Professor, Cardiothoracic Radiology, Mayo
Clinic Arizona, Phoenix, Arizona

PATRICIA M. DE GROOT, MD
Assistant Professor, Section of Thoracic
Imaging, Department of Diagnostic Radiology,
The University of Texas MD Anderson Cancer
Center, Houston, Texas

RACHAEL M. EDWARDS, MD
Resident, Department of Radiology, University
of Washington Medical Center, Seattle,
Washington

JEREMY J. ERASMUS, MD
Professor, Section of Thoracic Imaging,
Department of Diagnostic Radiology, The
University of Texas MD Anderson Cancer
Center, Houston, Texas

ARYEH FISCHER, MD
Department of Rheumatology, National Jewish Health, Denver, Colorado

TIMOTHY J. HARKIN, MD
Associate Professor, Division of Pulmonary, Critical Care and Sleep Medicine, Department of Medicine, Icahn School of Medicine at Mount Sinai, New York, New York

KIRK JORDAN, MD
Associate Professor, Department of Radiology, University of Texas Southwestern, Dallas, Texas

JEFFREY P. KANNE, MD
University of Wisconsin School of Medicine and Public Health, Madison, Wisconsin

LOREN KETAI, MD
Professor, Department of Radiology, University of New Mexico Health Science Center, Albuquerque, New Mexico

GREGORY KICSKA, MD, PhD
Assistant Professor, Department of Radiology, University of Washington Medical Center, Seattle, Washington

JANE P. KO, MD
Professor of Radiology, Thoracic Section, Department of Radiology, NYU Langone Medical Center, New York, New York

TILMAN L. KOELSCH, MD
Department of Radiology, National Jewish Health, Denver, Colorado

BRENT P. LITTLE, MD
Assistant Professor, Division of Cardiothoracic Imaging, Department of Radiology and Imaging Sciences, Emory University, Atlanta, Georgia

CONOR M. LOWRY, MD
Instructor of Radiology, Thoracic Section, Department of Radiology, NYU Langone Medical Center, New York, New York

DAVID A. LYNCH, MB
Professor, Department of Radiology, National Jewish Health, Denver, Colorado

CRISTOPHER A. MEYER, MD
University of Wisconsin School of Medicine and Public Health, Madison, Wisconsin

SAEED MIRSADRAEE, MD, PhD
Senior Clinical Lecturer in Radiology, Clinical Research Imaging Centre, Queen's Medical Research Institute, University of Edinburgh, Edinburgh, United Kingdom

DAVID P. NAIDICH, MD, FACR, FACCP
Professor, Department of Radiology, Center for Biological Imaging, NYU-Langone Medical Center, New York, New York

SUDHAKAR N.J. PIPAVATH, MD
Associate Professor, Department of Radiology, University of Washington Medical Center, Seattle, Washington

STEVEN L. PRIMACK, MD
Professor of Medicine, Division of Pulmonary Medicine; Professor of Radiology and Vice Chairman, Department of Radiology, Oregon Health and Science University, Portland, Oregon

J. CALEB RICHARDS, MD
Department of Radiology, National Jewish Health, Denver, Colorado

RODNEY SCHMIDT, MD, PhD
Professor, Department of Pathology, University of Washington Medical Center, Seattle, Washington

DANIELLE M. SEAMAN, MD
Duke University Medical Center, Durham, North Carolina

MARIA SHIAU, MD
Associate Professor, Department of Radiology, Center for Biological Imaging, NYU-Langone Medical Center, New York, New York

JOSHUA J. SOLOMON, MD
Department of Respiratory and Critical Care Medicine, National Jewish Health, Denver, Colorado

YUTAKA TSUCHIYA, MD
Department of Radiology, National Jewish
Health, Denver, Colorado; Department of
Respiratory Medicine, Showa University
Fujigaoka Hospital, Yokohama, Japan

EDWIN J.R. VAN BEEK, MD, PhD
SINAPSE Chair of Clinical Radiology, Clinical
Research Imaging Centre, Queen's Medical
Research Institute, University of Edinburgh,
Edinburgh, United Kingdom

Contents

> Computed tomography (CT) is central to the detection and diagnosis of a wide variety of pulmonary, cardiovascular, and other diseases of the chest. Successful interpretation of thoracic CT requires both an appreciation of the spectrum of normal appearances of the chest and a systematic approach to the characterization of thoracic pathology. This article provides an introduction to basic CT techniques and protocols, a review of normal CT anatomy, and an overview of commonly encountered abnormalities.

> Low-dose computed tomographic (LDCT) screening is now moving from clinical trials to clinical practice, following the report from the National Lung Screening Trial that LDCT screening for lung cancer can reduce the number of deaths from lung cancer by 20% in current and former smokers, ages 55 to 74 years, with a 30 pack-year smoking history. This article reviews the current evidence for screening, key elements of a successful lung cancer screening clinic, and reporting and management guidelines for LDCT screening findings.

> The development of widespread lung cancer screening programs has the potential to dramatically increase the number of thoracic computed tomography (CT) examinations performed annually in the United States, resulting in a greater number of newly detected, indeterminate solitary pulmonary nodules (SPNs). Additional imaging studies, such as fluorodeoxyglucose F 18 (FDG)–positron emission tomography (PET), have been shown to provide valuable information in the assessment of indeterminate SPNs. Newer technologies, such as contrast-enhanced dual-energy chest CT and FDG-PET/CT, also have the potential to facilitate diagnosis of potentially malignant SPNs.

> Primary lung cancer is the leading cause of cancer mortality in the world. Thorough clinical staging of patients with lung cancer is important, because therapeutic options and management are to a considerable degree dependent on stage at

presentation. Radiologic imaging is an essential component of clinical staging, including chest radiography in some cases, computed tomography, MRI, and PET. Multiplanar imaging modalities allow assessment of features that are important for surgical, oncologic, and radiation therapy planning, including size of the primary tumor, location and relationship to normal anatomic structures in the thorax, and existence of nodal and/or metastatic disease.

Thoracic imaging is widely used to detect lower respiratory tract infections, identify their complications, and aid in differentiating infectious from noninfectious thoracic disease. Less commonly, the combination of imaging findings and a clinical setting can favor infection with a specific organism. This confluence can occur in cases of bronchiectatic nontuberculous mycobacterial infections in immune-competent hosts, invasive fungal disease among neutropenic patients, *Pneumocystis jiroveci* pneumonia in patients with AIDS, and in cytomegalovirus infections in patients with recent hematopoietic cell transplantation. These specific diagnoses often depend on computed tomography scanning rather than chest radiography alone.

Chest radiography serves a crucial role in imaging of the critically ill. It is essential in ensuring the proper positioning of support and monitoring equipment, and in evaluating for potential complications of this equipment. The radiograph is useful in diagnosing and evaluating the progression of atelectasis, aspiration, pulmonary edema, pneumonia, and pleural fluid collections. Computed tomography can be useful when the clinical and radiologic presentations are discrepant, the patient is not responding to therapy, or in further defining the pattern and distribution of a radiographic abnormality.

Pulmonary vascular diseases encompass a large and diverse group of underlying pathologies ranging from venous thromboembolism to congenital malformations to inflammatory vasculitides. As a result, patients can present either acutely with dyspnea and chest pain or chronically with dyspnea on exertion, hypoxia, and right heart failure. Imaging, particularly with multidetector CT, plays a key role in the evaluation and management of patients with suspected pulmonary vascular disease and, given the widespread routine use of high-quality CT pulmonary angiography, it is imperative that radiologists be familiar these pathologies.

Occupational and environmental lung disease remains a major cause of respiratory impairment worldwide. Despite regulations, increasing rates of coal worker's pneumoconiosis and progressive massive fibrosis are being reported in the United States. Dust exposures are occurring in new industries, for instance, silica in hydraulic fracking. Nonoccupational environmental lung disease contributes to major respiratory disease, asthma, and COPD. Knowledge of the imaging patterns of occupational and environmental lung disease is critical in diagnosing patients with occult exposures and managing patients with suspected or known exposures.

contiguous high-resolution, 1-mm to 1.5-mm images. These images enable high-definition axial, coronal, and sagittal reconstructions, as well as advanced imaging techniques, including minimum intensity projection images and virtual bronchoscopy. Current indications most commonly include patients presenting with signs and symptoms of possible central airway obstruction, with or without hemoptysis. In addition to diagnosing airway abnormalities, computed tomography (CT) also serves a critical complementary role to current bronchoscopic techniques for both diagnosing and treating airway lesions. Advantages of CT include noninvasive visualization of the extraluminal extent of lesions, as well as visualization of airways distal to central airways obstructions. As discussed and illustrated later, thorough knowledge of current bronchoscopic approaches to central airway disease is essential for optimal correlative CT interpretation.

High-resolution chest computed tomography (CT) is one of the most useful techniques available for imaging bronchiolitis because it shows highly specific direct and indirect imaging signs. The distribution and combination of these various signs can further classify bronchiolitis as either cellular/inflammatory or fibrotic/constrictive. Emphysema is characterized by destruction of the airspaces, and a brief discussion of imaging findings of this class of disease is also included. Typical CT findings include destruction of airspace, attenuated vasculatures, and hyperlucent as well as hyperinflated lungs.

Standard imaging for the lungs allow excellent visualization of normal and abnormal pulmonary patterns. Computed tomography (CT), however, has limitations. The recognized patterns have limited specificity, do not always diagnose the pathology at a treatable stage, and do not provide physiologic information. Advances allow more physiologic approaches in lung imaging, namely, functional imaging. The main functional lung imaging modalities are CT and MRI. Contrast and noncontrast imaging approaches study pulmonary perfusion, dynamics of the flow in the pulmonary artery, and motion. Noble gases allow assessment of regional pulmonary ventilation. We discuss the role of novel imaging techniques in the functional lung assessment.

PROGRAM OBJECTIVE

The goal of the *Clinics in Chest Medicine* is to provide provide practitioners with state-of-the-art information that is clinically useful, concise, well referenced, and comprehensive.

TARGET AUDIENCE

All practicing physicians and healthcare professionals who provide patient care utilizing findings from *Chest Medicine Clinics of North America*.

LEARNING OBJECTIVES

Upon completion of this activity, participants will be able to:
1. Review methods of ICU and infection imaging.
2. Discuss methods of CT screening for and the staging of lung cancer.
3. Recognize the uses of central and small airway imaging in diseases such as emphysema.

ACCREDITATION

The Elsevier Office of Continuing Medical Education (EOCME) is accredited by the Accreditation Council for Continuing Medical Education (ACCME) to provide continuing medical education for physicians.

The EOCME designates this enduring material for a maximum of 15 *AMA PRA Category 1 Credit*(s)™. Physicians should claim only the credit commensurate with the extent of their participation in the activity.

All other health care professionals requesting continuing education credit for this enduring material will be issued a certificate of participation.

DISCLOSURE OF CONFLICTS OF INTEREST

The EOCME assesses conflict of interest with its instructors, faculty, planners, and other individuals who are in a position to control the content of CME activities. All relevant conflicts of interest that are identified are thoroughly vetted by EOCME for fair balance, scientific objectivity, and patient care recommendations. EOCME is committed to providing its learners with CME activities that promote improvements or quality in healthcare and not a specific proprietary business or a commercial interest.

The planning committee, staff, authors and editors listed below have identified no financial relationships or relationships to products or devices they or their spouse/life partner have with commercial interest related to the content of this CME activity:

Jeffrey B. Alpert, MD; Matthew R. Bentz, MD; Sonia L. Betancourt Cuellar, MD; Sanjeev Bhalla, MD; Katrina H. Busby, MD; Caroline Chiles, MD; Jared D. Christensen, MD; Jonathan H. Chung, MD; Kristopher W. Cummings, MD; Patricia M. de Groot, MD; Rachael M. Edwards, MD; Jeremy J. Erasmus, MD; Anjali Fortna; Timothy J. Harkin, MD; Kristen Helm; Kirk Jordan, MD; Loren Ketai, MD; Gregory Kicska, MD, PhD; Tilman L. Koelsch, MD; Brent P. Little, MD; Conor M. Lowry, MD; David A. Lynch, MB; Patrick Manley; Saeed Mirsadraee, MD, PhD; Palani Murugesan; David P. Naidich, MD, FACR, FACCP; Steven L. Primack, MD; J. Caleb Richards, MD; Rodney Schmidt, MD, PhD; Maria Shiau, MD; Joshua J. Solomon, MD; Yutaka Tsuchiya, MD; Edwin J.R. van Beek, MD, PhD.

The planning committee, staff, authors and editors listed below have identified financial relationships or relationships to products or devices they or their spouse/life partner have with commercial interest related to the content of this CME activity:

Brett W. Carter, MD has an employment affiliation with Amirsys, Inc; is a consultant/advisor for St. Jude Medical, Inc; and has research support from ACRIN.
Aryeh Fischer, MD is on the speakers' bureau for and is a consultant/advisor for Actelion Pharmaceuticals US, Inc; Gilead; InterMune; Boehringer Ingelheim GmbH; Bayer AG; and Seattle Genetics, Inc.; and has research support from InterMune.
Jeffrey P. Kanne, MD is a consultant/advisor for Parexel Informatics.
Jane P. Ko, MD receives royalties/patents from Elsevier B.V., is on the speakers' bureau for Siemens Corporation, and her spouse/partner has an employment affiliation with Alexion.
Cristopher A. Meyer, MD receives royalties/patents for film interpretation and lectures on occupational lung disease, and is a consultant/advisor for medicolegal expert testimony.
Sudhakar N.J. Pipavath, MD is a consultant/advisor for Boehringer Ingelheim GmbH.
Danielle M. Seaman, MD is a consultant/advisor for medicolegal expert testimony in the field of occupational lung disease, and receives research support from Bracco Diagnostic Inc.

UNAPPROVED/OFF-LABEL USE DISCLOSURE

The EOCME requires CME faculty to disclose to the participants:
1. When products or procedures being discussed are off-label, unlabelled, experimental, and/or investigational (not US Food and Drug Administration [FDA] approved); and
2. Any limitations on the information presented, such as data that are preliminary or that represent ongoing research, interim analyses, and/or unsupported opinions. Faculty may discuss information about pharmaceutical agents that is outside of

FDA-approved labelling. This information is intended solely for CME and is not intended to promote off-label use of these medications. If you have any questions, contact the medical affairs department of the manufacturer for the most recent prescribing information.

TO ENROLL

To enroll in the *Chest Medicine Clinics* Continuing Medical Education program, call customer service at 1-800-654-2452 or sign up online at http://www.theclinics.com/home/cme. The CME program is available to subscribers for an additional annual fee of USD $225.

METHOD OF PARTICIPATION

In order to claim credit, participants must complete the following:

1. Complete enrolment as indicated above.
2. Read the activity.
3. Complete the CME Test and Evaluation. Participants must achieve a score of 70% on the test. All CME Tests and Evaluations must be completed online.

CME INQUIRIES/SPECIAL NEEDS

For all CME inquiries or special needs, please contact elsevierCME@elsevier.com.

CLINICS IN CHEST MEDICINE

THE CLINICS ARE AVAILABLE ONLINE!
Access your subscription at:
www.theclinics.com

Preface

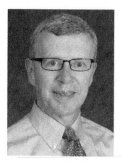 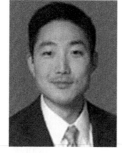

David A. Lynch, MB   Jonathan H. Chung, MD

Editors

Since the last issue of *Clinics in Chest Medicine* dedicated to chest imaging, published in 2008, the field has expanded at a rapid pace. For example, lung cancer screening with low-dose chest CT has been shown to reduce lung cancer mortality and is supported by major US insurance providers; quantitative imaging has come to the forefront as a means to assess chest imaging, and the temporal resolution of CT has improved to the point that even nongated CT scans are virtual cardiac CTs. In this issue, we are fortunate to have an accomplished team of international leaders in thoracic imaging, who have provide up-to-date authoritative reviews of important topics for the pulmonologist.

This issue begins with a thoughtful and informative general review on chest CT by Dr Brent Little. This is followed by three articles related to lung cancer. Drs Jared D. Christensen and Caroline Chiles present a timely appraisal of the current status of CT screening for lung cancer. A comprehensive review of the radiologist's role in evaluation of solitary pulmonary nodules is provided by Drs Jeffrey B. Alpert, Conor M. Lowry, and Jane P. Ko. Drs Patricia M. de Groot, Brett W. Carter, Sonia L. Betancourt Cuellar, and Jeremy J. Erasmus share their extensive experience with the imaging and staging of lung cancer.

Chest imaging plays an important role in acute pulmonary disease. Drs Loren Ketai, Kirk Jordan, and Katrina H Busby review the radiologist's role in the setting of pulmonary infection with wonderful examples of common and uncommon infections. Drs Matthew R. Bentz, and Steven L. Primack present a well-illustrated guide to the imaging evaluation of the critically ill patient. Drs Kristopher Cummings and Sanjeev Bhalla provide a highly informative and detailed review on pulmonary vascular diseases, including acute pulmonary embolism.

Imaging is of paramount importance in the diagnosis of diffuse lung diseases. Drs Danielle Seaman, Cristopher A. Meyer, Jeffrey P. Kanne provide a wide-ranging article on the imaging of common and uncommon occupational and environmental lung diseases. We are deeply grateful to our coauthors Drs Tilman Koelsch, Yutaka Tsuchiya, Aryeh Fischer, Joshua J. Solomon, and Caleb Richards, who respectively have provided articles on the idiopathic interstitial pneumonias, connective tissue disease, and cystic and nodular lung disease. These are complemented by the thoughtful review on large airways disease by Drs Maria Shiau, Timothy J. Harkin, and David P. Naidich, and by the analysis of the value of CT in diagnosis and differential diagnosis of small airways diseases by Drs Rachael M. Edwards, Gregory Kicska, Rodney Schmidt, and Sudhakar NJ. Pipavath. Drs Edwin van Beek and Saeed Mirsadraee conclude the issue by describing the

Clin Chest Med 36 (2015) xv–xvi
http://dx.doi.org/10.1016/j.ccm.2015.03.001
0272-5231/15/$ – see front matter © 2015 Published by Elsevier Inc.

state-of-the-art evaluation of regional and global pulmonary function by CT and MRI.

It has been our great honor to work with this outstanding group of authors. We have learned a great deal from reading their contributions. We offer our sincere thanks to all of them for their time and effort. We would also like to thank Casey Jackson and Patrick Manley at Elsevier, who were very helpful in ensuring compliance with deadlines and with production of this high-quality issue. We hope that this comprehensive review of the current state of chest imaging will advance the care of patients with acute and chronic lung diseases.

David A. Lynch, MB
National Jewish Health
Department of Radiology
1400 Jackson Street
Denver, CO 80206, USA

Jonathan H. Chung, MD
National Jewish Health
Department of Radiology
1400 Jackson Street
Denver, CO 80206, USA

E-mail addresses:
LynchD@NJHealth.org (D.A. Lynch)
chungj@njhealth.org (J.H. Chung)

Erratum

An error was made in the March 2015 issue of Chest Medicine Clinics on page 1. Dr Vijaya Knight's affiliation was incorrectly listed as "Program in Cell Biology, Department of Medicine, National Jewish Health, Denver, CO 80206, USA." It is correct as "Division of Pathology, Department of Medicine, National Jewish Health, Denver, CO 80206, USA."

Clin Chest Med 36 (2015) xvii
http://dx.doi.org/10.1016/j.ccm.2015.03.002
0272-5231/15/$ – see front matter Published by Elsevier Inc.

Approach to Chest Computed Tomography

Brent P. Little, MD

KEYWORDS

- Chest CT • Computed tomography • Thoracic imaging

KEY POINTS

- Chest computed tomography (CT) scan protocols are tailored to answer particular clinical questions. Contrast bolus administration, scan range, slice thickness, and CT tube settings are some of the parameters specified for each protocol.
- Postprocessing techniques such as 3-dimensional volume-rendering and maximum intensity projection provide additional ways of visualizing CT data sets and can supplement review of the axial images.
- Competent review of chest CT requires knowledge of normal CT anatomy and a systematic approach to detecting and characterizing thoracic pathology. Appreciation of the major categories of abnormal findings in each anatomic region is essential and provides a starting point for more advanced investigation of the CT appearances of specific diseases.
- Knowledge of a variety of common technical limitations and CT artifacts is essential in avoiding examination misinterpretation and for providing feedback about examination protocol and execution.

INTRODUCTION: DEFINITIONS AND NATURE OF THE PROBLEM

Computed tomography (CT) has become an essential tool in the diagnosis and treatment of a tremendous variety of diseases, with a dramatic increase in utilization since the development of the first CT scanners in the 1970s. Progress in scanner technology and advances in characterization of thoracic diseases have made CT a powerful diagnostic tool. The many contemporary indications for thoracic CT include characterization of pulmonary nodules and lung cancer, pulmonary metastatic disease, diseases of the aorta and pulmonary arteries, infections, postoperative complications, and interstitial lung disease. Electrocardiogram (ECG)-gated cardiac CT has also become a potent tool for evaluation of coronary artery disease and other diseases of the heart.

The complex anatomy of the thorax and the wide range of thoracic diseases with sometimes overlapping CT appearances can make interpretation challenging. The proliferation of CT scan indications and associated scan types can also create confusion in the selection of appropriate examination protocol. The following provides an introduction to the acquisition and review of chest CT, including a review of basic CT techniques and protocols, normal CT anatomy, and an organized approach for reviewing chest CT.

IMAGING TECHNIQUES
Basic Physics of Computed Tomography

CT arose from seminal work performed in the early 1970s by Godfrey Hounsfield, an English electrical engineer, with mathematical foundations pioneered in the 1950s by Allan Cormack; the 2 shared the Nobel Prize in Medicine in 1979 for their work.[1] For CT, the patient is centered on a table within a gantry containing a radiation source. A fan-shaped X-ray beam is directed toward the opposite side of the gantry, where detectors register radiation transmitted through the "slice" of tissue.[2] In modern scanners,

Disclosure: None.

Division of Cardiothoracic Imaging, Department of Radiology and Imaging Sciences, Emory University, Atlanta, GA 30309, USA

E-mail address: brent.p.little@emory.edu

the source and detectors rotate around the patient, providing data on the attenuation (the loss of photons due to interactions with tissue) of the beam across the range of angles subtended by the rotation. The scanner uses an algorithm to reconstruct the attenuation and position data, rendering a stack of images corresponding to the irradiated tissue. These images portray both the spatial location and the relative "density" or "attenuation" of objects within each CT slice.[3] Different materials have characteristic, reproducible units of CT attenuation, given in Hounsfield units (HU). CT machines are calibrated to assign water an attenuation value of 0, with higher attenuation materials (such as soft tissue and bone) yielding positive HU values, and lower attenuation materials (such as air) corresponding to negative HU values.[4] Typical CT attenuation values are shown in **Table 1** and **Fig. 1**.

Early generation scanners used an *axial* technique. In this technique, the table remains stationary during acquisition of a single slice, after which imaging briefly stops and the table moves as the patient is positioned for the next contiguous slice. Later generations of scanners provided a "helical" or "spiral" technique, with continuous motion of the table and patient while the gantry rotates around the patient. In this technique, a "volumetric" acquisition of the entire thorax can be obtained in one breath-hold, and the resulting images can be reformatted in multiple dimensions.[5] Most CT examinations are now performed with helical technique, with the exception of some high-resolution chest CT (HRCT) studies and prospectively gated cardiac CT examinations.

Scan Protocol

The selection of appropriate CT scan protocol is guided by the clinical question to be answered,

Table 1
Typical computed tomography attenuation values in Hounsfield units

Substance or Organ	Typical HU Value
Air	−1000
Normal lung	−700 to −900
Fat	−100
Water	0
Acute blood	50 to 80
Muscle	50
Intravenous contrast	300
Bone (cortex)	>1000

Data from Huda W, Slone RM. Review of radiologic physics. Baltimore (MD): Williams & Wilkins; 1995; and Seeram E. Computed tomography: physical principles, clinical applications & quality control. Philadelphia: Saunders; 1994.

in conjunction with patient history. Important considerations include the administration and timing of intravenous contrast, the craniocaudal scan range, and the desired scan slice thickness. A contrast-enhanced examination for a general indication such as evaluation of lung cancer or infection can be performed with a standard rate of injection (typically 2–3 mL/s), with images acquired from the thoracic inlet to the upper abdomen; the adrenal glands are often included in studies performed for cancer staging. Vascular examinations, including evaluation of the aorta and pulmonary arteries, usually require a fast injection (4–5 mL/s) with thin slices acquired over the entire chest.[6] HRCT is usually performed without contrast, with thin (1–2 mm) slices obtained from the lung apices to the lung bases.[7] Cardiac CT is typically performed with a high rate of contrast injection, thin slices, and an ECG-gated acquisition with limited scan range through the heart.

Patient Preparation, Positioning, and Scan Execution

After consent for intravenous contrast is obtained (if administered), the patient is positioned on the scan table with the body centered within the CT gantry. When possible, the patient's arms are placed above the head for chest CT; this avoids scatter and beam-hardening artifact from the bones and soft tissues of the arm. Next, a "scout topogram" of the patient is obtained (**Fig. 2**). Performed at very low radiation cost, this planar overview of the patient is used by the technologist to set the superior and inferior boundaries of the scan range to include the anatomy of interest. In addition, most CT scanners use the scout to estimate the patient tissue density at each position along the length of the scan range, increasing the CT tube current in areas of high tissue density (such as the abdomen) and decreasing in regions of low density (such as the lungs) to maintain optimal signal-to-noise ratio while minimizing radiation exposure, a technique known as "tube current modulation."[8]

Optimal timing of a CT intravenous contrast bolus relies on an accurate prediction of the time delay between the beginning of contrast administration and the desired contrast opacification of vessels or organs. For chest CT, an initial "localizer" image, obtained as a single axial CT image prescribed with the help of the scout image, is used to set a circular "region of interest" within the main pulmonary artery (for pulmonary CT angiography) or within the aorta (for arterial and general imaging) (**Fig. 3**). The scanner can be set to trigger the examination once a threshold contrast

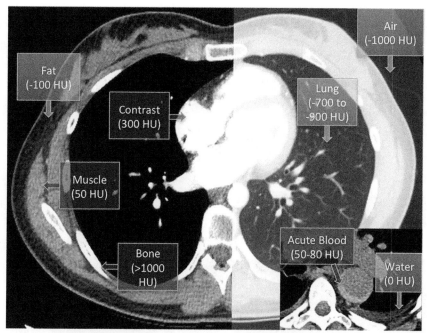

Fig. 1. Typical Hounsfield unit values at normal chest CT (*large image*). Inset in lower right corner shows a bright, crescentic acute aortic intramural hematoma with a simple fluid attenuation small left pleural effusion.

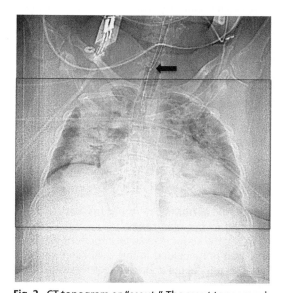

Fig. 2. CT topogram or "scout." The scout topogram is a planar image obtained at very low radiation cost. The technologist uses the scout to prescribe the superior and inferior extent of the CT scan range (*box*). The CT scanner also typically uses the scout to modulate the tube current appropriate to the tissue density at any point along the length of the patient (tube current modulation). Important findings may be present on the scout view but external to the scan range, such as this malpositioned nasogastric tube with tip overlying the high esophagus (*arrow*).

attenuation value is reached ("bolus tracking"). Alternatively, a small bolus of contrast (typically 20 mL) can be administered and used to calculate the delay time of the examination (a "test bolus").

Postprocessing

A variety of postprocessing techniques can be used to display CT information in helpful ways. Helical volumetric acquisition data can be processed to produce images reformatted in any spatial plane; coronal and sagittal reformatted images are often automatically produced at the scanner and sent to a picture archiving and communication system (PACS) for review. In addition, radiologists often use dedicated workstations or software integrated with PACS to perform additional reformatting, which is particularly helpful for review of vascular studies. Additional reformatting techniques, shown in **Fig. 4**, include the following.[9]

2-Dimensional multiplanar reformatting
Scans acquired with a volumetric, helical technique can be reformatted in any plane, most commonly the coronal and sagittal planes.

Maximum intensity projection
This technique projects the highest attenuation voxels of a "slab" of CT slices onto a 2-dimensional slice; the thickness and position of the slab can be selected by the radiologist or technologist. Maximum intensity projections (MIPs) can increase the sensitivity and efficiency of

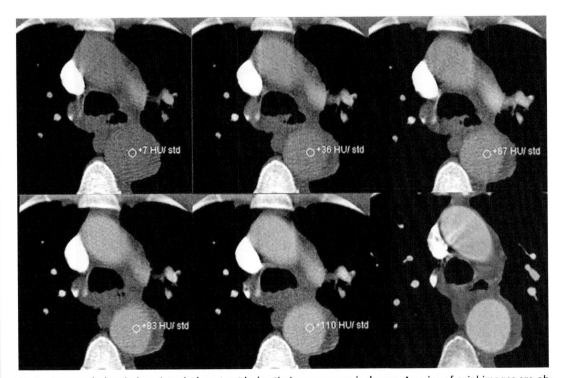

Fig. 3. Contrast bolus timing. A typical contrast bolus timing sequence is shown. A series of axial images are obtained with the table stationary, with a region of interest drawn over the desired vessel (in this case the descending aorta). In the bolus triggering method, shown here, the CT scanner monitors the attenuation within the region of interest and begins the scan automatically after a specified threshold is reached. The last (*bottom right*) panel shows the resulting CT angiography of the aorta, with the thrombosed false lumen of an aortic dissection seen within the descending aorta.

pulmonary nodule detection and can be helpful in illustrating the morphology and spatial extent of micronodular disease within the lungs.

Minimum intensity projection
This technique emphasizes the lowest attenuation pixel values in a "slab" of slices. Minimum intensity images (minIPs) are sometimes used for evaluation of the airways or the distribution of emphysema.

Three-dimensional volume rendering
Three-dimensional (3D) volume-rendered images can be used to display a volume of tissue in 3 dimensions, highlighting the spatial relationships between organs and vessels of interest.

IMAGING FEATURES AND DIFFERENTIAL DIAGNOSIS: REVIEWING CHEST COMPUTED TOMOGRAPHY
Review of the "Scout" Topogram

A planar image obtained at minimal radiation expenditure, the "scout" view or "topogram," provides an anatomic overview similar in appearance to a radiograph. The technologist uses the scout to plan the scan range of the examination, but the scout can also provide information either not present or difficult to appreciate in the axial CT images. The scout view can assist in assessing the following.

Lines, tubes, and other support apparatus
Sometimes the distal portion of a line or tube, such as a feeding or endotracheal tube, is captured in the scout view but not included in the range of axial image stack (see **Fig. 2**).

Pathologic abnormality in organs not fully included in the scan range
At times, the scout reveals an important finding in an organ not included in the axial scan range. A scout for a CT of the abdomen may illustrate pneumonia within a portion of the lung not included in the axial images, or a scout for a CT of the chest may show bowel obstruction or pneumoperitoneum not included in the axial images.

Findings at the "edge of the examination"
Findings at the edges of the axial image stack can be more obvious on the scout examination. For example, a traumatic C-spine fracture/dislocation may be much easier to appreciate on a lateral scout examination.

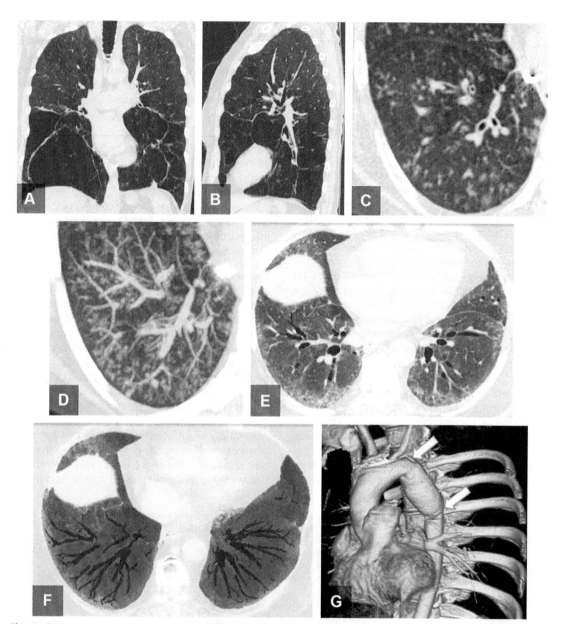

Fig. 4. Common postprocessing techniques. (*A, B*) Coronal and sagittal multiplanar reformatted images provide an effective demonstration of lower lobe predominant panacinar emphysema in α-1-antitrypsin deficiency. (*C, D*) Standard axial image in (*C*) shows numerous scattered pulmonary nodules; MIP with 1-cm slab thickness in (*D*) readily shows the centrilobular, tree-in-bud distribution of the nodules. (*E, F*) Standard axial projection in (*E*) shows patchy ground glass opacities and a suggestion of bronchiectasis; minIP in (*F*) shows the full extent of varicoid bronchiectasis in this case of a NSIP pattern of lung disease. (*G*) Volume-rendered image in a patient with traumatic aortic injury clearly shows the proximal and distal extent of the aortic injury (*arrows*).

Mediastinum

CT is a primary modality for evaluation of the mediastinum. Radiologists have classically divided the mediastinum into 3 main components—anterior, middle, and posterior. Although the original description of the components by famous chest radiologist, Ben Felson, includes the heart as part of the anterior mediastinum, other schemes include it as part of the middle mediastinum.[10] These categories are somewhat arbitrary, because masses can involve more than one mediastinal "compartment"; however, the schemes are helpful for organizing differential diagnosis of masses characterized at CT. Felson's original classification and the normal contents of the mediastinum are illustrated in **Fig. 5**. The heart and major thoracic vessels are treated separately in later discussion.

Both focal and diffuse mediastinal abnormalities can be characterized at CT. CT resolves even small mediastinal masses difficult or impossible to detect with chest radiographs. Size and exact location of a lesion are easily characterized, and extension to adjacent structures such as the great vessels or heart can be suspected based on encasement or loss of fat planes between a mass and adjacent anatomy. The attenuation characteristics (fat, fluid, soft tissue, calcification) of a mass are crucial to the differential diagnosis and may even be nearly pathognomonic of a particular entity, such as a combination of fat and calcium within a mediastinal teratoma.[10] Diffuse mediastinal pathologic abnormalities diagnosed at CT include postoperative mediastinitis or mediastinal hemorrhage, fibrosing mediastinitis, and mediastinal adenopathy. A few representative mediastinal pathologic abnormalities are shown in **Fig. 6**.

A variety of normal findings may mimic pathologic abnormality within the mediastinum. Residual thymic tissue, very common in patients in the early third decade and younger, can sometimes be seen in patients even in middle age. Thymic rebound hyperplasia or lymphoid hyperplasia can cause residual thymic tissue to expand, at times mimicking a

thymic neoplasm (see **Fig. 6**C).[11] Heart failure with mediastinal edema can cause haziness of the normally dark mediastinal fat and can cause mild enlargement of the mediastinal lymph nodes.[12] Fluid in a variety of pericardial recesses can mimic enlarged mediastinal lymph nodes.

Heart

Although ECG-gated CT has become the modality of choice for evaluation of the coronary arteries and the remainder of the heart, many important primary cardiac diseases and cardiac manifestations of lung disease can be diagnosed at nongated chest CT (see **Fig. 8**). An examination of the heart at standard, nongated chest CT should include the following.

Cardiac chambers

The internal diameter of the left ventricle (LV) is normally larger than the right ventricle, and the interventricular septum has convexity directed toward the right ventricle (**Fig. 7**).[13] Bowing of the interventricular septum to the left can be seen in acute right heart strain in the setting of pulmonary embolism (**Fig. 8**C), and in cases of chronic pulmonary hypertension. The atria are smooth, thin-walled chambers, normally of similar sizes, with a thin interatrial septum.

A variety of intracardiac masses can be seen, often presenting as filling defects within the cardiac chambers. Thrombi are the most common intracavitary mass, most often found at the left

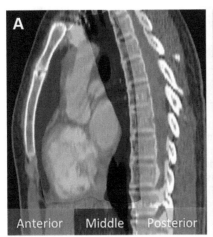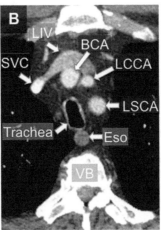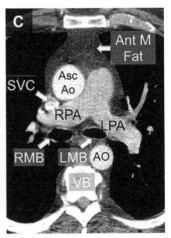

Fig. 5. Mediastinal classification and selected anatomy. (*A*) Felson's divisions of the mediastinum. In this classification scheme, the heart and all structures anterior to the posterior pericardial border are classified as within the anterior mediastinum, and the boundary between middle and posterior mediastinum is the posterior aspect of the first third of the vertebral bodies. (*B*) Anatomy of the upper mediastinum. BCA, brachiocephalic artery; Eso, esophagus; LCCA, left common carotid artery; LIV, left innominate vein; LSCA, left subclavian artery; SVC, superior vena cava; VB, vertebral body. (*C*) Anatomy at the level of the main pulmonary artery. Ant M Fat, anterior mediastinal fat; AO, descending aorta; Asc Ao, ascending aorta; LMB, left main bronchus; LPA, left pulmonary artery; RMB, right main bronchus; RPA, right pulmonary artery; VB, vertebral body.

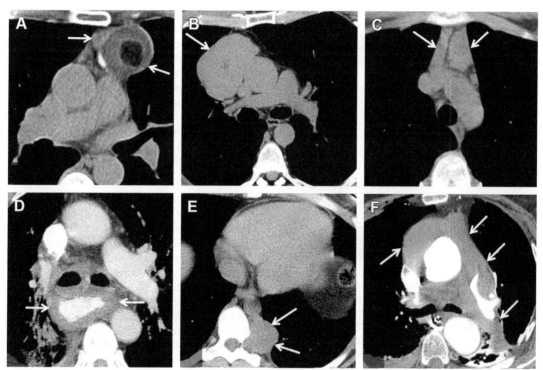

Fig. 6. Examples of mediastinal abnormalities at CT (*arrows*). (*A*) Anterior mediastinal mass contains fat, calcification, and soft tissue nodules; a benign cystic teratoma was confirmed at surgical resection. (*B*) Anterior mediastinal mass with homogenous soft tissue attenuation and small areas of central lower attenuation; a thymoma was pathologically proven. (*C*) Anterior mediastinal mass with a bilobed morphology in the anterior mediastinum, representing thymic rebound hyperplasia; note the central fatty cleft. (*D*) Middle mediastinal mass representing esophageal cancer. Circumferential thickening of a distended esophagus containing retained oral contrast is noted in the setting of partial obstruction distally. (*E*) Posterior mediastinal mass measured soft tissue attenuation and extended to the neural foramen, a typical appearance for a nerve sheath tumor; resection confirmed schwannoma. (*F*) Diffuse mediastinal abnormality representing hemorrhage in the setting of a type A aortic dissection with rupturing aneurysm; extensive high-attenuation acute hemorrhage is noted within the mediastinum.

ventricular apex, especially in the setting of aneurysm or wall thinning due to myocardial infarction, or in the left atrial appendage in patients with atrial fibrillation. Metastases are the most common tumor within the heart, with primary cardiac malignancies approximately 20 to 40 times less common.[14]

Myocardium

The normal left ventricular myocardium is of uniform thickness and enhances homogeneously on postcontrast imaging (see **Fig. 7**). Thinning and linear subendocardial fat or calcification of the LV wall signals a chronic myocardial infarct (see **Fig. 8**A), sometimes accompanied by an aneurysm, while hypoattenuation without thinning can be seen in acute infarction (see **Fig. 8**B). LV hypertrophy can be difficult to decisively diagnose at nongated CT, but is at times so striking that the diagnosis can be suggested. The right ventricular myocardium is normally thin, up to approximately

3 mm in thickness, barely noticeable at CT. Under conditions of chronically elevated right heart pressures, such as a left-to-right shunt like an atrial septal defect, the RV myocardium thickens and can become quite prominent at CT (see **Fig. 8**D).[12]

Coronary arteries

Although the lumens of the coronary arteries are not reliably assessed by routine nongated chest CT, the courses of the coronary arteries can be identified, and coronary calcification can be readily detected and qualitatively assessed for extent and severity at both noncontrast and contrast-enhanced CT.[15] Other incidental coronary findings at nongated CT include coronary or bypass graft aneurysms, and anomalous origins and courses of the coronary arteries.

Cardiac valves

Although motion often compromises evaluation of cardiac valves at nongated CT, abnormalities such

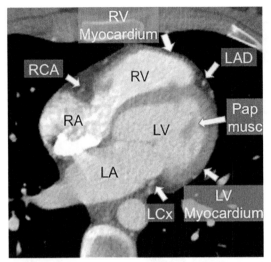

Fig. 7. Cardiac anatomy at nongated CT. The normal right ventricle (RV) is smaller than the LV, and the interventricular septum is convex rightward. The right atrium (RA) and left atrium (LA) are approximately the same size, and it is common for intravenous contrast to swirl in the RA. The LV myocardium enhances homogeneously, with uniform wall thickness. Two papillary muscle bundles, one of which is shown (pap musc), can be seen connecting to the mitral valve through chordae tendineae. Portions of the right coronary artery (RCA), left main coronary artery (not shown), left anterior descending artery (LAD), and left circumflex coronary artery (LCx) are often seen, where not obscured by cardiac motion.

as calcification, valve thickening, or even congenital diseases such as a bicuspid valve are often identifiable.[16] Occasionally, valve vegetations or tumors can be detected at nongated CT.

Pericardium

The normal pericardium is 3 mm or less in thickness and does not show noticeable enhancement. A pericardial effusion is a common finding at chest CT, and even a small amount of fluid within the pericardium can be identified at CT. Calcification and thickening of the pericardium can be seen in cases of prior or chronic pericarditis, sometimes resulting in constrictive physiology. Thickening and nodularity of the pericardium can also be seen in a malignant pericarditis.[16]

Large Thoracic Vessels

Aortic and pulmonary artery pathologic abnormalities are common indications for chest CT, and incidental findings in these and other thoracic vessels are not uncommon in chest CT performed for other reasons. Basic normal anatomy of the large thoracic vessels is shown in **Fig. 5.**

Aorta and arch vessels

The normal aorta has a thin, smooth wall and tapers as it descends to the left of the spine. Although normal aortic diameters vary with age, sex, and body surface area, the largest study of the aortic diameter at nongated CT supports an upper limit of normal of the ascending aorta of 4.1 cm, and for the descending aorta of 3.0 cm.[17] Calcified and noncalcified arterial plaque, aneurysms, dissections, thrombi, and other arterial pathologic abnormality can readily be identified at CT.

Pulmonary arteries

The normal right and left main pulmonary arteries arise from the central main pulmonary artery and gradually decrease in caliber as they branch into lobar (and interlobar), segmental, and subsegmental arteries. Many radiologists consider a main pulmonary artery diameter larger than 3.0 to 3.2 cm (or a diameter larger than that of the ascending aorta) *potentially* abnormal, suggesting elevated pulmonary arterial/right heart pressures. However, the specificity of this threshold has been a source of controversy, because many normal patients without pulmonary hypertension have measurements exceeding this threshold.[18] Pulmonary emboli, pulmonary artery aneurysms, and pulmonary arteriovenous malformations are some of the pathologic abnormalities well demonstrated at chest CT.

Major thoracic veins

The subclavian and jugular veins join to form an innominate vein on each side, which in turn drain into the superior vena cava. Contrast-enhanced examination allows detection of stenosis, usually accompanied by distended venous collaterals, and venous thrombi. However, mixing of contrast with unopacified blood often creates artifactual filling defects within these veins, and these should not be confused with venous thrombosis.

Thoracic Lymph Nodes

CT provides an accurate depiction of sizes and locations of thoracic lymph nodes and can guide surgical and semi-invasive techniques of nodal biopsy. Nodal location should be reported according to the revised International Society for the Study of Lung Cancer nodal map.[19] Orthogonal measurements in long and short axis of representative lymph nodes are standardly obtained. A 1-cm short-axis measurement is generally accepted as the threshold for deeming a lymph node "enlarged" at chest CT, with several notable exceptions. For subcarinal lymph nodes, 1.5 cm is typically used as an upper threshold of normal.

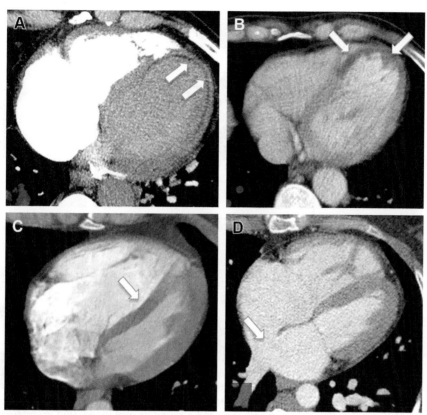

Fig. 8. Sample of cardiac abnormalities at nongated chest CT. (*A*) Chronic left ventricular infarct. Thinning of the left ventricular apex and lateral wall with subendocardial fat attenuation in the same distribution (*arrows*). (*B*) Acute left ventricular infarct with thrombus. Hypoenhancement of the myocardium at the LV apex is noted (*arrows*), and there is a small apical thrombus. (*C*) Acute right heart strain in pulmonary embolism. The normal rightward bowing of the interventricular septum has reversed (*arrow*) and the right ventricle and atrium are enlarged. Note the normal thickness of the right ventricular myocardium, suggesting an acute process. (*D*) Inferior sinus venosus atrial septal defect. A large defect is present in the interatrial septum (*arrow*); note hypertrophy of the right ventricular myocardium, in keeping with chronically elevated right heart pressures.

Cardiophrenic angle, internal mammary, and anterior peridiaphragmatic lymph nodes are normally inconspicuous at CT, and any visible lymph nodes in these locations can be viewed as potentially abnormal.

Large and Small Airways

CT allows evaluation of a variety of diseases of the trachea, bronchi, and bronchioles. Examination of the airways with lung windows allows assessment of the anatomy, patency, and wall thickness of the airways, while soft tissue windows allow further characterization of the morphology and attenuation (soft tissue, calcification, or other attenuation) of any airway thickening, nodules/masses, stenosis, or foreign bodies. Coronary and sagittal reformatted series can aid in characterization of the extent of disease; volume-rendered images and virtual bronchoscopy can be helpful in visualizing stenosis, endobronchial masses, and other abnormalities.

The normal trachea is a thin-walled structure with a smooth anterior and lateral cartilaginous component and a thin posterior membranous component (**Fig. 9**A). At inspiration, the normal trachea is usually ovoid. At expiration, the posterior membranous trachea can flatten or bow anteriorly in healthy normal subjects[20]; however, tracheal collapse greater than 70% at expiration compared with inspiration has been proposed as suggestive for tracheomalacia.[21] The upper limit of normal tracheal diameter in the coronal and sagittal planes is 25 and 27 mm in men and 21 and 23 mm in women; a tracheal diameter of greater than 3 cm and mainstem bronchial diameter greater than 2.4 cm are seen in tracheomegaly.[22] Normal bronchi have thin, cartilaginous walls with diameters similar to adjacent arteries. A bronchial diameter greater than the adjacent artery is a

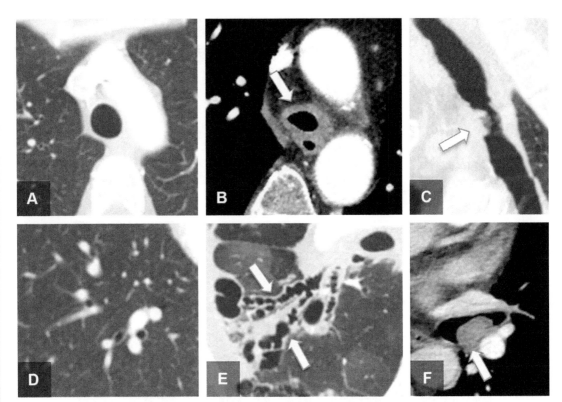

Fig. 9. Normal airways and samples of airway pathologic abnormality. (*A*) Normal trachea at inspiration. The normal trachea at inspiration has a thin, smooth wall and a round or oval shape. (*B*) Circumferential tracheal thickening (*arrow*)—granulomatosis with polyangiitis (GPA). Thickening and nodularity of the trachea can be seen in many infections, malignancies, and systemic conditions including GPA. (*C*) Focal tracheal mass—squamous cell carcinoma of the trachea. An irregular, polypoid mass (*arrow*) causes thickening and significant narrowing of the mid trachea. (*D*) Normal segmental bronchi (right lower lobe). Bronchial walls should be thin and smooth, and bronchial diameter should approximate that of the adjacent artery. (*E*) Bronchiectasis—cystic fibrosis. Varicoid and cystic bronchiectasis (*arrows*), bronchial wall thickening, and air trapping are seen in this patient with cystic fibrosis. (*F*) Endobronchial mass—carcinoid. Ovoid soft tissue mass with smooth borders (*arrow*) arises from the bronchial wall at the level of the distal left mainstem bronchus.

hallmark of bronchiectasis; however, many elderly patients without clinical evidence of airways disease have been noted to have bronchial-arterial ratios well in excess of 1:1.[23]

The small airways, the bronchioles, are noncartilaginous airways with walls composed mainly of smooth muscle and epithelium. Normal bronchioles have thin (<1 mm) walls at CT and taper smoothly in caliber as they course outward toward the lung periphery, becoming diminutive and difficult to appreciate in the outer 1 to 2 cm of the lung, especially in routine CT performed at slice thicknesses of greater than 2 mm (see **Fig. 9**D). A bronchial diameter larger than the adjacent pulmonary artery can signify bronchiectasis (see **Fig. 9**E).[7]

CT can depict focal or segmental thickening or nodularity of the airways seen in airway malignancies, infection, and systemic conditions, such as amyloidosis or granulomatosis with polyangiitis (see **Fig. 9**B, C). Asthma, smoking, chronic

bronchitis, infections, and many other airway diseases can cause diffuse bronchial wall thickening noticeable at CT. The presence, severity, and distribution of bronchiectasis can be characterized (see **Fig. 9**E), and endobronchial masses can be readily detected (see **Fig. 9**F). The full spectrum of airway diseases at CT is presented elsewhere in this volume.

Lungs: Overall Approach

Evaluation of the lung parenchyma is central to any chest CT evaluation. This section introduces an approach to characterizing lung abnormalities at chest CT.

Normal lung

Normal lung at inspiration displays relatively homogeneous low attenuation, with average Hounsfield unit values of approximately −700 to −900.[24] A slight gravitational gradient in lung opacity is a normal finding, and high attenuation in the posterior subpleural lungs, representing atelectasis, is common.[23]

Increase in lung opacity

An increase in lung opacity can be focal, multifocal, or diffuse and occurs in a large number of pulmonary diseases.

- ○ *Nodules* are round or ovoid focal opacities less than 3 cm in diameter; *masses* are similar focal opacities with diameters 3 cm or greater. The size, shape, border, attenuation, and location/distribution of nodules and masses, as well as the presence or absence of cavitation, are all important descriptors. Nodules and masses may be solid, "ground glass," or mixed attenuation; solitary or multiple; borders can be smooth, lobulated, or spiculated. Solid nodules may be any of a variety of attenuations, including soft tissue, calcium, fluid, and fat.
- ○ *Consolidation* is a patchy or regional area of increased lung opacity that obscures vessels and bronchial walls (**Fig. 10**A).[25] Consolidation can be focal (a lobe, segment, or portion of a segment), multifocal, or diffuse. The many causes of consolidation include infectious or organizing pneumonia, pulmonary edema, pulmonary adenocarcinoma or lymphoma, sarcoidosis, and numerous other diseases. Although usually soft tissue attenuation, consolidation can be high attenuation, such as in metastatic calcification or amiodarone toxicity, and can be low attenuation, such as in necrotizing pneumonia, or even fat attenuation, such as lipoid pneumonia.
- ○ *Ground glass opacity* is defined as hazy parenchymal opacity that does not obscure intervening vessels and airway walls (see **Fig. 10**B). Ground glass opacity can be focal, regional, or diffuse, and nodules can be either entirely or partly ground glass opacity. Similar to consolidation, the causes of ground glass opacity are numerous and include infection, edema, hemorrhage, alveolar damage, and certain diffuse lung diseases such as nonspecific interstitial pneumonitis (NSIP), desquamative interstitial pneumonitis, and lipoid pneumonia.[26]

Decrease in lung opacity

Similar to increased lung opacity, a decrease in opacity can be focal or diffuse.

- ○ *Cysts* are round, ovoid, or at times irregular air collections within the lung parenchyma with

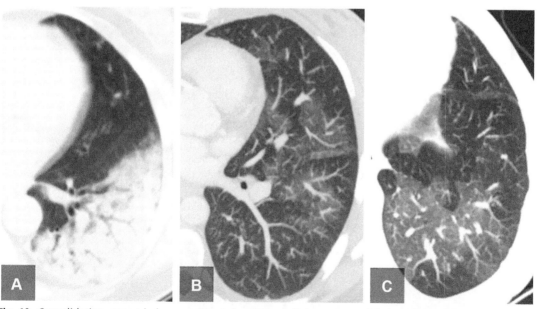

Fig. 10. Consolidation, ground glass opacity, and mosaic perfusion pattern. (*A*) Consolidation in a patient with organizing pneumonia. Air bronchograms are seen, and the opacity obscures the underlying vessels and bronchial walls. (*B*) Ground glass opacity in a patient with pulmonary edema. Hazy opacity does not obscure the intervening lung architecture. Note the normal uniformity of vessel diameters across regions of lung. (*C*) Mosaic perfusion pattern in a case of bronchiolitis obliterans. Lucent regions represent air trapping, and vessels in these regions have smaller diameters because of reflex vasoconstriction. Higher attenuation regions represent normal lung, and vessel diameters in these regions are larger because of shunting of blood flow from the areas of air trapping. Pulmonary vascular diseases such as pulmonary embolism can give a similar pattern of mosaic perfusion.

well-defined walls. The location, distribution, and morphology of cysts are important for differential diagnosis. Cysts can be an incidental finding, such as in a postinfectious pneumatocele, and can also be seen in a variety of diffuse cystic lung diseases such as Langerhans cell histiocytosis and lymphangioleiomyomatosis.

- *Emphysema* usually manifests at CT as a regional or diffuse decrease in lung attenuation without well-defined walls. Within areas of emphysema, vessel diameters are typically small, and a paucity of vessels is often noted. Although cysts tend to displace vessels, areas of emphysema contain linear branching opacities representing the centrilobular bronchovascular bundles; in cross-section, the bundle takes the form of a central nodular opacity within lobules, called the "central dot sign."
- *Blebs* (measuring less than 1 cm) and *bullae* (1 cm and larger) are focal air collections with very thin walls that often occur in the setting of emphysema.

Mosaic attenuation

Mosaic attenuation refers to alternating geographic regions of opacity and lucency within the lung parenchyma (see **Fig. 10**C).[27] The diameter of vessels within the lucent areas compared with that of vessels within the more opaque areas is paramount for determining the nature of the abnormality. A uniform diameter of vessels in both regions suggests that the higher attenuation is abnormal, corresponding to the ground glass opacity seen in infiltrative processes such as infection and pulmonary edema. A nonuniform vessel diameter with smaller caliber of vessels in areas of lucent lung signifies that the lucent areas are abnormal, representing either small airway disease with air trapping, or small vessel disease. The mechanisms are different: air trapping causes hypoxemic vasoconstriction in affected lobules, while small vessel diseases such as pulmonary embolism and chronic pulmonary hypertension have primary vascular effects, shunting flow toward other portions of the vascular bed.[28] On expiratory imaging, areas of normal lung should increase in attenuation, whereas areas of air trapping will maintain the same low level of attenuation.

Spatial distribution of disease

Both the craniocaudal and the central/peripheral extent of disease are important to determine formulating a differential diagnosis of diffuse lung disease (**Fig. 11**). Although the craniocaudal distribution can often be discerned from the axial images, coronal and sagittal reformatted images

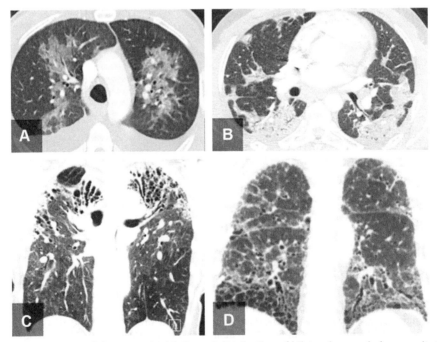

Fig. 11. Spatial distribution of disease at CT. (*A*) Central distribution of bilateral ground glass opacity in a case of pulmonary edema. (*B*) Peripheral distribution of disease in an instance of organizing pneumonia; eosinophilic pneumonia can also present as peripheral ground glass or consolidation. (*C*) Upper lung distribution in sarcoidosis. Note the upper lobe volume loss and traction bronchiectasis. (*D*) Lower lung distribution in UIP pattern of lung disease. Note the honeycombing and traction bronchiectasis and bronchiololectasis.

can be very helpful in confirming more subtle distributions of disease. The central/peripheral predominance of disease is readily assessed on axial images.

- Central distribution (see **Fig. 11**A) suggests diseases related to the bronchovascular bundles; examples include edema and bronchopneumonia in the acute setting, and perilymphatic diseases such as sarcoidosis or silicosis, lymphoma, or Kaposi sarcoma in the chronic setting.
- Peripheral distribution (see **Fig. 11**B) can be seen in acute diseases such as pulmonary infarction, septic emboli, and aspiration; in the subacute or chronic setting, this distribution can be seen in organizing or eosinophilic pneumonia, pulmonary fibrosis, and other diseases.
- Upper lobe distribution (see **Fig. 11**C) is seen in many perilymphatic and airway centric diseases such as sarcoidosis, silicosis, cystic fibrosis, tuberculosis, and Langerhans cell histiocytosis.
- Lower lobe distribution (see **Fig. 11**D) classically occurs in a usual interstitial pneumonitis (UIP) pattern of fibrosis and can also occur in gravitationally dependent processes such as aspiration and hematogenous metastatic disease.

Lung volumes

Lung volumes can be calculated with segmentation software running on PACS or a dedicated workstation. However, in daily practice, lung volumes can be quickly assessed via the scout image or coronal or sagittal reformatted images. Low lung volumes with poor diaphragmatic excursion can be appreciated in cases of severe fibrosis. Hyperexpanded lungs with a flattened diaphragm or prominent retrosternal clear space can be appreciated in cases of obstructive lung disease.

Lungs: Findings at High-Resolution Chest Computed Tomography

Several important pulmonary findings are best characterized with HRCT technique, performed with thin (0.625–2 mm) slices and reformatted with a high-spatial resolution image filter. The *secondary lobules* are 1- to 2.5-cm polygonal units of lung bounded by very thin (0.1 mm) walls, called the *interlobular septa*.[7] Venules and lymphatics course along the septa, indistinguishable from the septa themselves. Normal interlobular septa are usually difficult or impossible to appreciate, even at HRCT; thickening of the septa is abnormal and can be seen in infiltrative processes (such as

pulmonary edema, infection, lymphangitic carcinomatosis, and sarcoidosis) and pulmonary fibrosis. *Centrilobular core structures*—arterioles, bronchioles, and lymphatics—course along the center of the lobule and are supported by a fine centrilobular interstitium. Centrilobular arterioles measure approximately 1 mm and are often visible at HRCT as a central dot or tube within a lobule, while the other components are usually not visible.[29] A fine supporting interstitial meshwork called the *intralobular septa* runs throughout the secondary lobule, only visible when it is thickened, such as in pulmonary fibrosis.

Important findings at thin-section CT relevant to the secondary lobule include the following.

Nodules

With HRCT, the small nodules of diffuse lung diseases can be characterized as 1 of 3 distinct patterns.[30]

- *Random* (**Fig. 12**A): Nodules distributed throughout the lungs without predilection for any particular anatomic structure. Nodules with this pattern neither spare nor cluster along the pleural surfaces (including fissures) or interlobular septa. Examples of diseases producing this pattern are hematogenous metastases, miliary tuberculosis, and fungal infection.
- *Perilymphatic* (see **Fig. 12**B): Nodules favoring the axial lymphatics, clustering along the bronchovascular bundles centrally, and the peripheral lymphatics, including interlobular septa and subpleural/fissural intersititium. This pattern is often seen in sarcoidosis, silicosis and other pneumoconioses, and lymphangitic carcinomatosis.
- *Centrilobular* (see **Fig. 12**C): Nodules clustered along the core centrilobular structures, sparing the fissures and remainder of the subpleural lung, not touching the pleura, often occurring in small clusters. Centrilobular nodules can occur with either "tree-in-bud" or "pure centrilobular" morphology. The "tree-in-bud" pattern, most commonly seen in infectious bronchiolitis or aspiration, is caused by impacted bronchioles and alveoli, resembling branches and buds of a tree in springtime (see **Fig. 12**C).[31] The "pure centrilobular" pattern usually occurs as evenly spaced, indistinct ground glass nodules positioned within the center of the secondary lobule without associated branching opacities and can be seen in hypersensitivity pneumonitis and respiratory bronchiolitis. Because the centrilobular arteriole follows the course

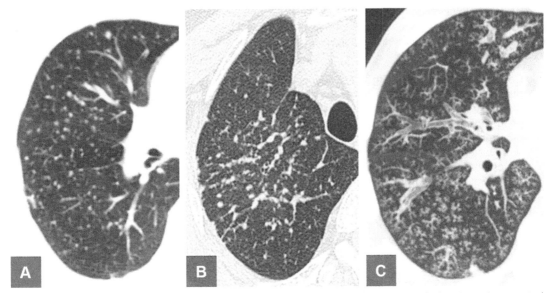

Fig. 12. CT patterns of small nodules. (*A*) Random distribution in a case of metastatic cholangiocarcinoma. Nodules neither spare nor cluster along the pleural surface (including fissures). (*B*) Perilymphatic distribution in a case of sarcoidosis. Nodules follow both the central lymphatics (bronchovascular bundles) and the peripheral lymphatics (pleural surfaces and interlobular septa). (*C*) Centrilobular nodules ("tree-in-bud" subtype) in a patient with cystic fibrosis. Nodules spare the pleura/fissures and occur in clusters.

of the bronchiole, small vessel diseases can also produce a pure centrilobular or tree-in-bud pattern of nodules; examples include vasculitis, endovascular metastases, or talc (excipient) emboli from crushed tablets in intravenous drug abuse, and the rare pulmonary capillary hemangiomatosis.

Linear/reticular opacities and honeycombing

- *Interlobular septal thickening* (**Fig. 13**A) manifests as linear or polygonal opacities occurring at 1 to 2.5-cm intervals, corresponding to the walls of the secondary pulmonary lobule. Often most noticeable at the periphery of the lung apex or base, interlobular septal thickening can be seen in any process causing infiltration or congestion of the venules, lymphatics, or interstitium at the periphery of the lobules. Smooth thickening is often caused by pulmonary edema, hemorrhage, or infection, while nodular thickening can be seen in sarcoidosis, pneumoconioses, and lymphangitic carcinomatosis, and irregular thickening can be seen in fibrosis.
- *Intralobular septal thickening* (see **Fig. 13**B) are irregular lines along the periphery of the lung between the interlobular septa. This type of septal thickening is often seen in interstitial lung diseases such as UIP and NSIP.
- *Honeycombing* (see **Fig. 13**C) refers to stacked rows of thick-walled cysts along the lung periphery and is often accompanied by irregular interlobular and intralobular septal thickening and architectural distortion. Although honeycombing can be seen in any disease involving significant fibrosis, a basilar predominant honeycombing is a hallmark of a UIP pattern of lung disease.[32]
- *Bronchiectasis and bronchiolectasis* (see **Fig. 13**D) manifest as an enlargement of the airway diameter relative to the adjacent artery that can be seen in diseases primarily affecting the airways, such as cystic fibrosis, chronic aspiration or infection, and bronchiolitis obliterans. When caused by fibrosis, such morphology is called *traction bronchiectasis/bronchiolectasis* and is usually accompanied by architectural distortion, reticulation, or honeycombing.

Pleura

Chest CT is an excellent modality for examination of the pleura. At CT, the normally very thin pleura is usually not visible. Pleural thickening or nodularity is abnormal and can be seen in inflammatory processes such as empyemas, or in pleural malignancy such as mesothelioma or metastatic disease. An uncomplicated transudative pleural effusion measures close to water attenuation (usually 0–10 HU) and should layer dependently

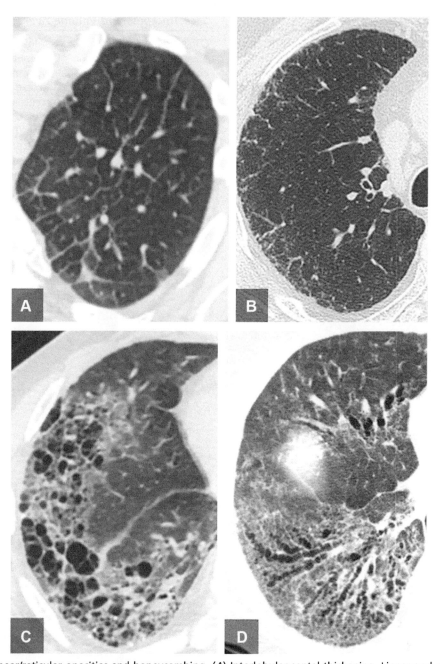

Fig. 13. Linear/reticular opacities and honeycombing. (*A*) Interlobular septal thickening. Linear and polyhedral opacities represent thickening interlobular septa in a patient with interstitial pulmonary edema, highlighting the 1 to 2.5-cm spacing of the secondary pulmonary lobule. (*B*) Intralobular and interlobular septal thickening. Irregular linear subpleural opacities in keeping with fibrosis in a patient with biopsy-proven UIP. (*C*) Honeycombing. Multiple contiguous rows of thick-walled cysts in this UIP pattern of fibrosis in rheumatoid lung disease. (*D*) Traction bronchiectasis and bronchiolectasis. Varicoid dilation of bronchi and bronchioles in a case of NSIP. Note that the involved airways have larger diameters than the adjacent vessels.

if loculation is not present. Empyemas and other exudative fluid collections can measure higher than water attenuation and are often accompanied by pleural thickening and enhancement.

Nondependent or lobulated margins of pleural fluid suggest the presence of loculation. High-attenuation fluid can be seen in an acute to sub-acute hemothorax.

Soft Tissues and Bones

A variety of primary bone and soft tissue diseases and manifestations of systemic disease can be characterized at CT reviewed with bone window settings and are beyond the scope of this article.

PEARLS AND PITFALLS: TECHNICAL CONSIDERATIONS AND ARTIFACTS

A variety of technical pitfalls and imaging artifacts can compromise chest CT interpretation, including the following.

Slice Thickness and Volume Averaging

CT slices with thickness less than 2 mm are desired for the evaluation of interstitial lung disease; thicker slices can cause "volume averaging" of important anatomy and pathologic abnormality with the adjacent lung, compromising detection and characterization of small nodules, reticulation, honeycombing, and other findings (**Fig. 14**A, B). For example, thick slices can cause small nodules or reticulation to be interpreted erroneously as ground glass opacity. Ground glass opacities, especially small ground glass nodules, may be

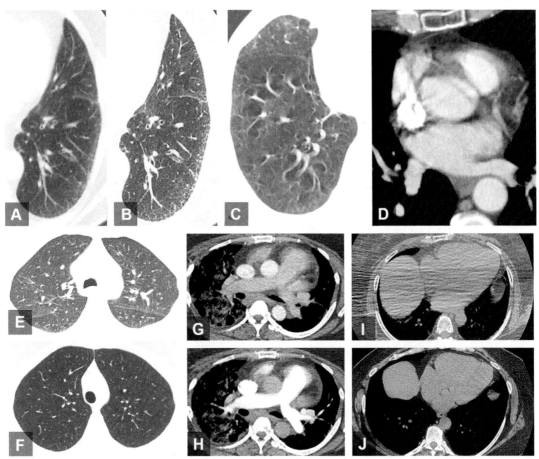

Fig. 14. Technical pitfalls at chest CT. (*A, B*) Volume averaging at larger slice thickness. At 5-mm slice thickness in (*A*), a band of apparent ground glass opacity is seen in the lateral periphery of the left lower lobe; at 1.25-mm slice thickness, fine reticular opacities representing fibrosis are readily identified. (*C, D*) Motion artifact. In (*C*), respiratory motion causes blurring and doubling of vessels; in (*D*), pulsation artifact from the aorta creates an artifactual linear opacity at the edge of the ascending aorta resembling a dissection. In addition, linear streaks radiating outward from the superior vena cava represent beam-hardening artifact from high intravenous contrast concentration in the vessel. (*E, F*) Expiratory versus inspiratory technique. An examination obtained at expiration (*E*) can increase lung opacity and cause dependent atelectasis, at times obscuring or mimicking pathologic abnormality. At inspiration (*F*), atelectasis resolves and lungs are normal in attenuation. (*G, H*) Problems with the contrast bolus. Suboptimal opacification of the pulmonary arteries in (*G*), and optimal opacification in (*H*). (*I, J*) Image noise and streak artifact. Examination in (*I*) was performed with the patient's arms at the patient's sides, causing a band of beam-hardening artifact across the image; the image in (*J*) was obtained with the patient's arms over the head, away from the CT beam.

obscured by volume averaging at larger slice thicknesses.

Motion Artifact

Patient respiratory motion can create artifact ranging from mild to severe and can lead to blurring of vessels, lung parenchyma, and other important anatomy and can obscure or mimic abnormalities such as nodules and pulmonary emboli (see **Fig. 14**C, D). Cardiac motion and aortic pulsation can blur vessel walls and make assessment of the pulmonary arteries and aorta problematic. At times, aortic motion can even mimic aortic dissection.

Inadequate Inspiration or Expiration

An incomplete inspiration or a scan acquired at expiration can lead to patchy atelectasis, obscuring nodules or mimicking ground glass opacity because of infiltrative diseases (see **Fig. 14**E, F). When an expiratory examination is desired for assessment of air trapping, an inadequate expiration can decrease sensitivity.

Problems with the Contrast Bolus

Although an intravenous contrast bolus injected at a relatively low rate (2–3 mL/s) may be adequate for a routine chest evaluation, a faster injection timed for the pulmonary arteries is desired for adequate vessel opacification, and a high rate of injection timed from the aorta is required for a thoracic CT angiogram (see **Fig. 14**G, H). Poor contrast opacification caused by improper timing of the examination, or by a patient deep breath or Valsalva at the time of scanning, can compromise evaluation of vessels and lead to a nondiagnostic examination.

Noise and Beam-Hardening Artifact

Image "noise" is perceived as graininess or streakiness that can compromise the diagnostic accuracy of an examination. Both CT scanner settings and patient factors can play a role.[3] A large body habitus can impair the transmission of radiation through the thorax and lead to a low signal-to-noise ratio; on the other hand, if CT scanner settings such as tube current and peak voltage are set too low, a noisy scan may result. A high concentration of contrast within the superior vena cava and the innominate veins can create "beam-hardening" artifact, potentially obscuring portions of the adjacent lung and vessels (see **Fig. 14**D). When a patient's arms are positioned at the patient's side for thoracic CT, the resulting streak and noise can compromise evaluation of portions of the anatomy of interest (see **Fig. 14**I, J).

CURRENT CONTROVERSIES
Radiation Dose Concerns and Dose Reduction

CT has become the leading source of medical imaging radiation, now responsible for approximately 68% of all medical imaging radiation exposure.[33,34] Although the long-term risks to adults of radiation exposure from CT imaging are still not well understood, much scholarly work and media attention have been given to this topic over the past few years, with ongoing calls for the reduction of CT radiation exposure.[35]

Effective radiation doses are specified in millisieverts (mSv), a unit incorporating both the estimated amount of administered radiation and the tissue sensitivities of the irradiated organs. Although a typical dose for a posteroanterior chest radiograph has been estimated at 0.02 mSv, the average dose for a standard chest CT was 7 mSv in one large analysis of literature from several countries, including the United States, equivalent to 350 posterioranterior chest radiographs.[36] Although this number seems large, it is important to note that average "background" radiation doses from ambient sources such as radon, cosmic rays, and radioisotopes in food averages 3 mSv a year and is higher at high altitudes.

Several groups have warned of an increased cancer risk due to radiation from CT. Brenner and Hall[37] controversially estimated in 2007 that 1.5% to 2.0% of all cancers in the United States may be attributable to CT radiation exposure, while other estimates have been much lower.[38] In the pediatric population, 2 large longitudinal studies spanning approximately 10 years provide evidence for a small absolute increase in risk of cancer from CT scans in children and young adults.[39,40] However, projections of cancer risk to adults from CT scans rely on studies of survivors of the Hiroshima and Nagasaki atomic bomb blasts, who incurred radiation doses much higher than a patient undergoing even multiple CTs; extrapolation from these doses of greater than 100 mSv in estimating cancer risk has been controversial and at the moment is not yet supported by direct evidence.[41] In addition, the benefits of performing CT for diagnosis, surveillance, or treatment planning are difficult to quantify but need to be weighed against any potential risks.

Despite incomplete knowledge of the long-term effects of radiation exposure from CT, the potential risks have spawned extensive dose reduction efforts in the imaging community. Advances in scanner hardware and software, lower-dose protocols and scanner settings, improved internal quality improvement programs, and national quality initiatives such as the American College of Radiology

CT Dose Index Registry have enabled lower dose scanning while maintaining diagnostic quality.[33,42]

SUMMARY

CT scan protocols can be tailored to answer particular clinical questions. Contrast bolus administration, scan range, slice thickness, and CT tube settings are some of the parameters specified for each protocol.

Postprocessing techniques such as 3D volume-rendering and maximum intensity projection provide additional ways of visualizing CT data sets and can supplement review of the axial images.

Competent review of chest CT requires knowledge of normal CT anatomy and a systematic approach to detecting and characterizing thoracic pathology. Appreciation of the major categories of abnormal findings in each anatomic region is essential and provides a starting point for more advanced investigation of the CT appearances of specific diseases.

Knowledge of a variety of common technical limitations and CT artifacts is essential in avoiding examination misinterpretation and for providing feedback about examination protocolling and execution.

REFERENCES

1. Hounsfield GN. Computerized transverse axial scanning (tomography). 1. Description of system. Br J Radiol 1973;46(552):1016–22.
2. Mahesh M. Search for isotropic resolution in CT from conventional through multiple-row detector. Radiographics 2002;22(4):949–62.
3. Goldman LW. Principles of CT and CT technology. J Nucl Med Technol 2007;35(3):115–28 [quiz: 129–30].
4. Huda W, Slone RM. Review of radiologic physics. Baltimore (MD): Williams & Wilkins; 1995.
5. Fuchs T, Kachelriess M, Kalender WA. Technical advances in multi-slice spiral CT. Eur J Radiol 2000; 36(2):69–73.
6. Bae KT. Intravenous contrast medium administration and scan timing at CT: considerations and approaches. Radiology 2010;256(1):32–61.
7. Kazerooni EA. High-resolution CT of the lungs. AJR Am J Roentgenol 2001;177(3):501–19.
8. Duong PA, Little BP. Dose tracking and dose auditing in a comprehensive computed tomography dose-reduction program. Semin Ultrasound CT MR 2014;35(4):322–30.
9. Beigelman-Aubry C, Hill C, Guibal A, et al. Multi-detector row CT and postprocessing techniques in the assessment of diffuse lung disease. Radiographics 2005;25(6):1639–52.
10. Whitten CR, Khan S, Munneke GJ, et al. A diagnostic approach to mediastinal abnormalities. Radiographics 2007;27(3):657–71.
11. Araki T, Sholl LM, Gerbaudo VH, et al. Imaging characteristics of pathologically proven thymic hyperplasia: identifying features that can differentiate true from lymphoid hyperplasia. AJR Am J Roentgenol 2014;202(3):471–8.
12. Bruzzi JF, Remy-Jardin M, Delhaye D, et al. When, why, and how to examine the heart during thoracic CT: Part 2, clinical applications. AJR Am J Roentgenol 2006;186(2):333–41.
13. Bruzzi JF, Remy-Jardin M, Delhaye D, et al. When, why, and how to examine the heart during thoracic CT: Part 1, basic principles. AJR Am J Roentgenol 2006;186(2):324–32.
14. Araoz PA, Eklund HE, Welch TJ, et al. CT and MR imaging of primary cardiac malignancies. Radiographics 1999;19(6):1421–34.
15. McKie SJ, Hardwick DJ, Reid JH, et al. Features of cardiac disease demonstrated on CT pulmonary angiography. Clin Radiol 2005;60(1):31–8.
16. Bogaert J, Centonze M, Vanneste R, et al. Cardiac and pericardial abnormalities on chest computed tomography: what can we see? Radiol Med 2010; 115(2):175–90.
17. Wolak A, Gransar H, Thomson LE, et al. Aortic size assessment by noncontrast cardiac computed tomography: normal limits by age, gender, and body surface area. JACC Cardiovasc Imaging 2008;1(2): 200–9.
18. Corson N, Armato SG 3rd, Labby ZE, et al. CT-based pulmonary artery measurements for the assessment of pulmonary hypertension. Acad Radiol 2014;21(4):523–30.
19. Walker CM, Chung JH, Abbott GF, et al. Mediastinal lymph node staging: from noninvasive to surgical. AJR Am J Roentgenol 2012;199(1):W54–64.
20. O'Donnell CR, Litmanovich D, Loring SH, et al. Age and sex dependence of forced expiratory central airway collapse in healthy volunteers. Chest 2012; 142(1):168–74.
21. Ridge CA, O'Donnell CR, Lee EY, et al. Tracheobronchomalacia: current concepts and controversies. J Thorac Imaging 2011;26(4):278–89.
22. Chung JH, Kanne JP, Gilman MD. CT of diffuse tracheal diseases. AJR Am J Roentgenol 2011; 196(3):W240–6.
23. Hansell DM. Thin-section CT of the lungs: the Hinterland of normal. Radiology 2010;256(3):695–711.
24. Rosenblum LJ, Mauceri RA, Wellenstein DE, et al. Density patterns in the normal lung as determined by computed tomography. Radiology 1980;137(2): 409–16.
25. Hansell DM, Bankier AA, MacMahon H, et al. Fleischner Society: glossary of terms for thoracic imaging. Radiology 2008;246(3):697–722.

26. Collins J, Stern EJ. Ground-glass opacity at CT: the ABCs. AJR Am J Roentgenol 1997;169(2):355–67.

27. Stern EJ, Muller NL, Swensen SJ, et al. CT mosaic pattern of lung attenuation: etiologies and terminology. J Thorac Imaging 1995;10(4):294–7.

28. Webb WR, Müller NL, Naidich DP. High-resolution CT of the lung. 4th edition. Philadelphia: Wolters Kluwer/Lippincott Williams & Wilkins; 2009.

29. Gotway MB, Reddy GP, Webb WR, et al. High-resolution CT of the lung: patterns of disease and differential diagnoses. Radiol Clin North Am 2005;43(3): 513–42, viii.

30. Raoof S, Amchentsev A, Vlahos I, et al. Pictorial essay: multinodular disease: a high-resolution CT scan diagnostic algorithm. Chest 2006;129(3): 805–15.

31. Rossi SE, Franquet T, Volpacchio M, et al. Tree-in-bud pattern at thin-section CT of the lungs: radiologic-pathologic overview. Radiographics 2005;25(3):789–801.

32. Lynch DA, Godwin JD, Safrin S, et al. High-resolution computed tomography in idiopathic pulmonary fibrosis: diagnosis and prognosis. Am J Respir Crit Care Med 2005;172(4):488–93.

33. Litmanovich DE, Tack DM, Shahrzad M, et al. Dose reduction in cardiothoracic CT: review of currently available methods. Radiographics 2014;34(6): 1469–89.

34. Schauer DA, Linton OW. NCRP Report No. 160, Ionizing Radiation Exposure of the Population of the United States, medical exposure–are we doing less with more, and is there a role for health physicists? Health Phys 2009;97(1):1–5.

35. Amis ES Jr, Butler PF, Applegate KE, et al. American College of Radiology white paper on radiation dose in medicine. J Am Coll Radiol 2007;4(5):272–84.

36. Mettler FA Jr, Huda W, Yoshizumi TT, et al. Effective doses in radiology and diagnostic nuclear medicine: a catalog. Radiology 2008;248(1):254–63.

37. Brenner DJ, Hall EJ. Computed tomography–an increasing source of radiation exposure. N Engl J Med 2007;357(22):2277–84.

38. Meer AB, Basu PA, Baker LC, et al. Exposure to ionizing radiation and estimate of secondary cancers in the era of high-speed CT scanning: projections from the Medicare population. J Am Coll Radiol 2012;9(4):245–50.

39. Mathews JD, Forsythe AV, Brady Z, et al. Cancer risk in 680,000 people exposed to computed tomography scans in childhood or adolescence: data linkage study of 11 million Australians. BMJ 2013;346: f2360.

40. Pearce MS, Salotti JA, Little MP, et al. Radiation exposure from CT scans in childhood and subsequent risk of leukaemia and brain tumours: a retrospective cohort study. Lancet 2012;380(9840): 499–505.

41. Meinel FG, Nance JW Jr, Harris BS, et al. Radiation risks from cardiovascular imaging tests. Circulation 2014;130(5):442–5.

42. Raman SP, Mahesh M, Blasko RV, et al. CT scan parameters and radiation dose: practical advice for radiologists. J Am Coll Radiol 2013;10(11):840–6.

Low-Dose Computed Tomographic Screening for Lung Cancer

Jared D. Christensen, MD[a], Caroline Chiles, MD[b],*

KEYWORDS

- Computed tomography (CT) • Lung cancer • Screening

KEY POINTS

- Screening with low-dose computed tomography (LDCT) has been shown to detect earlier-stage lung cancers and to reduce lung cancer–specific mortality by 20% in high-risk patients.
- The ideal lung cancer screening clinic includes a nurse navigator and representatives from primary care medicine, diagnostic radiology, pulmonary medicine, smoking cessation, thoracic oncology, radiation oncology, and thoracic surgery.
- Potential risks of LDCT screening for lung cancer include false-positive findings that initiate further workup, radiation exposure, overdiagnosis, patient anxiety, and increased costs to the patient.
- The likelihood of malignancy is higher for part-solid and nonsolid nodules than for solid nodules.
- The Lung CT Screening Reporting and Data System (Lung-RADS) provides a method of describing and categorizing nodules found at LDCT screening and includes management guidelines for nodule follow-up.
- LDCT screening for lung cancer provides an opportunity to detect other diseases, including chronic obstructive pulmonary disease (COPD), interstitial lung disease, coronary artery calcification, and extrapulmonary malignancy.

INTRODUCTION

Lung cancer is the leading cause of cancer-related mortality in the United States and the world, accounting for more deaths than colorectal, breast, and prostate cancer combined.[1] Despite advances in clinical care and diagnostic imaging, most patients diagnosed with lung cancer present with advanced-stage disease, in part accounting for a poor 5-year survival rate of only 15.9% and approximately 160,000 deaths in the United States annually.[1] Early diagnosis facilitates the treatment of lung cancer in its earliest, most curable stage. Screening with low-dose computed tomography (LDCT) has been shown to detect earlier-stage lung cancers and to reduce lung cancer–specific mortality by 20% in high-risk patients.[2]

THE EVIDENCE FOR SCREENING

The most informative study to have evaluated the effectiveness of imaging for lung cancer screening is the National Lung Screening Trial (NLST).[2] Eligibility criteria for this multicenter, randomized controlled trial are listed in **Box 1**. Patients were randomized to annual screening with either chest radiography (CXR) or LDCT, and all patients received a total of 3 screening examinations: a baseline study followed by 2 annual screening examinations. A positive result was the detection of

Disclosures: None.
[a] Department of Radiology, Duke University Medical Center, Box 3808, Durham, NC 27710, USA; [b] Department of Radiology, Wake Forest University Health Sciences Center, Medical Center Boulevard, Winston-Salem, NC 27157, USA
* Corresponding author.
E-mail address: cchiles@wakehealth.edu

Clin Chest Med 36 (2015) 147–160
http://dx.doi.org/10.1016/j.ccm.2015.02.002

Inclusion criteria

Age 55 to 74 years

Thirty or more pack-years smoking history

If former smoker, quit 15 or less years ago

Exclusion criteria

History of lung cancer

Treatment or evidence of any other cancer in the past 5 years, except for nonmelanoma skin cancer or carcinoma in situ

Prior lung resection

Signs or symptoms that could be attributable to malignancy (eg, weight loss, hemoptysis)

Acute respiratory infection treated with antibiotics within 12 weeks before eligibility assessment

Chest computed tomography examination in the past 18 months

Medical conditions that pose a significant risk of mortality during the trial period

either a noncalcified pulmonary nodule measuring at least 4 mm in diameter or another finding possibly attributable to lung cancer. Among the 53,454 participants enrolled in this study, there were significantly fewer lung cancer deaths among those screened with LDCT than among those randomized to CXR (356 deaths vs 443 deaths), with a relative reduction in lung cancer–specific mortality of 20.3% over a median of 6.5 years of follow-up ($P = .004$). In addition to reduced lung cancer mortality, the NLST also found a stage shift to earlier-stage disease in that 47.5% of the cancers detected in the LDCT screening group at the first annual repeat screen were at the earliest stage (IA), compared with only 15% at the time of diagnosis in a nonscreening population.[3–5]

Although the NLST was the first randomized trial to show a significant reduction in lung cancer mortality following computed tomographic (CT) screening, several other studies are ongoing. One of the largest is the Dutch-Belgian Nederlands-Leuvens Longkanker Screenings onderzoek (NELSON) trial, which is expected to report final results in late 2015.[6,7] The NELSON study differs from the NLST in several ways. First, the NELSON trial is a true comparison of CT screening versus no screening, which should provide more definitive quantification both of lung cancer–specific mortality reduction in screened patients and of the risks

associated with screening. The NELSON study participants become eligible for screening at a younger age (50 years), and study participants include smokers with a shorter smoking history (the equivalent of approximately 15 or more pack-years) and former smokers with a shorter interval since quitting (10 years or less).[7,8] Screening was performed at baseline, at year 1, and at year 3. Furthermore, the study incorporates volumetrics in nodule measurement and growth assessment, which may facilitate differentiation between benign nodules and suspicious nodules that require further evaluation.[9,10] The NELSON trial team has reported, during 3 screening rounds, a sensitivity of 84.6%, specificity of 98.6%, positive predictive value of 40.4%, and negative predictive value of 99.8%.[11] This positive predictive value is much higher than that achieved by other screening trials and could significantly affect cost-effectiveness analysis. The NELSON trial has demonstrated an even higher percentage of stage IA lung cancers than the NLST, with 74.1% of lung cancers in the second round of screening and 64.9% of lung cancers in the third round of screening diagnosed in this earliest stage.[11] The results from the NELSON study and other ongoing trials will be helpful in answering some of the questions raised by the NLST.

SETTING UP A LUNG CANCER SCREENING CLINIC
Key Personnel

American College of Radiology (ACR) Practice Parameters recommend a multidisciplinary approach to CT lung screening. The ideal lung cancer screening clinic includes a nurse navigator and representatives from primary care medicine, diagnostic radiology, pulmonary medicine, smoking cessation, thoracic oncology, radiation oncology, and thoracic surgery. Perhaps the most important individual in establishing a lung cancer screening clinic is the nurse navigator. This individual is responsible for ensuring that all elements of the screening process occur: verifying patient eligibility, reviewing the potential risks and benefits of screening with the patient, performing a CT screen with a low-radiation-dose technique, communicating study results to the patient, and scheduling either follow-up of patients with positive results or repeat annual LDCT for patients with negative or benign findings. Referrals for lung cancer screening largely come from primary care, so it is important to include primary care physicians and nurse practitioners in establishing a screening practice. Effective communication between screening clinic personnel and primary care providers can facilitate appropriate patient referrals.

The ability to track patients with positive screen results is essential to the success of a lung cancer screening clinic. This tracking can be achieved with a database or by incorporating screening results into the electronic medical record to ensure timely follow-up and management. Including hospital administration and information technology specialists during the clinic design can facilitate this process.

Who Should Be Screened?

Current eligibility criteria for lung cancer screening, as defined by the US Preventive Services Task Force (USPSTF) and the National Comprehensive Cancer Network (NCCN), are shown in **Table 1**.[12,13] The major differences between the 2 sets of eligibility criteria are age at which to stop screening (upper limit of 80 years in the USPSTF, 74 years in NCCN) and the inclusion of a second, lower-risk group recommended for screening in the NCCN guidelines. Although the differences are minor, most medical societies have endorsed the USPSTF eligibility criteria.

Shared Decision Making

Shared decision making in the setting of lung cancer screening is a collaborative process in which the patient and the health care provider discuss the risks and benefits of the procedure as they relate to that particular patient. Core elements of this process, as defined by the American Cancer Society, are included in **Table 2**.[14]

Risks and Benefits of Low-Dose Computed Tomography for Lung Cancer Screening

Potential risks and benefits of screening for lung cancer are listed in **Box 2**. An inherent risk of all screening tests is the potential for both false-negative and false-positive results. The sensitivity of the screening test should be sufficiently high to ensure that a cancer is not missed, whereas the specificity must be high enough to minimize the number of false-positive results. In the NLST, the sensitivity and specificity of LDCT screening were 93.8% and 73.4%, respectively.[15] Although 24.2% of LDCT screens were positive, most of these represented false-positive results, because only 3.6% of patients with positive results actually had lung cancer.[2]

The false-positive rate can be influenced by study design. The NELSON trial reported each screening CT result as negative, positive, or indeterminate. A CT scan demonstrating a nodule with a volume greater than 500 mm^3 (approximately 10 mm diameter) was considered positive, whereas a CT scan demonstrating a nodule between 50 and 500 mm^3 in volume (between approximately 5 and 10 mm in diameter) was considered indeterminate. Scans with indeterminate results were repeated at 6 to 8 weeks or 3 to 4 months, depending on screening round, which allowed calculation of nodule growth rates. An indeterminate scan result was then reclassified

Table 1 Lung cancer screening recommendations: patient eligibility		
Organization	**Recommendation**	**Criteria**
US Preventive Services Task Force (USPSTF)[13]	Grade B[a]	Age 55–80 y $\geq$30 pack-year smoking history; if former smoker, quit within previous 15 y
National Comprehensive Cancer Network (NCCN)[12]	Category 1[b]	Age 55–74 y $\geq$30 pack-year smoking history; if former smoker, quit within previous 15 y
	Category 2A[c]	Age $\geq$50 y $\geq$20 pack-year smoking history and one additional risk factor excluding second-hand smoke, such as history of lung cancer in a first-degree relative, personal history of malignancy, carcinogen exposure (ie, radon), or pulmonary disease (eg, COPD or pulmonary fibrosis)

[a] USPSTF grade B: High certainty that the net benefit is moderate or moderate certainty that the net benefit is moderate to substantial; recommend providing the service.
[b] NCCN category 1: Based on high-level evidence; uniform NCCN consensus.
[c] NCCN category 2A: Based on a lower level of evidence; uniform consensus that intervention is appropriate.

Table 2
Core elements of shared decision making, per the American Cancer Society guidelines

Element	Description
Benefit	Screening with LDCT has been shown to substantially reduce the risk of dying from lung cancer.
Limitations	LDCT does not detect all lung cancers or all lung cancers early, and not all patients who have a lung cancer detected by LDCT avoid death from lung cancer.
Harms	There is a significant chance of a false-positive result, which requires additional periodic testing and, in some instances, an invasive procedure to determine whether or not an abnormality is lung cancer or some non-lung cancer–related incidental finding. Fewer than 1 in 1000 patients with a false-positive result experience a major complication resulting from a diagnostic workup. Death within 60 d of a diagnostic evaluation has been documented but is rare and most often occurs in patients with lung cancer.

Data from Wender R, Fontham ET, Barrera E Jr, et al. American Cancer Society lung cancer screening guidelines. CA Cancer J Clin 2013;63:107–17.

as a positive result if a nodule demonstrated a volume doubling time less than 400 days.[11] This approach resulted in a much lower false-positive rate of only 2% to 3% (depending on the screening round), of which 34% to 46% cases showed true-positive results.

The false-positive rate is also affected by the threshold used for defining a positive screen result. Gierada and colleagues[16] demonstrated that raising the threshold from 4 to 5 mm in the NLST would have resulted in a missed or delayed diagnosis in only 1% of lung cancers and would have avoided 15.8% of the false-positive results. Raising the threshold even further to 6 mm would have resulted in a missed or delayed diagnosis of lung cancer in 3% and would have avoided 36.8% of the false-positive results.

Box 2
Potential risks and benefits of CT lung screening

Risks

  False-positive screen results, requiring unnecessary testing and procedures

  False-negative screen results

  Overdiagnosis

  Testing anxiety

  Radiation exposure and induced carcinogenesis

  Cost

Benefits

  Reduced lung cancer mortality

  Reduced disease-related morbidity

  Reduced treatment-related morbidity

When positive results are obtained on screening studies, additional testing is often required. Despite the high false-positive rate in the NLST, most patients with a positive screening examination result were managed noninvasively with follow-up imaging; only 9.4% of patients required invasive testing. Of those patients who underwent invasive testing, the rate of major complications was 0.06% for those without cancer and 11.2% for those with lung cancer. This result suggests that, although LDCT screening has a higher rate of false-positive results compared with other screening modalities, the number of invasive tests performed is low, complications from such procedures are rare, and the risks of additional testing are primarily incurred by patients who do have lung cancer.[1]

False-negative cases are those reported as negative but in which a diagnosis of lung cancer is made before the repeat annual LDCT. This occurrence is uncommon; in both the NLST and NELSON trial, less than 1% of the negative results were false negative.[2,11]

Overdiagnosis occurs when screening identifies histologically confirmed lung cancer that would not have resulted in a patient's death if left untreated, which can occur when a lung cancer is indolent or slow growing, as well as when a patient's death from other comorbidities occurs first. Potential harmful effects of overdiagnosis include the psychological stress that accompanies a diagnosis of cancer, as well as the morbidity and mortality that may accompany unnecessary medical procedures. Overdiagnosis is inherent in any screening test. A recent analysis modeling NLST data estimates the rate of overdiagnosis for lung cancer using LDCT to be 18.5%.[17] Although this rate may initially seem high, reported overdiagnosis rates for other screening examinations are higher, ranging from 29% to 44% for prostate specific antigen screening for prostate cancer and 30% to 54% for mammography for breast cancer screening.[18–20]

Despite the low radiation dose associated with lung cancer screening CT, radiation-induced malignancy remains a concern because the screening examination is expected to be repeated annually and may generate additional imaging follow-up. The technical parameters used for screening in the NLST yielded a mean effective radiation dose of 1.4 mSv (standard deviation = 0.5 mSv) across all scanners.[21] This dose can be compared with an average effective dose of 7 to 8 mSv for a diagnostic chest CT or 10 to 15 mSV for a diagnostic chest CT angiogram for possible pulmonary embolism.[22] Investigators in the ITA-LUNG (Italian Lung) screening trial not only reported a similar mean effective radiation dose of 1.2 to 1.4 mSv for LDCT but also pointed out that screening patients often undergo additional imaging examinations to evaluate positive findings.[23] They calculated a mean effective dose of 6.2 to 6.8 mSv during 4 years of screening, with 77.4% of the dose attributed to annual LDCT and the remaining 22.6% attributed to follow-up examinations, such as CT, Positron Emission Tomography (PET) with 18F-fluorodeoxyglucose (18F-FDG), or CT-guided fine-needle aspiration biopsy.

To date, there are no outcomes data regarding radiation-induced malignancies derived from patients undergoing LDCT screening. Models of NLST data estimate that 1 cancer death per 2500 patients screened may be attributable to radiation, indicating that the potential benefit of preventing lung cancer deaths is greater than the potential radiation risk.[24,25] The mean latency period from radiation exposure to development of cancer is longer than 30 years for standard-dose screening examinations and is projected to be even longer for LDCT screening techniques. The average age of patients who underwent screening in the NLST was 62 years; thus, the risk of radiation-induced carcinogenesis is extremely low when screening is performed in an appropriate population.

Performing the Low-Dose Computed Tomographic Screening Examination

The goal of screening for lung cancer with CT is to obtain images that provide visualization of lung nodules while delivering radiation doses that are as low as reasonably achievable. The inherent contrast between lung nodules and the lung parenchyma allows scanning techniques that are significantly different from diagnostic CT of the chest, with markedly lower radiation doses. The typical NLST participant was scanned with a kilovoltage peak (kVp) of 120, and an effective milliamperes × seconds/table pitch (mAs) of 40. It has been suggested that a body mass index (BMI)-based protocol could be used to minimize radiation exposure.[26] Current NCCN guidelines recommend a kVp of 100 to 120 and less than or equal to 40 mAs for patients whose BMI is less than 30 and a kVp of 120 and less than or equal to 60 mAs for patients with a BMI greater than 30.[12] Iterative reconstruction is a new technique for radiation reduction in MDCT (multi-detector computed tomography). Research is on-going to determine its impact on nodule detection before it is incorporated into LDCT screening protocols.

The scans are obtained in full inspiration, without intravenous or oral contrast media. Axial images, with slice thicknesses of 1 to 2.5 mm, are the standard for viewing images; however, it is helpful to reconstruct the images into thicker slices, such as 5 to 8 mm, with maximum intensity projection (MIP), for viewing in axial, coronal, or sagittal planes. On the thicker slices, pulmonary vessels are more likely to be in the imaging plane, so that it is easier to distinguish pulmonary nodules from pulmonary arteries or veins.

FINDINGS ON LOW-DOSE COMPUTED TOMOGRAPHIC SCREENING EXAMINATIONS
Lung Nodules

The likelihood that a nodule represents lung cancer is determined by its size, consistency, and growth rate. The diameter or volume should be measured on lung window settings. For nodules that are not spherical, 2 measurements should be made, of the long axis and the orthogonal short axis. The diameter is then recorded as the mean of these 2 measurements. Using the mean nodule diameter, the ACR Lung-RADS version 1.0 considers the following to be suspicious for lung cancer: solid nodules 8 mm and larger and part-solid nodules 6 mm and larger with a solid component measuring 6 to 8 mm.[27] When comparison CT scans are available, new solid nodules 6 to 8 mm in size or growing solid nodules less than 8 mm are also considered suspicious, as are part-solid nodules with a new or growing solid component.[27] The NELSON trial determined that the probability of lung cancer was high (15.2%) for nodules 10 mm and larger in diameter.[28]

Features that suggest a benign cause include fat attenuation or calcification that is complete, central, popcorn, or lamellar (**Fig. 1**). Perifissural or subpleural nodules that are triangular or polygonal

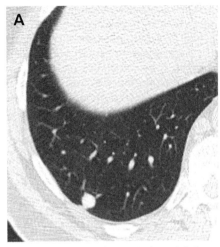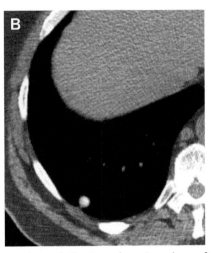

Fig. 1. This solid nodule seen on lung windows (*A*) shows complete calcification when viewed on soft-tissue windows (*B*), suggesting a benign cause.

in shape may represent benign subpleural lymph nodes (**Fig. 2**).[29]

The consistency of the nodule should be recorded as solid, part-solid, or nonsolid (ground glass). The likelihood of malignancy is higher for part-solid and nonsolid nodules than for solid nodules, likely attributable to noncalcified granulomas, which account for most solid nodules. In the Early Lung Cancer Action Project (ELCAP), Henschke and colleagues[30] determined that the likelihood of malignancy was only 7% for solid nodules but was 63% for part-solid nodules and 18% for nonsolid nodules (**Figs. 3–5**).

A growing nodule with a volume doubling time of less than 400 days causes concern for malignancy (see **Fig. 3**). The NELSON trial demonstrated a 9.9% (range, 3.7%–43.3%) likelihood of malignancy in nodules with volume doubling times shorter than 400 days.[28] Nodules that have not grown in size for 2 years are likely benign.

A large number of nodules seen at lung cancer screening cannot be readily categorized as either benign or malignant and require further investigation, usually with repeat LDCT.

Incidental Findings

Incidental findings are defined as abnormalities discovered on an imaging examination that are unrelated to the purpose of the examination. In the case of LDCT screening for lung cancer, the CT scan may reveal abnormalities in the lower neck, the thorax, and the upper abdomen. Some of these abnormalities are clinically significant findings, whereas others are unlikely to be significant. Examples of incidental findings unlikely to be clinically significant include pleural plaques, lymph nodes smaller than 1 cm in short axis, renal cysts, and small nodules within the thyroid and adrenal glands. Reporting these findings can lead to unnecessary patient anxiety and costs associated with workups. On the other hand, LDCT may reveal findings that are likely to be clinically significant and potential contributors to morbidity and mortality in the screening population.

The leading causes of mortality within the NLST were cardiovascular disease (24.8%), lung cancer (24.1%), other neoplasms (22.3%), and respiratory illness (10.4%).[2] The NLST was designed to compare the ability of screening with LDCT to

Fig. 2. This 6-mm solid nodule (*arrow*) adjacent to the minor fissure has a high likelihood of benignity because of its size, morphology, and location. This nodule was unchanged after 7 years of follow-up.

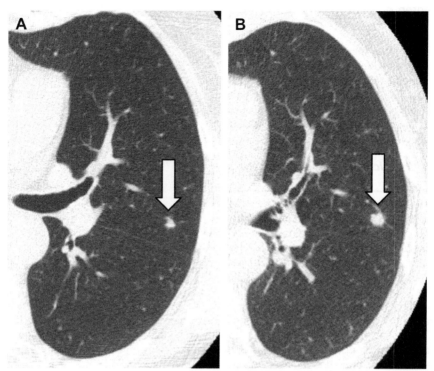

Fig. 3. This 4- × 5-mm solid nodule (*arrow*) in the left upper lobe has a low likelihood of malignancy on initial screening (*A*). However, interval growth on a repeat annual LDCT screen (*B*) reclassified this nodule (*arrow*) as suspicious (Lung-RADS category 4A).

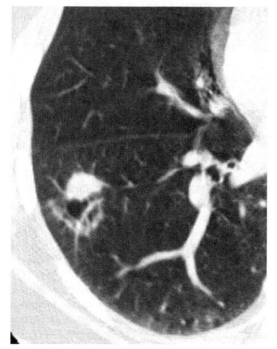

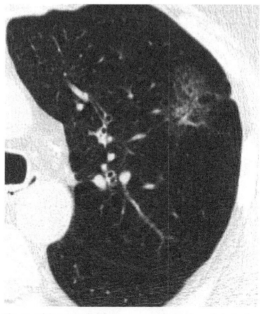

Fig. 4. This part-solid nodule in the right lower lobe has a high likelihood of malignancy because of its size and consistency. A solid component larger than 8 mm categorizes this nodule as suspicious (Lung-RADS 4B). Appropriate management includes diagnostic chest CT, 18F-FDG-PET-CT or tissue sampling.

Fig. 5. This nonsolid (pure ground glass) nodule in the left upper lobe is considered to have a benign appearance in the Lung-RADS system (Category 2). Although Lung-RADS recommends continued annual screening for all nonsolid nodules smaller than 20 mm, the NCCN guidelines manage nonsolid nodules 5 to 10 mm in diameter with repeat LDCT in 6 months.

reduce mortality from lung cancer, as compared with screening with CXR, in a high-risk cohort. It was not designed to identify or intervene in other disease conditions. It is possible that recognition of other diseases at the time of CT screening could reduce morbidity or mortality by earlier diagnosis and intervention.

Emphysema/Chronic Obstructive Pulmonary Disease

Although chronic obstructive pulmonary disease (COPD) is a common condition within any population of older, heavy smokers, it remains an under-reported illness, even in volunteers within lung cancer screening programs. Within the NELSON trial, pulmonary function testing identified COPD in 38% (437 of 1140) of participants.[31] Only 3.6% of the population reported physician-diagnosed emphysema, and 8.2% reported physician-diagnosed bronchitis. The investigators also developed a diagnostic model, using CT measures of emphysema and air trapping, body mass index, pack-years, and smoking status. Their model was 63% sensitive and 88% specific in predicting which patients would have spirometric evidence of COPD, defined as the ratio of forced expiratory volume in the first second to forced vital capacity of less than 70%. Emphysema can be evaluated on the inspiratory CT images as areas of decreased attenuation with ill-defined walls (**Fig. 6**). A threshold of −950 HU (Hounsfield units) is commonly used to define areas of emphysema for quantitative analysis.

Some heavy smokers exhibit an airway-predominant COPD phenotype on LDCT screening.[32,33] Airway wall thickness and diameter can be assessed on axial images (**Fig. 7**). The NELSON trial added expiratory CT to the screening protocol in a subset of patients. The expiratory

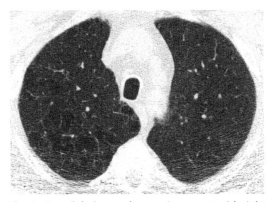

Fig. 6. Centrilobular emphysema is present, with right upper lobe predominance, on LDCT performed for lung cancer screening.

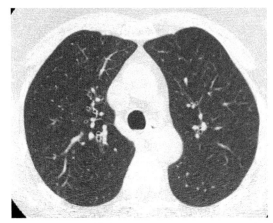

Fig. 7. Airway wall thickening is present, suggesting an airway-predominant COPD phenotype.

images enable quantification of air trapping, which can be assessed by determining the ratio of mean lung density on expiratory images to that on inspiratory images.[34]

The value of CT identification of COPD at lung cancer screening is 2-fold. First, it may prompt pulmonary function testing in previously undiagnosed patients with COPD, facilitating appropriate clinical management and reducing COPD exacerbations. Second, COPD is a risk factor for lung cancer and may factor into decisions about lung cancer risk, nodule management, and appropriate screening intervals.[35,36]

Smoking-Related Interstitial Lung Disease

In addition to identifying COPD, the LDCT scans of heavy cigarette smokers may reveal smoking-related interstitial lung diseases, including desquamative interstitial pneumonia (DIP), respiratory bronchiolitis–related interstitial lung disease, pulmonary Langerhans cell histiocytosis, and idiopathic pulmonary fibrosis.[37,38] These diseases overlap, and features of one disease or of multiple diseases may be present in the same patient.[39]

Interstitial lung abnormalities are common in the lung cancer screening population, occurring in approximately 9.7%.[40] Jin and colleagues[40] retrospectively reviewed the LDCT scans of 884 participants in the NLST and recognized nonfibrotic patterns of interstitial lung abnormalities, including ground glass opacity, consolidation, and mosaic attenuation in 52 (5.9%). The ground glass opacities likely represented respiratory bronchiolitis and, to a lesser extent, DIP. A fibrotic pattern (ground glass with reticular pattern, reticular pattern, or honeycombing) was less common, occurring in 19 (2.1%). An additional 15 patients (1.7%) displayed mixed patterns of fibrotic and nonfibrotic interstitial lung abnormalities. At 2-year follow-up, the nonfibrotic patterns had improved in 49% of cases but had progressed in 11%. Conversely, none of the fibrotic patterns had improved at 2-year follow-up, and 37% of cases demonstrated progression.

Coronary Artery Calcification

There were more deaths from cardiovascular disease than from lung cancer in the NLST (956 vs 930).[2] As advancing age and smoking are risk factors for atherosclerosis, the eligibility criteria for lung cancer screening also produce a population at risk of coronary artery disease. Coronary artery calcification is visible on the nongated unenhanced LDCT images obtained for screening, albeit at a lower spatial resolution than on a dedicated electrocardiogram-gated cardiac CT image (**Fig. 8**). Several investigators have shown that coronary artery calcification as measured on lung cancer screening CT image is associated with cardiovascular events and deaths.[41–43] Within a case-cohort study of 958 subjects in the NELSON trial, multivariate-adjusted hazard ratios for coronary events, as compared with Agatston scores of 0 for coronary artery calcification, were 1.38 for Agatston scores of 1 to 100, 3.04 for scores of 101 to 1000, and 7.77 for scores greater than 1000.[41]

Extrapulmonary Malignancy

Rampinelli and colleagues[44] reported finding an asymptomatic extrapulmonary malignancy with a frequency of 1 case per 200 individuals screened

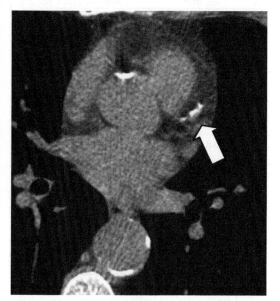

Fig. 8. Atherosclerotic calcification is visible within the left anterior descending coronary artery (*arrow*) on LDCT performed for lung cancer screening.

for lung cancer for 5 consecutive years. Renal cancers and lymphomas were the most frequent extrapulmonary cancers detected. The frequency of detecting extrapulmonary findings depends not only on the screening year (baseline vs annual follow-up) but also on the anatomy included within the screening CT. Extrapulmonary malignancies are detected more commonly on the baseline examination and at a lower rate on subsequent screens. Current screening protocols extend from the lower neck to the upper abdomen, so that the lung apices through the lung bases are completely included. In a 1999 to 2001 lung cancer screening trial at the Mayo Clinic, the screening CT included both the chest and abdomen and extended from the level of the sternal notch to the iliac crests.[45] Swensen and colleagues[45] diagnosed 18 extrapulmonary malignancies in 1520 participants during a 3-year interval, for a detection rate of 1.2%. The most commonly encountered tumors were renal cell carcinoma, breast cancer, lymphoma, and gastric tumor.

The advantages of identifying extrapulmonary malignancy at an early stage must be weighed against the risks and costs associated with working up lesions with a low likelihood of clinical significance. There are currently no accepted guidelines for the reporting and management of incidental findings specifically in the setting of lung cancer screening.

UNDERSTANDING THE LOW-DOSE COMPUTED TOMOGRAPHIC REPORT: THE AMERICAN COLLEGE OF RADIOLOGY LUNG CT SCREENING REPORTING AND DATA SYSTEM

The NLST implemented strict structured reporting for screening examinations; however, reporting criteria have not been mandated in clinical practice and variability among programs is common. In an effort to minimize confusion in report interpretation, the ACR Lung Cancer Screening Committee developed the Lung-RADS to facilitate standardized reporting, uniform management, and outcomes monitoring. Version 1.0 was released in April 2014.[27] The format adopts many of the conventions found in the ubiquitous Breast Imaging Reporting and Data System (BIRADS). Both the ACR Lung-RADS and NCCN Guidelines provide management recommendations for LDCT screening findings (**Tables 3–5**). Unfortunately, the 2 systems are discordant in some areas, although the recommendations typically only differ in the follow-up imaging interval.

Few published data are available regarding outcomes associated with the use of Lung-RADS

Table 3
American College of Radiology CT Lung Reporting and Data System categories and modifiers

Category	Descriptor	Comment
0	Incomplete	Incomplete evaluation; awaiting comparison examinations
1	Negative	No nodules; definitely benign nodules
2	Benign	Nodules with a very low likelihood of cancer due to size or lack of growth
3	Probably benign	Findings with a low likelihood of representing cancer; however, short-term follow-up is recommended
4A	Suspicious	Findings requiring additional diagnostic imaging evaluation (eg, follow-up LDCT or PET-CT)
4B	Suspicious	Findings requiring additional diagnostic imaging evaluation and/or tissue sampling (eg, diagnostic chest CT, PET-CT, or biopsy)
4X	Suspicious	Additional features or findings that increase the probability for malignancy (evaluation per 4B category)
Modifiers	**Descriptor**	**May Be Added to Categories 0–4**
S	Other	Significant or potentially significant findings unrelated to lung cancer
C	Prior lung cancer	For use in patients with prior diagnosis of lung cancer undergoing screening

Abbreviation: GGN, Ground-glass nodule.

Data from American College of Radiology (ACR) Lung CT Screening Reporting and Data System (Lung-RADS) Version 1.0. Available at: http://www.acr.org/Quality-Safety/Resources/LungRADS. Accessed September 4, 2014.

Table 4
Lung cancer screening management guidelines: differences between ACR Lung-RADS v. 1.0 and NCCN v. 1.2015 recommendations on baseline screening LDCT

Screening Finding	ACR Lung-RADS	Screening Finding	NCCN
Solid nodules			
<6 mm	Continue annual LDCT	<6 mm	Annual LDCT for 2 y
≥6 to <8 mm	6 mo LDCT	6–8 mm	3 mo LDCT
≥8 to <15 mm	3 mo LDCT; PET-CT	>8 mm	Consider PET-CT
≥15 mm	Chest CT; PET-CT; tissue sampling		
Part-solid nodules			
<6 mm total diameter	Continue annual LDCT	<6 mm	Annual LDCT for 2 y
≥6 mm with solid component <6 mm	6 mo LDCT	6–8 mm	3 mo LDCT
≥6 mm with solid component ≥6 to <8 mm	3 mo LDCT; PET-CT	>8 mm	Consider PET-CT
Solid component ≥8 mm	Chest CT; PET-CT; tissue sampling		
Nonsolid nodules (GGN)			
<20 mm	Continue annual LDCT	≤5 mm	LDCT in 12 mo
		>5 to 10 mm	LDCT in 6 mo
		>10 mm	LDCT in 3–6 mo
≥20 mm	6 mo LDCT		

Abbreviation: GGN, ground-glass nodule.

Data from National Comprehensive Cancer Network (NCCN) Lung Cancer Screening Guidelines Version 1.2015. Available at: http://www.nccn.org/professionals/physician_gls/pdf/lung_screening.pdf. Accessed October 12, 2014; and American College of Radiology (ACR) Lung CT Screening Reporting and Data System (Lung-RADS) Version 1.0. Available at: http://www.acr.org/Quality-Safety/Resources/LungRADS. Accessed September 4, 2014.

Table 5
Lung cancer screening management guidelines: differences between ACR Lung-RADS v. 1.0 and NCCN recommendations v. 1.2015 for new or growing nodules

Screening Finding	ACR Lung-RADS	Screening Finding	NCCN
Solid nodules			
New <4 mm	Continue annual LDCT		
New 4 to <6 mm	6 mo LDCT		
Growing <8 mm or new 6 to <8 mm	3 mo LDCT; PET-CT	6–8 mm with growth on 6-mo follow-up CT	Surgical excision
New or growing and ≥8 mm	Chest CT; PET-CT; tissue sampling	>8 mm with growth on 3-mo follow-up CT	Surgical excision
Part-solid nodules			
New <6 mm total diameter	6 mo LDCT		
≥6 mm with new or growing solid component <4 mm	3 mo LDCT	6–8 mm with growth on 6-mo follow-up CT	Surgical excision
New or growing ≥4 mm solid component	3 mo LDCT; PET-CT may be used if solid component ≥8 mm	>8 mm with growth on 3-mo follow-up CT	Surgical excision
Nonsolid nodules (GGN)			
		≤5 mm with growth or development of solid component at 12-mo follow-up CT	LDCT in 3–6 mo or consider surgical excision
		>5 to 10 mm with growth or development of solid component at 6-mo follow-up CT	Surgical excision
		>10 mm with growth or development of solid component at 3-mo follow-up CT	Surgical excision
≥20 mm and unchanged or slowly growing	Continue annual LDCT		
≥20 mm and new	6 mo LDCT		

Abbreviation: GGN, ground-glass nodule.

Data from National Comprehensive Cancer Network (NCCN) Lung Cancer Screening Guidelines Version 1.2015. Available at: http://www.nccn.org/professionals/physician_gls/pdf/lung_screening.pdf. Accessed October 12, 2014; and American College of Radiology (ACR) Lung CT Screening Reporting and Data System (Lung-RADS) Version 1.0. Available at: http://www.acr.org/Quality-Safety/Resources/LungRADS. Accessed September 4, 2014.

reporting. A single retrospective study evaluating the use of Lung-RADS in comparison with the NLST screening reporting criteria found an increase in the positive predictive value by a factor of 2.5 (from 6.9%–17.3%) without an increase in false-negative results[46]; this is largely attributable to an increase in the size threshold for a positive result from 4 to 6 mm for solid nodules. Similar findings were reported by an analysis of I-ELCAP data.[47] Both the NCCN and ACR have since adopted 6 mm as the minimum nodule size for a positive CT screening result.

FINANCIAL ISSUES

At present, LDCT for lung cancer screening is not covered by most third-party payers, meaning most patients who qualify for screening must pay for the service out of pocket. With advertised costs of $99 to $1000, screening remains out of reach for many patients.[48] Since the results of the NLST, more than 30 major medical societies have endorsed LDCT for lung cancer screening. The recent USPSTF grade B recommendation for lung cancer screening using LDCT in asymptomatic adults aged 55 to 80 years who have a 30 pack-year smoking history and currently smoke or have quit within the past 15 years requires all new private insurers under the Affordable Care Act to cover LDCT for lung cancer screening for high-risk patients.[49] On November 10, 2014, the Centers for Medicare and Medicaid Services issued a proposed decision memo stating that evidence was sufficient to provide coverage for a lung cancer screening counseling and shared decision-making visit and, for appropriate beneficiaries, annual screening for lung cancer with LDCT.[50]

SUMMARY

Early detection of lung cancer through the use of LDCT is an effective, evidence-based strategy for improving the health of high-risk patients. Results from the prospective, randomized controlled NLST demonstrate that LDCT screening significantly reduces the mortality from lung cancer and is appropriate with careful patient selection and follow-up. Secondary analyses of NLST data as well as the results of currently ongoing trials will aid in further refining screening guidelines.

REFERENCES

1. Siegel R, Ma J, Zou Z, et al. Cancer statistics, 2014. CA Cancer J Clin 2014;64:9–29.
2. National Lung Screening Trial Research Team, Aberle DR, Adams AM, et al. Reduced lung-cancer mortality with low-dose computed tomographic screening. N Engl J Med 2011;365:395–409.
3. Aberle DR, DeMello S, Berg CD, et al. Results of the two incidence screenings in the National Lung Screening Trial. N Engl J Med 2013;369:920–31.
4. Detterbeck FC, Postmus PE, Tanoue LT. The stage classification of lung cancer: diagnosis and management of lung cancer, 3rd ed: American College of Chest Physicians evidence-based clinical practice guidelines. Chest 2013;143:e191S–210S.
5. Shepherd FA, Crowley J, Van Houtte P, et al. The International Association for the Study of Lung Cancer lung cancer staging project: proposals regarding the clinical staging of small cell lung cancer in the forthcoming (seventh) edition of the tumor, node, metastasis classification for lung cancer. J Thorac Oncol 2007;2:1067–77.
6. van der Aalst CM, van Iersel CA, van Klaveren RJ, et al. Generalisability of the results of the Dutch-Belgian randomised controlled lung cancer CT screening trial (NELSON): does self-selection play a role? Lung Cancer 2012;77:51–7.
7. van Iersel CA, de Koning HJ, Draisma G, et al. Risk-based selection from the general population in a screening trial: selection criteria, recruitment and power for the Dutch-Belgian randomised lung cancer multi-slice CT screening trial (NELSON). Int J Cancer 2007;120:868–74.
8. Pedersen JH, Ashraf H, Dirksen A, et al. The Danish randomized lung cancer CT screening trial–overall design and results of the prevalence round. J Thorac Oncol 2009;4:608–14.
9. Heuvelmans MA, Oudkerk M, de Bock GH, et al. Optimisation of volume-doubling time cutoff for fast-growing lung nodules in CT lung cancer screening reduces false-positive referrals. Eur Radiol 2013;23:1836–45.
10. Xu DM, Gietema H, de Koning H, et al. Nodule management protocol of the NELSON randomised lung cancer screening trial. Lung Cancer 2006;54:177–84.
11. Horeweg N, Scholten ET, de Jong PA, et al. Detection of lung cancer through low-dose CT screening (NELSON): a prespecified analysis of screening test performance and interval cancers. Lancet Oncol 2014;15(12):1342–50.
12. National Comprehensive Cancer Network (NCCN) Lung Cancer Screening Guidelines Version 1.2015. Available at: http://www.nccn.org/professionals/physician_gls/pdf/lung_screening.pdf. Accessed October 12, 2014.
13. Moyer VA, U.S. Preventive Services Task Force. Screening for lung cancer: U.S. Preventive Services Task Force recommendation statement. Ann Intern Med 2014;160:330–8.
14. Wender R, Fontham ET, Barrera E Jr, et al. American Cancer Society lung cancer screening guidelines. CA Cancer J Clin 2013;63:107–17.

15. National Lung Screening Trial Research Team, Church TR, Black WC, et al. Results of initial low-dose computed tomographic screening for lung cancer. N Engl J Med 2013;368:1980–91.

16. Gierada DS, Pinsky P, Nath H, et al. Projected outcomes using different nodule sizes to define a positive CT lung Cancer screening examination. J Natl Cancer Inst 2014;106–12.

17. Patz EF Jr, Pinsky P, Gatsonis C, et al. Overdiagnosis in low-dose computed tomography screening for lung cancer. JAMA Intern Med 2014;174:269–74.

18. Loeb S, Bjurlin MA, Nicholson J, et al. Overdiagnosis and overtreatment of prostate cancer. Eur Urol 2014;65:1046–55.

19. Gotzsche PC, Nielsen M. Screening for breast cancer with mammography. Cochrane Database Syst Rev 2011;(1):CD001877.

20. Etzioni R, Penson DF, Legler JM, et al. Overdiagnosis due to prostate-specific antigen screening: lessons from U.S. prostate cancer incidence trends. J Natl Cancer Inst 2002;94:981–90.

21. Larke FJ, Kruger RL, Cagnon CH, et al. Estimated radiation dose associated with low-dose chest CT of average-size participants in the National Lung Screening Trial. AJR Am J Roentgenol 2011;197:1165–9.

22. Mettler FA Jr, Huda W, Yoshizumi TT, et al. Effective doses in radiology and diagnostic nuclear medicine: a catalog. Radiology 2008;248:254–63.

23. Mascalchi M, Mazzoni LN, Falchini M, et al. Dose exposure in the ITALUNG trial of lung cancer screening with low-dose CT. Br J Radiol 2012;85:1134–9.

24. Einstein AJ, Henzlova MJ, Rajagopalan S. Estimating risk of cancer associated with radiation exposure from 64-slice computed tomography coronary angiography. JAMA 2007;298:317–23.

25. Berrington de Gonzalez A, Kim KP, Berg CD. Low-dose lung computed tomography screening before age 55: estimates of the mortality reduction required to outweigh the radiation-induced cancer risk. J Med Screen 2008;15:153–8.

26. Manowitz A, Sedlar M, Griffon M, et al. Use of BMI guidelines and individual dose tracking to minimize radiation exposure from low-dose helical chest CT scanning in a lung cancer screening program. Acad Radiol 2012;19:84–8.

27. American College of Radiology (ACR) Lung CT Screening Reporting and Data System (Lung-RADS) Version 1.0. Available at: http://www.acr.org/Quality-Safety/Resources/LungRADS. Accessed September 4, 2014.

28. Horeweg N, van Rosmalen J, Heuvelmans MA, et al. Lung cancer probability in patients with CT-detected pulmonary nodules: a prespecified analysis of data from the NELSON trial of low-dose CT screening. Lancet Oncol 2014;15(12):1332–41.

29. Ahn MI, Gleeson TG, Chan IH, et al. Perifissural nodules seen at CT screening for lung cancer. Radiology 2010;254:949–56.

30. Henschke CI, Yankelevitz DF, Mirtcheva R, et al. CT screening for lung cancer: frequency and significance of part-solid and nonsolid nodules. AJR Am J Roentgenol 2002;178:1053–7.

31. Mets OM, Buckens CF, Zanen P, et al. Identification of chronic obstructive pulmonary disease in lung cancer screening computed tomographic scans. JAMA 2011;306:1775–81.

32. Han MK, Agusti A, Calverley PM, et al. Chronic obstructive pulmonary disease phenotypes: the future of COPD. Am J Respir Crit Care Med 2010;182:598–604.

33. Friedlander AL, Lynch D, Dyar LA, et al. Phenotypes of chronic obstructive pulmonary disease. COPD 2007;4:355–84.

34. Mets OM, Zanen P, Lammers JW, et al. Early identification of small airways disease on lung cancer screening CT: comparison of current air trapping measures. Lung 2012;190(6):629–33.

35. Tammemagi MC, Katki HA, Hocking WG, et al. Selection criteria for lung-cancer screening. N Engl J Med 2013;368:728–36.

36. Tammemagi CM, Pinsky PF, Caporaso NE, et al. Lung cancer risk prediction: prostate, lung, colorectal and ovarian cancer screening trial models and validation. J Natl Cancer Inst 2011;103:1058–68.

37. Hidalgo A, Franquet T, Gimenez A, et al. Smoking-related interstitial lung diseases: radiologic-pathologic correlation. Eur Radiol 2006;16:2463–70.

38. Hansell DM, Nicholson AG. Smoking-related diffuse parenchymal lung disease: HRCT-pathologic correlation. Semin Respir Crit Care Med 2003;24:377–92.

39. Heyneman LE, Ward S, Lynch DA, et al. Respiratory bronchiolitis, respiratory bronchiolitis-associated interstitial lung disease, and desquamative interstitial pneumonia: different entities or part of the spectrum of the same disease process? AJR Am J Roentgenol 1999;173:1617–22.

40. Jin GY, Lynch D, Chawla A, et al. Interstitial lung abnormalities in a CT lung cancer screening population: prevalence and progression rate. Radiology 2013;268:563–71.

41. Jacobs PC, Gondrie MJ, van der Graaf Y, et al. Coronary artery calcium can predict all-cause mortality and cardiovascular events on low-dose CT screening for lung cancer. AJR Am J Roentgenol 2012;198:505–11.

42. Mets OM, Vliegenthart R, Gondrie MJ, et al. Lung cancer screening CT-based prediction of cardiovascular events. JACC Cardiovasc Imaging 2013;6:899–907.

43. Shemesh J, Henschke CI, Shaham D, et al. Ordinal scoring of coronary artery calcifications on low-dose CT scans of the chest is predictive of death

from cardiovascular disease. Radiology 2010;257: 541–8.

44. Rampinelli C, Preda L, Maniglio M, et al. Extrapulmonary malignancies detected at lung cancer screening. Radiology 2011;261:293–9.

45. Swensen SJ, Jett JR, Hartman TE, et al. Lung cancer screening with CT: Mayo Clinic experience. Radiology 2003;226:756–61.

46. McKee BJ, Regis SM, McKee AB, et al. Performance of ACR Lung-RADS in a Clinical CT Lung Screening Program. J Am Coll Radiol 2015;12:273–6.

47. Henschke CI, Yip R, Yankelevitz DF, et al, International Early Lung Cancer Action Program Investigators. Definition of a positive test result in computed tomography screening for lung cancer: a cohort study. Ann Intern Med 2013;158:246–52.

48. Munden RF, Godoy MC. Lung cancer screening: state of the art. J Surg Oncol 2013;108:270–4.

49. Patient Protection and Affordable Care Act. (Public Law 111–148), 2010. Available at: https://www.healthcare.gov/where-can-i-read-the-affordable-care-act/. Accessed September 4, 2014.

50. Proposed decision memo for screening for lung cancer with low dose computed tomography (LDCT) (CAG-00439N). Available at: http://www.cms.gov/medicare-coverage-database/details/nca-proposed-decision-memo.aspx?NCAId=274. Accessed September 4, 2014.

Imaging the Solitary Pulmonary Nodule

Jeffrey B. Alpert, MD*, Conor M. Lowry, MD, Jane P. Ko, MD

KEYWORDS

- Solitary pulmonary nodule • Solitary lung nodule • Pulmonary nodule • Lung cancer
- Lung cancer screening • Screening chest CT • PET/CT

KEY POINTS

- Discovery of a solitary pulmonary nodule (SPN) often results in a diagnostic dilemma that requires consideration of both clinical risk factors and imaging features to estimate the likelihood of malignancy.
- Patient risk factors, such as age, smoking, and underlying malignancy, may influence the likelihood of malignancy, and imaging features, such as nodule density, composition, shape, size, and growth rate, all aid in determining the malignant potential of an indeterminate SPN.
- In addition to multidetector chest CT, imaging, such as contrast-enhanced chest CT and fluoro-deoxyglucose F 18 (FDG)–positron emission tomography (PET), can provide greater diagnostic value. Newer imaging modalities, such as contrast-enhanced dual-energy CT (DECT) and FDG-PET/CT, are increasingly available and able to provide greater data more efficiently.

INTRODUCTION

Lung cancer mortality remains the highest among all other common types of cancers combined, with a reported 5-year mortality as high as 84%.[1,2] Indeterminate lung nodules are frequently detected incidentally on thoracic CT performed for clinical indications or for screening. A review of 8 large lung cancer screening programs revealed a prevalence of at least 1 lung nodule on chest CT ranging from 8% to 51%, with the prevalence of malignancy among these nodules varying from 1% to 12%.[3–8] Although results from the National Lung Screening Trial indicate that lung cancer screening using low-dose chest CT results in a relative reduction in lung cancer mortality of 20%, the positive predictive value (PPV) of low-dose CT screening is approximately 5%.[9–11] Therefore, a large number of lung nodules detected on screening studies ultimately prove benign, and the uncertainty of an indeterminate lung nodule may produce increased medical costs and patient risk and anxiety. Both clinical acumen and an understanding of currently available imaging are necessary for management of the newly discovered lung nodule to ensure accurate and timely diagnosis of a potential lung cancer.

Multidisciplinary groups, such as the Fleischner Society and the American College of Chest Physicians, have issued evidence-based recommendations for management of solid and subsolid lung nodules, which incorporate clinical risk factors, the utility and timeliness of imaging examinations, the benefits and risks of intervention, and patient preference (**Tables 1** and **2**).[12–14] The American College of Radiology has published appropriateness criteria to assist in the imaging evaluation of an incidentally discovered SPN.[15] The objective of this article is to review the methods of radiologic detection and characterization of the pulmonary nodule, highlighting the strengths and the pitfalls associated with noninvasive evaluation.

Disclosures: Dr J.B. Alpert is Speaker honorarium, Siemens Medical, which is unrelated to this work.
Thoracic Section, Department of Radiology, NYU Langone Medical Center, 660 First Avenue, 7th Floor, New York, NY 10016, USA
* Corresponding author.
E-mail address: Jeffrey.alpert@nyumc.org

Clin Chest Med 36 (2015) 161–178
http://dx.doi.org/10.1016/j.ccm.2015.02.003

Table 1
Current Fleischner Society recommendations for imaging follow-up and management of small incidentally detected lung nodules

Nodule Size (mm)[a]	Low-Risk Patient[b]	High-Risk Patient[c]
≤4	No follow-up needed[d]	Follow-up CT at 12 mo; if unchanged, no further follow-up[e]
>4–6	Follow-up CT at 12 mo; if unchanged, no further follow-up[e]	Initial follow-up CT at 6–12 mo then at 18–24 mo if no change[e]
>6–8	Initial follow-up CT at 6–12 mo then at 18–24 mo if no change	Initial follow-up CT at 3–6 mo then at 9–12 and 24 mo if no change
>8	Follow-up CT at approximately 3, 9, and 24 mo; dynamic contrast-enhanced CT, PET, and/or biopsy	Same as for low-risk patient

Note. Newly detected indeterminate nodule in persons 35 years of age or older.
  [a] Average of length and width.
  [b] Minimal or absent history of smoking and of other known risk factors.
  [c] History of smoking or of other known risk factors.
  [d] The risk of malignancy in this category (<1%) is substantially less than that in a baseline CT scan of an asymptomatic smoker.
  [e] Nonsolid nodules (GGNs) or PSNs may require longer follow-up to exclude indolent adenocarcinoma.
  From MacMahon H, Austin JH, Gamsu G, et al. Guidelines for management of small pulmonary nodules detected on CT scans: a statement from the Fleischner Society. Radiology 2005;237:398; with permission.

DEFINITIONS AND DIFFERENTIAL DIAGNOSIS

The SPN is defined as a spherical opacity measuring up to 3 cm in greatest diameter that is surrounded by lung parenchyma.[15,16] The differential diagnosis of the SPN is broad, ranging from primary lung cancer to various benign entities, such as infectious pneumonia and granulomatous disease (**Table 3**). Benign neoplasia, such as hamartoma, and vascular entities, such as pulmonary arteriovenous malformation, may produce solid nodules. Diagnostic considerations for the subsolid lung nodule include entities such as hemorrhage, infarction, organizing pneumonia, and focal fibrosis. After discovery of an SPN, the likelihood of malignancy depends on several clinical factors, including age, exposure to tobacco smoke and other carcinogens, underlying pulmonary fibrosis, and personal or family history of lung or other primary malignancy.[17] Lung cancer diagnoses have shifted from smoking-related squamous cell lung carcinoma to adenocarcinoma involving younger patients, with greater attention to the role of genetic mutations in the development of lung cancer.[18]

IMAGING TECHNIQUES FOR NODULE EVALUATION
Chest Radiography

Chest radiography remains the most frequently used first-line imaging tool for diagnosis of cardiopulmonary disease. The sensitivity and specificity of chest radiographs, however, are well known to be inferior to CT for lung nodule detection.[10,19] Suboptimal patient positioning and poor inspiratory lung volumes can hinder detection of lung nodules. Even without technical limitations, overlying bones, such as ribs, clavicles, scapula, and spine, in addition to the heart, hilum, and diaphragm, obscure portions of the lung. Due to numerous overlying bones, the lung apex is one of the most difficult areas to detect a lung nodule on chest radiograph (**Fig. 1**). A nodule in the retrocardiac or hilar region is often difficult to visualize on the frontal radiograph, although the lateral projection assists in evaluation of these areas.

Technical advances, such as bone-suppression software and dual-energy subtraction, have been developed to enhance the sensitivity of chest radiographs, and computer-aided detection (CAD) software has been shown to improve radiologists' detection of lung nodules on radiographs.[20,21] A study by Freedman and colleagues[22] showed a significant improvement in radiologists' ability to detect lung nodules on chest radiographs using bone-suppression software, improving sensitivity for detection of suspicious lung nodules from 49.5% to 66.3%. Approximately 75% of nodules detected with computer assistance were obscured more than 50% by overlying bones.

Solid lung nodules are more evident than subsolid lesions on chest radiographs, which are particularly difficult to visualize. The determination

Table 2
Current Fleischner Society recommendations for management of subsolid lung nodules discovered at CT

Nodule Type	Management Recommendations	Additional Remarks
Solitary pure GGNs		
≤5 mm	No CT follow-up required	Obtain contiguous 1-mm-thick sections to confirm that nodule is truly a pure GGN
>5 mm	Initial follow-up CT at 3 mo to confirm persistence then annual surveillance CT for a minimum of 3 y	FDG-PET is of limited value, potentially misleading, and therefore not recommended
Solitary PSNs	Initial follow-up CT at 3 mo to confirm persistence. If persistent and solid component <5 mm, then yearly surveillance CT for a minimum of 3 y. If persistent and solid component ≥5 mm, then biopsy or surgical resection	Consider PET/CT for PSNs >10 mm
Multiple subsolid nodules		
Pure GGNs ≤5 mm	Obtain follow-up CT at 2 and 4 y	Consider alternate causes for multiple GGNs ≤5 mm
Pure GGNs >5 mm without a dominant lesion(s)	Initial follow-up CT at 3 mo to confirm persistence and then annual surveillance CT for a minimum of 3 y	FDG-PET is of limited value, potentially misleading, and therefore not recommended
Dominant nodule(s) with part-solid or solid component	Initial follow-up CT at 3 mo to confirm persistence. If persistent, biopsy or surgical resection is recommended, especially for lesions with >5 mm solid component	Consider lung-sparing surgery for patients with dominant lesion(s) suspicious for lung cancer

Note. These guidelines assume meticulous evaluation, optimally with contiguous thin sections (1 mm) reconstructed with narrow and/or mediastinal windows to evaluate the solid component and wide and/or lung windows to evaluate the non-solid component of nodules, if indicated. When electronic calipers are used, bidimensional measurements of both the solid and ground-glass components of lesions should be obtained as necessary. The use of a consistent low-dose technique is recommended, especially in cases for which prolonged follow-up is recommended, particularly in younger patients. With serial scans, always compare with the original baseline study to detect subtle indolent growth.

From Naidich DP, Bankier AA, MacMahon H, et al. Recommendations for the management of subsolid pulmonary nodules detected at CT: a statement from the Fleischner Society. Radiology 2013;266:306; with permission.

of nodule calcification can also be challenging on chest radiograph, and the ability of radiologists to confidently detect calcium in an SPN by chest radiograph is considered low.[23] When a small nodule less than 7 mm is visualized, however, it is more likely to be calcified than those larger than 7 mm (**Fig. 2**).[24]

When an SPN is initially discovered on chest radiograph, prior chest radiographs play an important role in demonstrating stability over time. If a solid nodule is unchanged over 2 years, the nodule is typically considered benign,[25] although faint opacities representing subsolid lesions may require longer follow-up. When temporal stability cannot be established with prior examinations, follow-up chest radiographs may be considered if clinical symptoms suggest an infectious or inflammatory etiology. If a nodule persists on follow-up radiographs, patients typically proceed to CT for confirmation of the nodule and more sensitive evaluation of nodule features. If clinical symptoms are absent or discordant with initial chest radiograph findings, the clinician may prefer to proceed directly to CT for better assessment of the lungs.

Table 3
Differential diagnosis of the solitary pulmonary nodule

	Benign		Malignant
Infectious	Pneumonia; abscess	Primary lung cancer, solid	Adenocarcinoma
	Granuloma		Squamous cell carcinoma
Noninfectious	Rheumatoid nodule		Small cell carcinoma
	Wegener granuloma		Carcinoid
	Sarcoidosis		Lymphoma
	Hemorrhage; lung infarct[a]	Primary lung cancer,	Adenocarcinoma
	Organizing pneumonia[a]	subsolid	Minimally invasive
			adenocarcinoma
	Lipoid pneumonia		AIS
Neoplastic	Hamartoma		AAH
	Sclerosing hemangioma	Solitary lung metastasis	
Vascular	Pulmonary arteriovenous		
	malformation		
Congenital	Bronchial atresia		
	Bronchogenic cyst		
Miscellaneous	Intrapulmonary lymph		
	node		
	Mucus-impacted airway		
	Focal scar; fibrosis[a]		
	Round atelectasis		

[a] Frequently subsolid.

Computed Tomography

Multidetector CT allows more detailed characterization of the SPN using thinner data obtained with higher spatial and temporal resolution. Axial chest CT images are typically generated with 5 mm of Z-axis data. Raw data are reconstructed using high- or low-frequency algorithms for evaluation of lungs or soft tissues, respectively. A high-frequency reconstruction algorithm (or lung kernel) maximizes spatial resolution for depiction of fine margins or internal features of the lung parenchyma, although image noise in increased. A low-frequency algorithm (or soft tissue kernel) reduces image noise and, therefore, aids in tissue attenuation characterization, such as differentiating soft tissue from fat and calcification, at the expense of lower spatial resolution.[17] Reconstructed data should be viewed using appropriate window settings for the tissue of interest. For example, evaluation of the lungs and bones should be performed using data reconstructed with a high-frequency algorithm and viewed with corresponding lung and bone window settings. The mediastinum should be assessed on

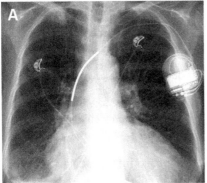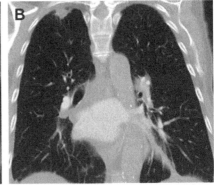

Fig. 1. Lung cancer. (*A*) Frontal radiograph in a 67-year-old woman. A large nodular opacity at the right apex is partially obscured by overlying ribs and clavicle. (*B*) Reformatted coronal CT image in lung window demonstrates the irregular nodule with mild peripheral calcification on the right, subsequently diagnosed as adenocarcinoma.

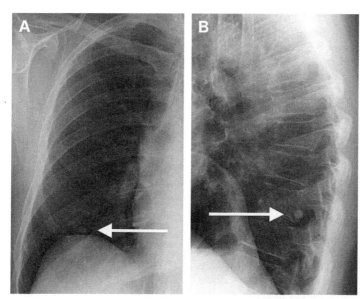

Fig. 2. Calcified nodule. Frontal (*A*) and lateral (*B*) radiographs of a 44-year-old man. A dense 7-mm nodule projects over the right lower lobe (*arrows*). The density suggests a calcified nodule, which was a stable finding over several years and subsequently confirmed as densely calcified on a subsequent chest CT.

low-frequency reconstructed images and viewed in soft tissue windows.

Increasingly, thin-section 1-mm axial lung window images are reconstructed to complement 5-mm images; these thin-section images have greater spatial resolution than thicker sections at the expense of higher image noise. In a study of more than 500 patients with subcentimeter SPNs, Lee and colleagues[26] found that lung nodules were significantly larger when measured on 1-mm axial images versus when measured on 5-mm images. A significant difference in nodule density and the presence of calcification occurred when viewed on 5-mm and 1-mm images. For instance, an apparent ground-glass lung nodule on 5-mm images may prove solid density when viewed on thin 1-mm images (**Fig. 3**), and a small focus of calcification identified on 1-mm images may not be appreciated on 5-mm images due to volume averaging with adjacent lung parenchyma. Thin 1-mm images can be used to create multiplanar reformatted images in the coronal and sagittal planes to better evaluate nodule shape and size. Other postprocessing techniques, such as

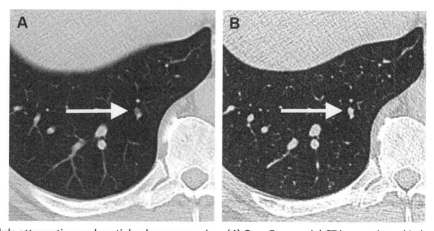

Fig. 3. Nodule attenuation and partial volume averaging. (*A*) On a 5-mm axial CT image viewed in lung window, a 5-mm nodule (*arrow*) in the posterior basal right lower lobe appears as ground-glass attenuation. (*B*) Corresponding 1-mm axial CT image more accurately demonstrates the solid attenuation of the nodule (*arrow*) with greater spatial resolution.

maximum intensity projection images, also aid in nodule detection.[27] Advanced quantitative measurements, such as 3-D nodule volume and density, are facilitated by the high spatial resolution of thin-section images. Thin-data sets can also be utilized by CAD software, which has been shown to assist radiologists in identifying both solid and ground-glass lung nodules.[28]

Consideration of cumulative radiation dose to a patient is an important factor in lung nodule management. Low-dose CT techniques have been developed for surveillance of indeterminate lung nodules. Dose-reduction techniques include lower tube currents of 40 to 80 mA-second (mAs), tube current modulation that adjusts tube current for varying soft tissue thickness, limiting the craniocaudal Z axis, and the use of lower kilovolt tube potentials (kVp). Although reducing patient radiation exposure produces increased image noise, evaluation of the high-contrast lungs is affected to a lesser degree than the adjacent mediastinum and soft tissues. With the use of low-dose CT techniques, attention to protocol consistency among follow-up examinations and awareness of increased image noise are both important considerations when evaluating a lung nodule over time.

Intravenous contrast is typically not required for CT evaluation of the pulmonary nodule, although it may be useful when a lesion is sizable and there is suspicion of malignancy. Contrast is also beneficial when a vascular cause, such as arteriovenous malformation, is suspected.

Computed tomography imaging features

Increased use of multidetector chest CT has lead to increased detection of lung nodules that may be as small as 1 to 2 mm.[12] Overall, the risk of primary malignancy among small solid lung nodules less than 4 mm is low, less than 1%, even among smokers, although the likelihood of malignancy is directly related to nodule size.[12] Imaging features, such as nodule density, composition, shape, margin, size and rate of growth, can all be used to determine the likelihood of malignancy.

Several methods have been developed to quantify the likelihood of malignancy among solitary lung nodules. Investigation by Gurney and colleagues[29,30] established likelihood ratios using Bayes theorem to quantify the probability of malignancy of both chest radiograph and clinical findings. Only 2 chest radiograph findings allowed reliable distinction of malignancy from benignity: nodule size and cavity wall thickness. Despite the utility of this analysis, other imaging methods, such as FDG-PET, were shown better predictors of malignancy.[31] More recently, a large study was conducted to determine the probability of

malignancy of lung nodules discovered on initial low-dose screening CT.[32] This study by McWilliams and colleagues reported predictors of malignancy that included clinical features, such as advanced age and family history of lung cancer, and imaging features, such as upper lobe location, larger nodule size, spiculated margins, and part-solid attenuation.

Nodule attenuation Although a majority of SPNs are solid, great attention in recent years has been directed toward to the subsolid lung nodule, a term that encompasses both the part-solid nodule (PSN), composed of both solid and nonsolid components, and the purely ground-glass nodule (GGN), with nonsolid density through which normal lung architecture remains visible (**Figs. 4 and 5**). A subsolid lung nodule may represent a benign etiology, such as focal inflammation or fibrosis. Greater than half of these lesions can be transient, even those that are large and contain solid components.[33] Persistent nodules have a high likelihood of representing slowly growing neoplasia. The literature has shown that an incidentally discovered GGN is more likely to represent malignancy than an incidental solid lung nodule, with a likelihood of malignancy of 59% to 73% compared with 7% to 9%.[3,34–36] It may be useful to note, however, that these studies were performed before the revised classification of adenocarcinoma, and, as a result, some of these persistent GGNs may now be characterized as

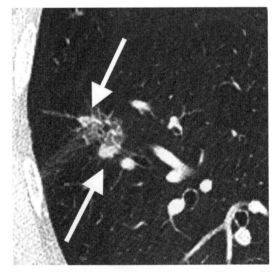

Fig. 4. Right upper lobe PSN in a 78-year-old nonsmoker. This nodule is composed of both solid (*arrows*) and ground-glass attenuation. Irregular nodule margins and spiculation are also noted. Surgical wedge resection and pathologic evaluation revealed lepidic predominant adenocarcinoma.

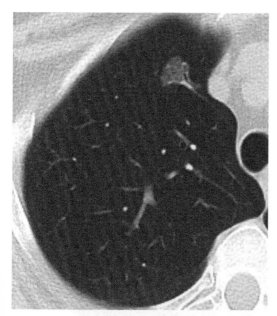

Fig. 5. Purely GGN. Newly discovered solitary right upper lobe GGN in a 66-year-old former smoker. This 1.5-cm lesion demonstrates no solid component and is, therefore, suspicious for AIS. For a purely GGN larger than 5 mm, initial follow-up imaging is currently recommended in 3 months. If persistent, annual CT at 1 year from the initial scan for a minimum of 3 years would comply with Fleischner Society management guidelines.

preinvasive neoplasia rather than true invasive malignancy.

A small persistent GGN up to 5 mm in size may represent a localized area of mildly atypical type II pneumocytes referred to as atypical adenomatous hyperplasia (AAH).[37] AAH is considered a precursor to adenocarcinoma in situ (AIS), which is characterized histopathologically by its lepidic noninvasive growth pattern and which typically appears on CT as a purely GGN measuring up to 3 cm in size. AIS is one of several lung cancer subtypes previously described as bronchioloalveolar carcinoma, a term applied to a heterogeneous group of neoplasms, which was reclassified in 2011 by the International Association for the Study of Lung Cancer, the American Thoracic Society, and European Respiratory Society.[37]

GGN attenuation has been correlated with lepidic growth of neoplastic cells indolently spreading along normal lung architecture without invasion. This has been elegantly outlined pathologically by Noguchi and colleagues,[38] describing a spectrum of adenocarcinoma that includes invasion of neoplastic cells and resultant structural collapse; tumor invasion strongly correlates with the size of a solid component seen on imaging.[39] PSNs have

been correlated with invasive adenocarcinoma, ranging from minimally invasive adenocarcinoma (MIA), which measures up to 3 cm with an invasive component up to 5 mm in size, to more advanced invasive adenocarcinoma subtypes, such as lepidic-predominant adenocarcinoma and invasive mucinous adenocarcinoma.[37,38]

A solid lung nodule may represent invasive adenocarcinoma, although other forms of primary lung malignancy, such as squamous cell carcinoma, small cell carcinoma, and carcinoid, are also diagnostic considerations. Benign etiologies may also account for a solid SPN, the most common being a granuloma, which can be indistinguishable from a malignant lesion.[40] Nodule features, such as margin, size, and growth, may be helpful in determining the likelihood of malignancy of a solid nodule, and the presence and distribution of calcification are useful for differentiating benign and malignant etiologies.

Four benign patterns of nodule calcification have been identified: diffuse, central, lamellated, and popcorn (**Fig. 6**). The first 3 patterns are typically associated with prior infection, such as tuberculosis or histoplasmosis, whereas popcorn calcification is frequently associated with chondroid calcification within a hamartoma (**Fig. 7**). Hamartomas are benign neoplasms that arise from fibrous connective tissue beneath the mucous membrane of the bronchial wall and have cartilage as the dominant mesenchymal tissue, forming lobules with cleftlike branching patterns and variable amounts of calcification.[41] In a study by Siegelman and colleagues,[41] 47 hamartomas were evaluated and were typically 2.5 cm or less in size with smooth margins, frequently containing focal fat and calcification. Fat attenuation was present in 38% of specimens, whereas 21% contained both fat and calcification. Calcification alone was seen in 4%, whereas the remaining 36% showed no CT evidence of fat or calcification. The presence of fat within an SPN is considered a reliable indicator of benignity; rarely, a pulmonary lipoma may be present, although fewer than 10 instances of intraparenchymal pulmonary lipoma have been reported in the literature.[42] Among patients with liposarcoma or renal cell carcinoma, a solitary fat-containing metastasis is possible.[43] Fat density can also be seen within an area of lipoid pneumonia. Slow growth can occur among hamartomas; recognizable growth is typically identified only if studied longer than 3 years.[44]

Indeterminate patterns of calcification, such as eccentric, stippled, or amorphous calcification, may be seen in malignant lesions (**Fig. 8**).[45] Calcification can be seen in up to 10% of lung cancers, often large and centrally located.[46] Eccentric

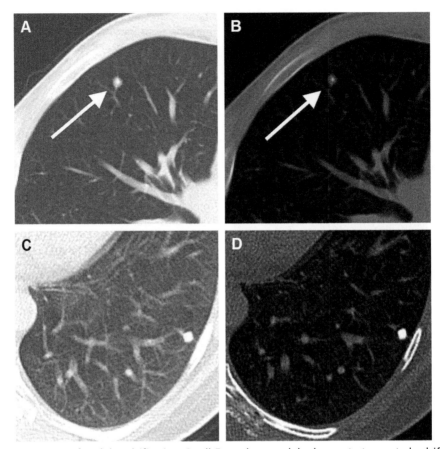

Fig. 6. Benign patterns of nodule calcification. Small 5-mm lung nodule demonstrates central calcification (*arrows*), which occupies a large portion of the lesion, as seen on 5-mm axial CT image in lung (*A*) and bone (*B*) windows. A diffusely calcified left lower lobe nodule is present in this patient with a history of tuberculosis exposure, seen on lung (*C*) and bone (*D*) windows.

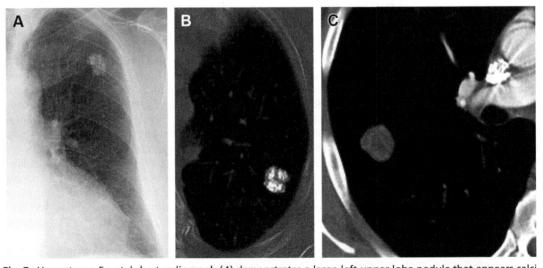

Fig. 7. Hamartoma. Frontal chest radiograph (*A*) demonstrates a large left upper lobe nodule that appears calcified. Axial CT image in bone window (*B*) demonstrates findings consistent with a hamartoma, due to the presence of a popcorn-like pattern of calcification. (*C*) As shown on axial soft tissue window, a right lower lobe hamartoma in a different patient contains visible fat density, another feature of hamartoma. No calcification is present.

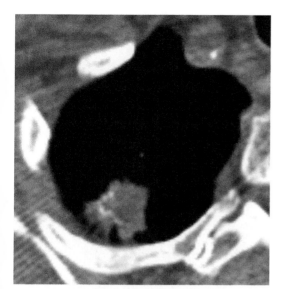

Fig. 8. Indeterminate calcification pattern. Stippled eccentric calcification is present at the lateral margin of an irregular right apical mass diagnosed as lung cancer.

calcification may reflect dystrophic calcification within a malignant nodule or a granuloma that has become engulfed by an adjacent malignant nodule. Stippled calcification can be seen among metastases from mucin-producing primary malignancies, such as breast, colon, and ovarian cancer.[47] Rarely, carcinoid or a solitary metastasis from a bone-producing tumor, such as osteosarcoma, can be entirely or partially calcified.[48] On contrast-enhanced chest CT, a high attenuation lesion may represent an avidly enhancing nodule

rather than calcification; in such instances, viewing the lesion with bone windows may be helpful.

Nodule morphology The shape and margin of a pulmonary nodule may be indicative of its behavior. A smoothly marginated nodule is often benign, although primary or metastatic malignant nodules can exhibit smooth margins in 20% to 30% of instances.[29] When located adjacent to a pleural or fissural surface, a smoothly marginated solid nodule may represent an intrapulmonary lymph node. Small series of pathologically proved intrapulmonary lymph nodes identified on CT have shown nearly all nodules located below the level of the carina within 15 mm of the pleural margin.[49–51] Intrapulmonary lymph nodes are usually triangular or oval in shape and frequently have a thin septal connection or pleural tag, which pathologically represents a dilated lymphatic channel.[51,52] In the absence of underlying malignancy, these nodules are typically considered benign; Ahn and colleagues[52] reported slight interval growth of only 7 of 159 perifissural lung nodules, which were followed over 2 years among a cohort of high risk lung cancer screening patients. After more than 7 years, none of the nodules seen on CT had reportedly developed into lung cancers. Still, metastatic involvement from underlying malignancy is possible and should prompt further evaluation.[51,53]

In contrast to a smooth nodule margin, an irregular, spiculated, or lobulated margin demonstrates a higher likelihood of malignancy, ranging from 33% to 100% (**Figs. 9** and **10**).[3,54,55] A lobulated contour is considered the result of uneven or

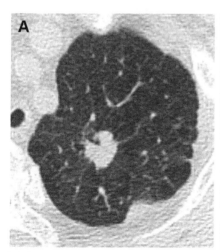
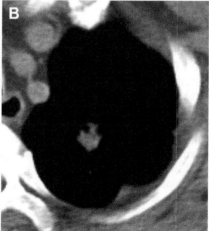

Fig. 9. Lobulated margins. Lobulated left upper lobe lung nodule shown in both lung (*A*) and soft tissue (*B*) windows. Mildly irregular margins of this proved adenocarcinoma are better seen on lung images, which are reconstructed using a high-frequency algorithm that enables higher spatial resolution. The soft tissue composition of the nodule is better evaluated on low-frequency algorithm images that minimize image noise.

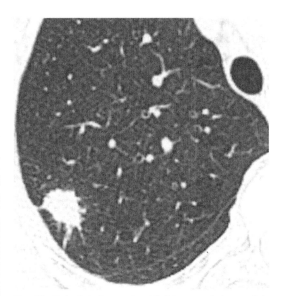

Fig. 10. Spiculated margins. Right upper lobe nodule in a 58-year-old nonsmoker, pathologically proved to represent adenocarcinoma. Mildly lobulated margins are also present.

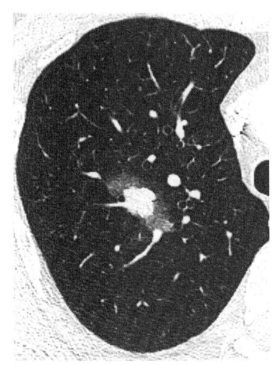

Fig. 11. Ground-glass halo. A halo of ground-glass attenuation nearly surrounds a lobulated right upper lobe nodule and is visible on axial lung window. Adenocarcinoma was diagnosed after surgical excision. In this instance, ground-glass opacity corresponded to extension of neoplastic cells into the adjacent interstitium.

asymmetric growth within a lung nodule.[56] Nodule spiculation may represent growth of abnormal cells along the lung interstitium, although inflammation may also produce an irregular or spiculated nodule margin.

A solid nodule surrounded by ground-glass attenuation, termed a halo sign, is more often seen with multiple lesions related to infection or inflammation, with the halo of ground-glass opacity attributed to inflammatory fluid and hemorrhage (**Fig. 11**). Hemorrhage from hypervascular metastases, however, such as melanoma or choriocarcinoma, and tumor infiltration of the interstitium surrounding a solid malignant nodule can also produce the CT halo sign.[57,58] In distinction, the reversed halo sign denotes a ground-glass attenuation nodule surrounded by a rim of solid consolidation (**Fig. 12**). The differential diagnosis of the reversed halo sign is equally broad, including solitary and multiple lesions, ranging from fungal and mycobacterial infection to granulomatosis, sarcoidosis, lung infarction, and cryptogenic organizing pneumonia. The imaging sign has also been described in instances of malignancy and subsequent treatment, including radiation therapy and radiofrequency ablation.[59]

Nodule cavitation is observed in both benign and malignant settings (**Fig. 13**). Necrotizing pneumonia related to *Staphylococcus*, *Klebsiella*, and *Pseudomonas* species as well as fungal and mycobacterial infection can produce nodule cavitation. Noninfectious granulomatous disease, such as Wegener granulomatosis and polyangiitis

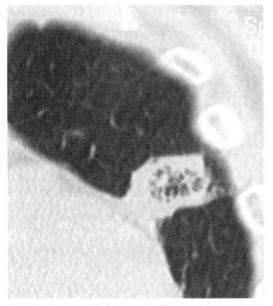

Fig. 12. Reversed halo sign. Reformatted coronal CT image in lung window illustrates the reversed halo sign, corresponding to a left upper lobe infarct in a patient with acute pulmonary embolism.

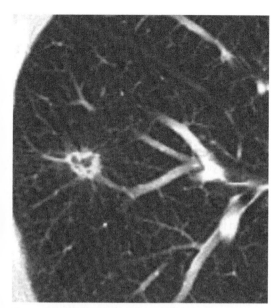

Fig. 13. Nodule cavitation. Solitary cavitary lung nodule in the right lower lobe, representing a single metastatic focus of colon carcinoma; cavity walls are slightly irregular and measure up to 6 mm in thickness. Nodule margins are also slightly irregular and spiculated.

and, uncommonly, sarcoidosis, are also possible causes. Areas of lung infarction can also occasionally cavitate. In general, benign cavities demonstrate thin and smooth walls, whereas thick or irregular walls are more indicative of malignancy, such as squamous cell carcinoma. Studies have shown that increasingly thick walls convey greater likelihood of malignancy; a lesion with wall thickness of 4 mm or less has a 92% likelihood of being benign, whereas 95% of lesions with wall thickness greater than 15 mm prove malignant, although considerable overlap between benign and malignant etiologies exists.[60]

Nodule size and growth Nodule size is an important predictor of the likelihood of malignancy. As Wahidi and colleagues[3] observed among 8 large lung cancer screening programs, the likelihood of a small lung nodule less than 5 mm in diameter representing malignancy is as low as 1%. Recently published data from the Dutch-Belgian Randomized Lung Cancer Screening Trial (Dutch acronym: NELSON) found no significantly increased risk of lung cancer between patients with small nodules less than 5 mm in diameter or less than or equal to 100 mm³ in volume and those patients without lung nodules.[61] In patients with underlying malignancy, however, these conclusions do not apply. In a study of 275 patients with a history of lung cancer who underwent lung nodule resection, Ginsberg and colleagues[62] discovered a

malignancy rate of 42% among nodules 5 mm or less in size. This highlights the increased risk of malignant nodules in patients with underlying malignancy. Regardless of risk, greater nodule size portends an increased likelihood of malignancy, with nodules between 5 to 10 mm demonstrating a 6% to 28% chance of malignancy. For nodules greater than 20 mm in diameter, the percentage of malignant nodules increases to 64% to 82%.[3]

For subsolid lung nodules, the relationship between size and likelihood of malignancy is less established. A GGN 5 mm or smaller in diameter probably reflects a focus of AAH whereas a nodule larger than 5 mm is more likely to represent AIS or invasive adenocarcinoma.[13]

Nodule growth can be an important indicator of malignant behavior. Growth is traditionally considered in terms of volumetric doubling time (VDT). Assuming that lung nodules are round, a doubling of volume reflects an increase in diameter of approximately 25% (based on the equation for volume $4/3\ \pi r^3$).[17] Rapidly enlarging nodules with a VDT of less than 20 days are typically considered benign, representing an area of inflammation or infection. Multiple studies have demonstrated a median VDT among malignant nodules of approximately 100 days.[63–65] Henschke and colleagues[63] reported a median VDT of 98 days calculated from linear bidimensional measurements among 111 lung cancers detected on screening chest CT; only 3% of cancers demonstrated a VDT greater than 400 days, all of which were subsolid. Half of all cancers had a VDT of less than 100 days; 55 were solid and 1 was subsolid. Studies have illustrated the effective use of CT volumetric software to assist in determination of nodule doubling times; a study of 63 nodules showed a median VDT of 117 days for malignant nodules and 947 days for benign nodules with a NPV of 98% (using a cutoff of 500 days for malignant behavior).[64] A study showed that 3-D semiautomated nodule volumetry detected nodule growth and enabled computation of growth rate earlier than with traditional visual assessment.[65] Such tools may prove especially useful for characterization of indolent, slowly growing low-grade neoplasia.

Solid lung nodules are traditionally considered benign when stable for more than 2 years, correlating with a VDT greater than 730 days. In distinction, subsolid nodules may double in size in as many as 1346 days.[66] Subsolid lung nodules are often difficult to accurately measure due to poorly perceived or irreproducible margins, high interobserver variability, and indolent growth. The presence of a new solid component within a previously purely GGN or a preexisting solid component that is increasing in size or density may reflect cellular invasion. Therefore, both nodule size and attenuation should be carefully evaluated when assessing subsolid nodules (**Fig. 14**).[67] Infrequently, the overall size of a nodule may decrease while the solid composition of the nodule increases, representing disease progression rather than regression. Given these reasons, a quantitative measure of mass that reflects the physical density and volume of a nodule has been investigated as a method to enable earlier detection of subsolid nodule growth with less variability than nodule diameter or volume.[68] Nodule mass has recently been used to differentiate invasive adenocarcinoma from MIA and AIS subtypes.[69]

Additional Computed Tomography Imaging Techniques

Most incidentally discovered lung nodules are initially evaluated without intravenous contrast. Nodule enhancement after intravenous contrast administration, however, can provide valuable information regarding malignant potential. Although less frequently used because of the widespread availability of PET/CT, nodule enhancement CT remains a useful alternative to further characterize the indeterminate SPN when PET/CT is unavailable. Yamashita and colleagues[70] assessed enhancement characteristics of 32 benign and malignant SPNs and found that all malignant nodules (n = 18) enhanced completely, whereas peripheral and capsular enhancement was identified among some other benign lesions, such as hamartoma and granuloma; enhancement attenuation between 20 and 60 Hounsfield units (HU) served as a good predictor of malignancy. A larger study found a significant difference in enhancement between benign and malignant nodules that was significantly related to central nodule vascularity, as determined pathologically.[71] Pitfalls can occur with contrast-enhanced CT technique, with false-positive results related to benign inflammation and infection and false-negative interpretations associated with necrotic or partially calcified malignant lesions.

DECT technology has the ability to assess nodule enhancement using a single contrast-enhanced CT acquisition, eliminating the need for precontrast imaging (**Fig. 15**). DECT capitalizes on the varying behavior of soft tissue and iodine at different photon energies and is typically performed with 2 radiation beams of 2 different kVp, emitted from 1 rapidly alternating CT tube or emitted from 2 separate CT tubes operating simultaneously. Prior investigation found noncontrast DECT unreliable for differentiating benign and malignant nodules using 2 separate acquisitions at 80 and 140 kVp settings.[72] Current DECT technique enables near-simultaneous acquisition of both kilovolt potentials. With this information, material decomposition generates iodine-enhanced and virtual noncontrast (VNC) images, made possible by the different behavior of iodine when exposed to 2 different kVp and allowing an estimation of contrast enhancement.[73] Assessing the clinical utility of DECT to evaluate SPNs, Chae and colleagues[74] found good agreement of CT density numbers between iodine-enhanced images and nodule enhancement as measured by pre- and postcontrast images as well as VNC and traditional noncontrast images.

Positron Emission Tomography Imaging

By assessing the metabolic activity of a lung nodule, FDG-PET and combined FDG-PET/CT are well-established methods for assessing indeterminate lesions greater than 1 cm in diameter, with sensitivity of 97% and sensitivity of 78%.[75]

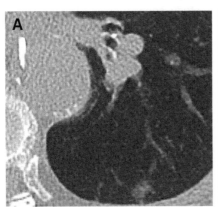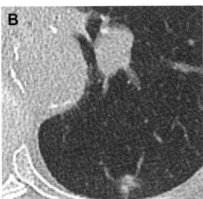

Fig. 14. Progression of a subsolid nodule. (*A*) A subtle subsolid nodule is identified in the periphery of the left lower lobe. (*B*) Nine months later, the nodule has a more distinct margin, and there has been an increase in nodule density. MIA was diagnosed after surgical excision.

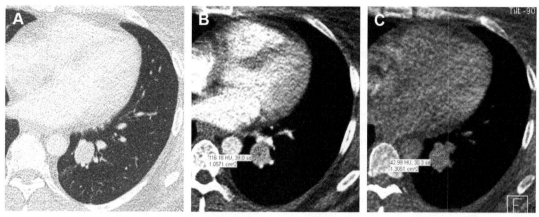

Fig. 15. DECT. (*A*) Round, smoothly marginated central left lower lobe lung nodule measures approximately 2 cm in diameter. (*B*) Contrast-enhanced DECT was performed; the nodule measures approximately 115 HU in density on the composite image created from high and low kVp image data. (*C*) VNC image created from material decomposition of DECT data shows noncontrast density measurement of 43 HU, indicating contrast enhancement of greater than 60 HU.

Christensen and colleagues[76] directly compared contrast-enhanced CT and FDG-PET in the characterization of indeterminate SPNs larger than 7 mm in size; 42 nodules were examined, and, using CT enhancement threshold of 15 HU and metabolic activity greater than the mediastinal blood pool on FDG-PET, both techniques were shown valuable. Nodule-enhancement CT showed sensitivity and specificity of 100% and 29%, respectively, with a PPV of 68% and negative predictive value (NPV) of 100%, whereas FDG-PET sensitivity and specificity were 96% and 76%, respectively, with a PPV of 86% and NPV of 93%. When directly comparing the 2 modalities, the higher specificity of FDG-PET (76% vs 29%) deemed it preferable to contrast-enhanced CT. CT remained a useful tool, however, due to its high NPV, lower cost, and greater convenience to patients.

PET/CT imaging combines assessment of metabolic activity with PET imaging and the visual assessment of nodule morphology on CT (**Fig. 16**). A study of 186 pathologically proved SPNs by Sim and colleagues[77] reported that PET/CT had an accuracy of 81% in diagnosing malignant nodules. The sensitivity and specificity were 87% and 50%, respectively, whereas the PPV and NPV were 91% and 40%. The study showed that although using a maximum standardized uptake value (SUV_{max}) threshold of 2.5, the likelihood of malignancy increased as SUV_{max} increased. False-negative results may be attributed to nodule size smaller than 7 mm, and carcinoid may occasionally produce false-negative results.[17,78,79] FDG uptake is also considered unreliable for evaluation of subsolid lung nodules, which may represent areas of infection, inflammation, or neoplasia.[78] A study of 53 pathologically

A   **B**

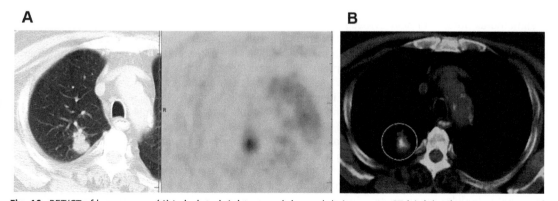

Fig. 16. PET/CT of lung cancer. (*A*) Lobulated right upper lobe nodule is seen on CT (*right*), whereas a corresponding area of increased FDG metabolism (SUV_{max} 12) is seen on the adjacent PET image (*left*). (*B*) Coregistration of PET and CT images indicate the right upper lobe nodule is metabolically active. Adenocarcinoma was diagnosed after surgical excision.

proved PSNs evaluated with PET/CT demonstrated a higher mean and SUV_{max} among benign PSNs than malignant PSNs, implying that malignant PSNs may demonstrate little if any SUV uptake.[80]

Nodule Biopsy

When noninvasive imaging modalities are unable to reliably characterize an indeterminate SPN as benign or malignant, minimally invasive transthoracic needle biopsy may be considered. Percutaneous needle aspiration provides overall diagnostic accuracy in approximately 75% of cases.[81,82] Accuracy is significantly related to lesion size (greater than 1 cm in diameter) and length of the needle path (40 mm or less).[82] Choi and colleagues[83] studied the utility of CT-guided percutaneous aspiration and core biopsy in 305 lung lesions smaller than 1 cm and reported that a final diagnosis was achieved in 88% of cases. Diagnostic accuracy of a malignant nodule was 95%, whereas sensitivity and specificity were 93% and 99%, respectively. Aspiration and core biopsy in combination had a higher diagnostic yield than aspiration alone. Complications, such as pneumothorax, occur in approximately 30% of instances and require thoracostomy tube placement in up to 5%.[82] Smaller nodule size and higher complication rate are not consistently associated with one another.[81] Factors, such as forced expiratory volume in the first second of expiration, the number of lung punctures performed, and the length of the needle path, however, have been shown to have a significant impact on the likelihood on pneumothorax; the likelihood of chest tube placement has been significantly associated with the number of lung punctures, for example.[82] A more shallow angle of needle entry with the pleura and lesion location adjacent to fissures has been reported in association with a higher pneumothorax rate.[84] In this investigation, the pneumothorax rate was not affected by the number of core samples or the time the introducer needle was present within the lung parenchyma using coaxial technique.

The role of transthoracic needle biopsy in evaluation of the subsolid lung nodule remains under debate. In a study of nearly 200 patients, De Filippo and colleagues[85] reported overall accuracy of needle aspiration of 95% for solid lung nodules and 67% for subsolid nodules. Another investigation found a sensitivity of 89% for malignant subsolid lung nodules undergoing transthoracic needle aspiration, with a specificity and PPV of 100%.[86] Although needle biopsy may be useful for determination of malignancy, particularly in

poor surgical candidates, there are diagnostic limitations. AIS, MIA, and more invasive adenocarcinoma subtypes manifesting as subsolid lung nodules cannot be reliably diagnosed with small biopsy samples or cytology alone; the lesion ideally should be sampled in its entirety to determine the full extent of invasion, if present.[87] Accordingly, current Fleischner Society guidelines for diagnosis and management of subsolid lung nodules place little emphasis on the role of needle biopsy.[13]

MANAGEMENT CONSIDERATIONS

Evidence-based recommendations from multidisciplinary groups, such as the American College of Chest Physicians (ACCP) and the Fleischner Society, provide crucial management guidelines for patients with indeterminate solid and subsolid lung nodules. Imaging, such as chest CT and FDG-PET, plays a central role in evaluation of these nodules. Current ACCP guidelines address large (>8 mm) and small (≤8 mm) solid nodules, as well as subsolid lung nodules, with emphasis on the clinical probability of malignancy. The risks and benefits of noninvasive and invasive procedures and the preferences of the patient are also important considerations.[14]

Fleischner Society guidelines for incidentally detected solid lung nodules are based on nodule size and patient risk factors (see **Table 1**).[12] For nodules up to 8 mm in diameter, surveillance chest CT is recommended based on the low likelihood of malignancy; the frequency of follow-up imaging depends on nodule size and the presence of risk factors, such as smoking, family history of malignancy, and environmental exposure. These guidelines are proposed in conjunction with clinical information, and recommendations do not apply in young patients under age 35, patients with underlying malignancy, or patients with suspected infection.[12]

Management guidelines for subsolid lung nodules vary compared with their solid counterparts, and Fleischner Society guidelines strongly emphasize the need to interpret imaging recommendations in light of clinical history (see **Table 2**).[13] Nodule size plays a smaller role in management of subsolid nodules. Management recommendations are heavily influenced by the presence and size of a solid component, based on the correlation between solid density, tissue invasion, and corresponding aggressive behavior. FDG-PET plays a limited role in evaluation of these lesions and is not recommended for purely GGNs but can be considered for PSN larger than 10 mm. Tissue sampling or resection is recommended more readily for subsolid nodules based on the higher likelihood of malignancy compared with solid nodules.[13] Continuing controversy surrounding these nodules indicates that modifications to management algorithms should be anticipated as information continues to emerge.

SUMMARY

Discovery of an SPN often results in a diagnostic dilemma. Patient risk factors, such as age, smoking, and underlying malignancy, may influence the perceived likelihood of malignancy, and imaging features, such as nodule density, shape, size, and growth rate, all aid in determining the malignant potential of an indeterminate lung nodule. In addition to multidetector chest CT, additional imaging techniques, such as FDG-PET and nodule enhancement, potentially facilitated by DECT, can provide greater diagnostic value. Ultimately, management of the solitary lung nodule depends on a combination of clinical risk and imaging features and requires a multidisciplinary approach.

REFERENCES

1. American Cancer Society. What are the key statistics about lung cancer? Available at: http://www.cancer.org/cancer/lungcancer-non-smallcell/detailedguide/non-small-cell-lung-cancer-key-statistics. Accessed December 1, 2014.

2. Harders SW, Madsen HH, Rasmussen TR, et al. High resolution spiral CT for determining the malignant potential of solitary pulmonary nodules: refining and testing the test. Acta Radiol 2011;52:401–9.

3. Wahidi MM, Govert JA, Goudar RK, et al. Evidence for the treatment of patients with pulmonary nodules: when is it lung cancer?: ACCP evidence-based clinical practice guidelines (2nd edition). Chest 2007;132:94S–107S.

4. Gohagan J, Marcus P, Fagerstrom R, et al. Baseline findings of a randomized feasibility trial of lung cancer screening with spiral CT scan vs chest radiograph: the Lung Screening Study of the National Cancer Institute. Chest 2004;126:114–21.

5. Henschke CI, McCauley DI, Yankelevitz DF, et al. Early Lung Cancer Action Project: overall design and findings from baseline screening. Lancet 1999;354:99–105.

6. Henschke CI, Yankelevitz DF, Libby DM, et al. Early lung cancer action project: annual screening using single-slice helical CT. Ann N Y Acad Sci 2001;952:124–34.

7. Swensen SJ, Jett JR, Sloan JA, et al. Screening for lung cancer with low-dose spiral computed tomography. Am J Respir Crit Care Med 2002;165:508–13.

8. Swensen SJ, Jett JR, Hartman TE, et al. Lung cancer screening with CT: Mayo Clinic experience. Radiology 2003;226:756–61.

9. National Lung Screening Trial Research Team, Aberle DR, Adams AM, et al. Reduced lung-cancer mortality with low-dose computed tomographic screening. N Engl J Med 2011;365:395–409.

10. Aberle DR, DeMello S, Berg CD, et al. Results of the two incidence screenings in the National Lung Screening Trial. N Engl J Med 2013;369:920–31.

11. Patz EF Jr, Pinsky P, Gatsonis C, et al. Overdiagnosis in low-dose computed tomography screening for lung cancer. JAMA Intern Med 2014;174:269–74.

12. MacMahon H, Austin JH, Gamsu G, et al. Guidelines for management of small pulmonary nodules detected on CT scans: a statement from the Fleischner Society. Radiology 2005;237:395–400.

13. Naidich DP, Bankier AA, MacMahon H, et al. Recommendations for the management of subsolid pulmonary nodules detected at CT: a statement from the Fleischner Society. Radiology 2013;266:304–17.

14. Gould MK, Donington J, Lynch WR, et al. Evaluation of individuals with pulmonary nodules: when is it lung cancer? Diagnosis and management of lung cancer, 3rd ed: American College of Chest Physicians evidence-based clinical practice guidelines. Chest 2013;143:e93S–120S.

15. Khan A. ACR appropriateness criteria on solitary pulmonary nodule. J Am Coll Radiol 2007;4:152–5.

16. Austin JH, Muller NL, Friedman PJ, et al. Glossary of terms for CT of the lungs: recommendations of the Nomenclature Committee of the Fleischner Society. Radiology 1996;200:327–31.

17. Truong MT, Ko JP, Rossi SE, et al. Update in the evaluation of the solitary pulmonary nodule. Radiographics 2014;34:1658–79.

18. Wahbah M, Boroumand N, Castro C, et al. Changing trends in the distribution of the histologic types of lung cancer: a review of 4,439 cases. Ann Diagn Pathol 2007;11:89–96.

19. Doo KW, Kang EY, Yong HS, et al. Comparison of chest radiography, chest digital tomosynthesis and low dose MDCT to detect small ground-glass opacity nodules: an anthropomorphic chest phantom study. Eur Radiol 2014;24:3269–76.

20. Schalekamp S, van Ginneken B, Koedam E, et al. Computer-aided detection improves detection of pulmonary nodules in chest radiographs beyond the support by bone-suppressed images. Radiology 2014;272:252–61.

21. Szucs-Farkas Z, Schick A, Cullmann JL, et al. Comparison of dual-energy subtraction and electronic bone suppression combined with computer-aided detection on chest radiographs: effect on human observers' performance in nodule detection. AJR Am J Roentgenol 2013;200:1006–13.

22. Freedman MT, Lo SC, Seibel JC, et al. Lung nodules: improved detection with software that suppresses the rib and clavicle on chest radiographs. Radiology 2011;260:265–73.

23. Berger WG, Erly WK, Krupinski EA, et al. The solitary pulmonary nodule on chest radiography: can we really tell if the nodule is calcified? AJR Am J Roentgenol 2001;176:201–4.

24. Ketai L, Malby M, Jordan K, et al. Small nodules detected on chest radiography: does size predict calcification? Chest 2000;118:610–4.

25. Nathan MH, Collins VP, Adams RA. Differentiation of benign and malignant pulmonary nodules by growth rate. Radiology 1962;79:221–32.

26. Lee HY, Goo JM, Lee HJ, et al. Usefulness of concurrent reading using thin-section and thick-section CT images in subcentimetre solitary pulmonary nodules. Clin Radiol 2009;64:127–32.

27. Kawel N, Seifert B, Luetolf M, et al. Effect of slab thickness on the CT detection of pulmonary nodules: use of sliding thin-slab maximum intensity projection and volume rendering. AJR Am J Roentgenol 2009; 192:1324–9.

28. Godoy MC, Kim TJ, White CS, et al. Benefit of computer-aided detection analysis for the detection of subsolid and solid lung nodules on thin- and thick-section CT. AJR Am J Roentgenol 2013;200:74–83.

29. Gurney JW. Determining the likelihood of malignancy in solitary pulmonary nodules with Bayesian analysis. Part I. Theory. Radiology 1993;186:405–13.

30. Gurney JW, Lyddon DM, McKay JA. Determining the likelihood of malignancy in solitary pulmonary nodules with Bayesian analysis. Part II. Application. Radiology 1993;186:415–22.

31. Dewan NA, Shehan CJ, Reeb SD, et al. Likelihood of malignancy in a solitary pulmonary nodule: comparison of Bayesian analysis and results of FDG-PET scan. Chest 1997;112:416–22.

32. McWilliams A, Tammemagi MC, Mayo JR, et al. Probability of cancer in pulmonary nodules detected on first screening CT. N Engl J Med 2013;369:910–9.

33. Koo CW, Miller WT, Kucharczuk JC. Focal ground-glass opacities in non-small cell lung carcinoma resection patients. Eur J Radiol 2012;81:139–45.

34. Li F, Sone S, Abe H, et al. Malignant versus benign nodules at CT screening for lung cancer: comparison of thin-section CT findings. Radiology 2004; 233:793–8.

35. Takashima S, Sone S, Li F, et al. Small solitary pulmonary nodules (< or =1 cm) detected at population-based CT screening for lung cancer: reliable high-resolution CT features of benign lesions. AJR Am J Roentgenol 2003;180:955–64.

36. Henschke CI, Yankelevitz DF, Mirtcheva R, et al. CT screening for lung cancer: frequency and significance of part-solid and nonsolid nodules. AJR Am J Roentgenol 2002;178:1053–7.

37. Travis WD, Brambilla E, Noguchi M, et al. International association for the study of lung cancer/american thoracic society/european respiratory society international multidisciplinary classification of lung adenocarcinoma. J Thorac Oncol 2011;6: 244–85.

38. Noguchi M, Morikawa A, Kawasaki M, et al. Small adenocarcinoma of the lung. Histologic characteristics and prognosis. Cancer 1995;75:2844–52.

39. Lee KH, Goo JM, Park SJ, et al. Correlation between the size of the solid component on thin-section CT and the invasive component on pathology in small lung adenocarcinomas manifesting as ground-glass nodules. J Thorac Oncol 2014;9:74–82.

40. Thiessen R, Seely JM, Matzinger FR, et al. Necrotizing granuloma of the lung: imaging characteristics and imaging-guided diagnosis. AJR Am J Roentgenol 2007;189:1397–401.

41. Siegelman SS, Khouri NF, Scott WW Jr, et al. Pulmonary hamartoma: CT findings. Radiology 1986;160: 313–7.

42. Parsons L, Shahir K, Rao N. Intraparenchymal pulmonary lipoma: pathologic-radiologic correlation of a rare presentation of a common neoplasm. Ann Diagn Pathol 2014;18:244–7.

43. Muram TM, Aisen A. Fatty metastatic lesions in 2 patients with renal clear-cell carcinoma. J Comput Assist Tomogr 2003;27:869–70.

44. Jensen KG, Schiodt T. Growth conditions of hamartoma of the lung: a study based on 22 cases operated on after radiographic observation for from one to 18 years. Thorax 1958;13:233–7.

45. Mahoney MC, Shipley RT, Corcoran HL, et al. CT demonstration of calcification in carcinoma of the lung. AJR Am J Roentgenol 1990;154:255–8.

46. Grewal RG, Austin JH. CT demonstration of calcification in carcinoma of the lung. J Comput Assist Tomogr 1994;18:867–71.

47. Seo JB, Im JG, Goo JM, et al. Atypical pulmonary metastases: spectrum of radiologic findings. Radiographics 2001;21:403–17.

48. Winer-Muram HT. The solitary pulmonary nodule. Radiology 2006;239:34–49.

49. Shaham D, Vazquez M, Bogot NR, et al. CT features of intrapulmonary lymph nodes confirmed by cytology. Clin Imaging 2010;34:185–90.

50. Matsuki M, Noma S, Kuroda Y, et al. Thin-section CT features of intrapulmonary lymph nodes. J Comput Assist Tomogr 2001;25:753–6.

51. Hyodo T, Kanazawa S, Dendo S, et al. Intrapulmonary lymph nodes: thin-section CT findings, pathological findings, and CT differential diagnosis from pulmonary metastatic nodules. Acta Med Okayama 2004;58:235–40.

52. Ahn MI, Gleeson TG, Chan IH, et al. Perifissural nodules seen at CT screening for lung cancer. Radiology 2010;254:949–56.

53. Taniguchi Y, Haruki T, Fujioka S, et al. Subpleural intra-pulmonary lymph node metastasis from colorectal cancer. Ann Thorac Cardiovasc Surg 2009;15:250–2.

54. Swensen SJ, Silverstein MD, Ilstrup DM, et al. The probability of malignancy in solitary pulmonary nodules. Application to small radiologically indeterminate nodules. Arch Intern Med 1997;157:849–55.

55. Swensen SJ, Brown LR, Colby TV, et al. Pulmonary nodules: CT evaluation of enhancement with iodinated contrast material. Radiology 1995;194:393–8.

56. Heitzman ER, Markarian B, Raasch BN, et al. Pathways of tumor spread through the lung: radiologic correlations with anatomy and pathology. Radiology 1982;144:3–14.

57. Pinto PS. The CT halo sign. Radiology 2004;230: 109–10.

58. Shrot S, Schachter J, Shapira-Frommer R, et al. CT halo sign as an imaging marker for response to adoptive cell therapy in metastatic melanoma with pulmonary metastases. Eur Radiol 2014;24:1251–6.

59. Godoy MC, Viswanathan C, Marchiori E, et al. The reversed halo sign: update and differential diagnosis. Br J Radiol 2012;85:1226–35.

60. Woodring JH, Fried AM, Chuang VP. Solitary cavities of the lung: diagnostic implications of cavity wall thickness. AJR Am J Roentgenol 1980;135:1269–71.

61. Horeweg N, van Rosmalen J, Heuvelmans MA, et al. Lung cancer probability in patients with CT-detected pulmonary nodules: a prespecified analysis of data from the NELSON trial of low-dose CT screening. Lancet Oncol 2014;15:1332–41.

62. Ginsberg MS, Griff SK, Go BD, et al. Pulmonary nodules resected at video-assisted thoracoscopic surgery: etiology in 426 patients. Radiology 1999;213: 277–82.

63. Henschke CI, Yankelevitz DF, Yip R, et al. Lung cancers diagnosed at annual CT screening: volume doubling times. Radiology 2012;263:578–83.

64. Revel MP, Merlin A, Peyrard S, et al. Software volumetric evaluation of doubling times for differentiating benign versus malignant pulmonary nodules. AJR Am J Roentgenol 2006;187:135–42.

65. Ko JP, Berman EJ, Kaur M, et al. Pulmonary Nodules: growth rate assessment in patients by using serial CT and three-dimensional volumetry. Radiology 2012;262:662–71.

66. Aoki T, Nakata H, Watanabe H, et al. Evolution of peripheral lung adenocarcinomas: CT findings correlated with histology and tumor doubling time. AJR Am J Roentgenol 2000;174:763–8.

67. Kakinuma R, Ohmatsu H, Kaneko M, et al. Progression of focal pure ground-glass opacity detected by low-dose helical computed tomography screening for lung cancer. J Comput Assist Tomogr 2004;28: 17–23.

68. de Hoop B, Gietema H, van de Vorst S, et al. Pulmonary ground-glass nodules: increase in mass as an early indicator of growth. Radiology 2010; 255:199–206.

69. Lim HJ, Ahn S, Lee KS, et al. Persistent pure ground-glass opacity lung nodules >/= 10 mm in diameter at CT scan: histopathologic comparisons and prognostic implications. Chest 2013;144:1291–9.

70. Yamashita K, Matsunobe S, Tsuda T, et al. Solitary pulmonary nodule: preliminary study of evaluation with incremental dynamic CT. Radiology 1995;194: 399–405.

71. Swensen SJ, Brown LR, Colby TV, et al. Lung nodule enhancement at CT: prospective findings. Radiology 1996;201:447–55.

72. Swensen SJ, Yamashita K, McCollough CH, et al. Lung nodules: dual-kilovolt peak analysis with CT–multicenter study. Radiology 2000;214:81–5.

73. Chae EJ, Song JW, Krauss B, et al. Dual-energy computed tomography characterization of solitary pulmonary nodules. J Thorac Imaging 2010;25: 301–10.

74. Chae EJ, Song JW, Seo JB, et al. Clinical utility of dual-energy CT in the evaluation of solitary pulmonary nodules: initial experience. Radiology 2008; 249:671–81.

75. Gould MK, Maclean CC, Kuschner WG, et al. Accuracy of positron emission tomography for diagnosis of pulmonary nodules and mass lesions: a meta-analysis. JAMA 2001;285:914–24.

76. Christensen JA, Nathan MA, Mullan BP, et al. Characterization of the solitary pulmonary nodule: 18F-FDG PET versus nodule-enhancement CT. AJR Am J Roentgenol 2006;187:1361–7.

77. Sim YT, Goh YG, Dempsey MF, et al. PET-CT evaluation of solitary pulmonary nodules: correlation with maximum standardized uptake value and pathology. Lung 2013;191:625–32.

78. Nomori H, Watanabe K, Ohtsuka T, et al. Evaluation of F-18 fluorodeoxyglucose (FDG) PET scanning for pulmonary nodules less than 3 cm in diameter, with special reference to the CT images. Lung Cancer 2004;45:19–27.

79. Erasmus JJ, McAdams HP, Patz EF Jr, et al. Evaluation of primary pulmonary carcinoid tumors using FDG PET. AJR Am J Roentgenol 1998;170:1369–73.

80. Tsushima Y, Tateishi U, Uno H, et al. Diagnostic performance of PET/CT in differentiation of malignant and benign non-solid solitary pulmonary nodules. Ann Nucl Med 2008;22:571–7.

81. Kothary N, Lock L, Sze DY, et al. Computed tomography-guided percutaneous needle biopsy of pulmonary nodules: impact of nodule size on diagnostic accuracy. Clin Lung Cancer 2009;10: 360–3.

82. Ohno Y, Hatabu H, Takenaka D, et al. CT-guided transthoracic needle aspiration biopsy of small (< or = 20 mm) solitary pulmonary nodules. AJR Am J Roentgenol 2003;180:1665–9.

83. Choi SH, Chae EJ, Kim JE, et al. Percutaneous CT-guided aspiration and core biopsy of pulmonary nodules smaller than 1 cm: analysis of outcomes of 305 procedures from a tertiary referral center. AJR Am J Roentgenol 2013;201:964–70.

84. Ko JP, Shepard JO, Drucker EA, et al. Factors influencing pneumothorax rate at lung biopsy: are dwell time and angle of pleural puncture contributing factors? Radiology 2001;218:491–6.

85. De Filippo M, Saba L, Concari G, et al. Predictive factors of diagnostic accuracy of CT-guided transthoracic fine-needle aspiration for solid noncalcified, subsolid and mixed pulmonary nodules. Radiol Med 2013;118:1071–81.

86. Maxwell AW, Klein JS, Dantey K, et al. CT-guided transthoracic needle aspiration biopsy of subsolid lung lesions. J Vasc Interv Radiol 2014;25:340–6, 346.e1.

87. Travis WD, Garg K, Franklin WA, et al. Evolving concepts in the pathology and computed tomography imaging of lung adenocarcinoma and bronchioloalveolar carcinoma. J Clin Oncol 2005;23:3279–87.

Staging of Lung Cancer

Patricia M. de Groot, MD*, Brett W. Carter, MD,
Sonia L. Betancourt Cuellar, MD, Jeremy J. Erasmus, MD

KEYWORDS

- NSCLC • Lung cancer • TNM staging

KEY POINTS

- Staging of lung cancer determines management and therapeutic options; therefore, accuracy of staging is essential.
- Clinical staging in patients presenting with lung cancer generally underestimates the extent of disease when compared with the pathologic stage.
- Radiologic imaging, including computed tomography (CT), MRI, and ^{18}F-fluoro-2-deoxy-D-glucose PET/CT, is an essential component of clinical staging and allows assessment of disease manifestations that are important for surgical, oncologic, and radiation therapy planning.
- The 7th edition of TNM Staging from the International Association for the Study of Lung Cancer/American Thoracic Society has been used since 2010 and the 8th edition is expected in 2015.
- Future staging classifications for lung cancer may include information about histology, biomarkers, and biochemical and demographic prognostic factors.

INTRODUCTION

Primary lung cancer is the leading cause of cancer mortality in the world, largely prefaced by the fact that patients with lung cancer often present with locally advanced or metastatic disease.[1] Imaging is important in the clinical staging and management of these patients because therapeutic options and mortality are to a considerable degree dependent on stage at presentation.

This article discusses the use of chest radiography, computed tomography (CT), MRI, and PET in the current TNM staging of non–small cell lung cancer (NSCLC). In addition, limitations, current controversies, and future directions in staging are briefly reviewed.

IMAGING TECHNIQUES

Clinical evaluation in patients presenting with lung cancer is required to provide an initial assessment of stage, although, in general, the clinical stage underestimates the extent of disease when compared with the pathologic stage. Radiologic imaging is an essential component of this clinical staging and allows assessment of disease manifestations that are important for surgical, oncologic, and radiation therapy planning, including size of the primary tumor, location and relationship to normal anatomic structures in the thorax, and existence of nodal and/or metastatic disease.

Numerous clinical guidelines have been promulgated by different organizations to aid in the evaluation of patients with lung cancer and assist in therapeutic decision-making. Silvestri and colleagues[2] have recently reviewed clinical lung cancer staging based on the American College of Chest Physicians (ACCP) 3rd edition of Evidence-Based Clinical Practice Guidelines for Diagnosis and Management of Lung Cancer, referenced in this article.

Chest Radiography

Chest radiography is commonly a first assessment modality for patients who present with

---

Disclosures: None.
Section of Thoracic Imaging, Department of Diagnostic Radiology, The University of Texas MD Anderson Cancer Center, 1515 Holcombe Boulevard, Unit 1478, Houston, TX 77030, USA
* Corresponding author.
E-mail address: pdegroot@mdanderson.org

Clin Chest Med 36 (2015) 179–196
http://dx.doi.org/10.1016/j.ccm.2015.02.004
0272-5231/15/$ – see front matter © 2015 Elsevier Inc. All rights reserved.

cardiopulmonary symptoms, including chest pain, cough, and dyspnea. However, although useful in ascertaining advanced disease, the limitations of chest radiography in accurately determining TNM descriptors in patients with potentially resectable disease typically mandate imaging with CT and/ or PET/CT and/or MRI. In assessing the value of multimodality staging for lung cancer, Farjah and colleagues[3] found that patients who underwent bimodality evaluation (CT plus PET or CT plus invasive staging), or trimodality staging (CT, PET, and invasive staging) had a significantly lower risk of death compared with single-modality assessment. Bimodality staging compared with single modality had a hazard ratio of 0.58 (99% confidence interval [CI], 0.56–0.60) and trimodality evaluation compared with single-modality had a hazard ratio of 0.49 (99% CI, 0.45–0.54).

Computed Tomography

A CT of the chest with administration of intravenous contrast material is recommended for evaluation of all patients with known or suspected primary lung cancer.[2] CT is used to assess most characteristics of the primary tumor (T descriptor), including size and location, but locoregional invasion can be difficult to determine. CT can demonstrate frank mediastinal or chest wall invasion, but it is not optimal in distinguishing the presence or extent of subtle involvement of the pleura, mediastinal structures, or chest wall.

Detection of nodal metastases is also performed with CT, using greater than 1 cm short-axis diameter as a threshold for suspected metastatic disease. CT is useful in determining the absence or presence of intrathoracic and extrathoracic metastatic disease, including contralateral lung nodules, pleural and pericardial nodules and effusions, bone metastases, or adrenal nodules/masses.

CT of the chest alone is sufficient for staging of patients with pure ground glass opacities and an otherwise normal study, and for patients with peripheral stage IA disease.[2] Otherwise, further imaging with ^{18}F-fluoro-2-deoxy-D-glucose (FDG) PET is recommended for NSCLC patients potentially eligible for curative treatment. When PET is unavailable or cannot be performed, a contrast-enhanced CT of the abdomen is recommended.[2]

MRI

MRI has superior soft tissue contrast compared with CT and is the optimal modality for evaluating subtle mediastinal or chest wall involvement by tumor. For paramediastinal tumors, MRI is useful in assessing tumor involvement of the heart, great vessels, and pericardium and is better than CT at

identifying myocardial or cardiac chamber invasion.[4] MRI is also effective in the evaluation of superior sulcus tumors. MRI is the first-line imaging modality in the investigation of brain metastases.[2,5] In addition, small lesions in the liver can be more frequently detected on contrast-enhanced MRI than CT,[6] and chemical shift MRI can be used to characterize adrenal nodules.

PET

FDG PET has poor intrinsic resolution and generally is not useful in evaluating the primary tumor, but the detection of nodal and distant metastases is improved compared with CT.[7,8] Furthermore, integrated FDG PET/CT is more accurate for nodal and metastatic disease staging than separately interpreted FDG PET and CT.[9] Accordingly, FDG PET and FDG PET/CT are now commonly used for staging in patients with NSCLC.[2,8] In most patients with NSCLC, whole-body FDG PET is recommended when no metastatic disease is detected on CT, as unexpected detection of nodal and/or distant metastases can affect management in up to 14% of patients.[10] In fact, it has been reported that unnecessary thoracotomy can be avoided in 1 of 5 patients through the use of FDG PET imaging.[7]

TNM STAGING: 7TH EDITION

The current 7th edition of the TNM staging system classification for NSCLC is founded entirely on anatomic information (Table 1).[11] Stage evaluation of patients with small cell lung cancer (SCLC) is similar but is not addressed here.[12] For the interested reader, the review by Jett and colleagues[13] on staging and management of SCLC provides an excellent resource.

Primary Tumor

The T descriptor is determined by the size, location, and extent of the primary tumor and is usually assessed by CT (Box 1). Descriptors T1 through T4 reflect prognosis and determine treatment options in patients with limited nodal metastasis and absence of distant metastasis.[14]

T Descriptor	5-year Survival (%)
pT1a N0M0	77
pT1b N0M0	71
pT2a N0M0	58
pT2b N0M0	49
pT2c N0M0	35
pT3 N0M0	38
pT4 (any N)	22

Table 1
IASLC 7th edition TNM stage grouping table

Seventh Edition T/M	N0 Stage	N1 Stage	N2 Stage	N3 Stage
T1a (≤2 cm)	IA	IIA	IIIA	**IIIB**
T1b (>2–3 cm)	IA	IIA	IIIA	**IIIB**
T2a (>3–5 cm)	IB	IIA	IIIA	**IIIB**
T2b (>5–7 cm)	IIA	IIB	IIIA	**IIIB**
T3 (>7 cm)	IIB	IIIA	IIIA	**IIIB**
T3 (invasion)	IIB	IIIA	IIIA	**IIIB**
T3 (same lobe nodules)	IIB	IIIA	IIIA	**IIIB**
T4 (extension)	IIIA	IIIA	**IIIB**	**IIIB**
T4 (ipsilateral lung nodules)	IIIA	IIIA	**IIIB**	**IIIB**
M1a (pleural/ pericardial effusion)	**IV**	**IV**	**IV**	**IV**
M1a (contralateral lung nodules)	**IV**	**IV**	**IV**	**IV**
M1b (distant metastases)	**IV**	**IV**	**IV**	**IV**

Bold denotes unresectable disease.
Reprinted with permission *courtesy of* the International Association for the Study of Lung Cancer. Copyright 2009 IASLC.

Variations in tumor measurements can alter the T descriptor and potentially overall stage. In particular, measurements of irregular lesions with spiculation are often inconsistent and interobserver agreement is low (**Fig. 1**).[15] Furthermore, there is no global standardization of the window or plane used for measurements, allowing for variation according to local or individual practice.[16] Although axial tumor dimensions are most commonly used, studies have shown that measurements in coronal and/or sagittal planes can yield different results.[17]

Measurement of the primary tumor can be difficult when the margins are obscured by postobstructive consolidation or atelectasis. Although the inclusion of FDG PET/CT information in target volume delineation improves tumor localization for radiation therapy and decreases the amount of normal tissue included in the planning target volume, the poor resolution of PET scanners precludes precise tumor measurement. T2-weighted magnetic resonance (MR) imaging can also often distinguish postobstructive processes, which have a higher signal intensity compared with the lung malignancy.[18] Diffusion-weighted sequences can be additionally helpful, because tumors have a higher signal intensity than atelectasis.[19]

Involvement of the pleura, chest wall, and mediastinum by the primary tumor and presence of one or more nodules in the same lung as the primary tumor are also part of the T descriptor. Additional nodules in the same lobe as the primary tumor have a T3 descriptor, while satellite nodules in other lobes of the same lung are designated T4. It is important to emphasize that these descriptors do not preclude resection. CT is useful in determining the presence of additional tumor nodules and frank mediastinal or chest wall invasion (**Fig. 2**). However, limited locoregional invasion can often not be definitively determined. Imaging features that suggest pleural involvement include greater than 3 cm contact between the tumor and adjacent pleural surface, elimination of the extrapleural fat plane, obtuse angles between the pleural surface and tumor, and contact with the pleura that exceeds tumor height.[20] MRI, despite superior soft tissue contrast resolution, does not provide high sensitivity or specificity for subtle pleural invasion. Findings indicative of chest wall invasion on MR include infiltration of the extrapleural fat plane on T1 sequences and hyperintense signal of the parietal pleura on T2 images.[21,22] Nonetheless, the presence and extent of invasion has implications for therapeutic management. For instance, the surgical approach can be altered to include en-bloc resection of the primary malignancy and chest wall when there is locoregional invasion rather than a lobectomy alone. In addition, centrally located tumors close to the spinal cord impose radiation dose-volume constraints, and determination of tumor margins is important and can affect the delivery of radiotherapy.

MR imaging can be used to successfully assess pericardial or myocardial invasion and is useful in evaluating superior sulcus tumors for involvement of the brachial plexus, regional vasculature, and adjacent spine and vertebra (**Fig. 3**).[23,24] This is important because involvement of the brachial plexus roots or trunks superior to the T1 nerve root, invasion of the trachea or esophagus, and greater than 50% invasion of a vertebral body are absolute contraindications to surgical resection.[23–26]

Although FDG PET and FDG PET/CT are generally not performed to determine the T descriptor, FDG uptake by the primary tumor has been reported to be potentially useful in modifying management in patients with resectable disease.[27] In this regard, subsolid nodules with 25% or more of ground glass component and maximum standardized uptake value (SUVmax) 2.9 or less rarely have lymphatic, vascular, or pleural invasion, and nodal metastasis or recurrence occurs in only 1%, raising the possibility that these patients can

Box 1
IASLC 7th edition TNM descriptors

T – Primary tumor

TX: Primary tumor cannot be assessed, *or* tumor proven by the presence of malignant cells in sputum or bronchial washings but not visualized by imaging or bronchoscopy

T0: No evidence of primary tumor

Tis: Carcinoma in situ

T1: Tumor 3 cm or less in greatest dimension, surrounded by lung or visceral pleura, without bronchoscopic evidence of invasion more proximal than the lobar bronchus (ie, not in the main bronchus)

   T1a: Tumor 2 cm or less in greatest dimension[a]

   T1b: Tumor more than 2 cm but not more than 3 cm in greatest dimension

T2: Tumor more than 3 cm but not more than 7 cm; or tumor with *any* of the following features[b]:

- Involves main bronchus, 2 cm or more distal to the carina
- Invades visceral pleura
- Associated with atelectasis or obstructive pneumonitis that extends to the hilar region but does not involve the entire lung

      T2a: Tumor more than 3 cm but not more than 5 cm in greatest dimension

      T2b: Tumor more than 5 cm but not more than 7 cm in greatest dimension

T3: Tumor more than 7 cm or one that directly invades any of the following: chest wall (including superior sulcus tumors), diaphragm, phrenic nerve, mediastinal pleura, parietal pericardium; *or* tumor in the main bronchus less than 2 cm distal to the carina[a] but without involvement of the carina; *or* associated atelectasis or obstructive pneumonitis of the entire lung or separate tumor nodule(s) in the same lobe as the primary.

T4: Tumor of any size that invades any of the following: mediastinum, heart, great vessels, trachea, recurrent laryngeal nerve, esophagus, vertebral body, carina; separate tumor nodule(s) in a different ipsilateral lobe to that of the primary.

N – Regional lymph nodes

NX: Regional lymph nodes cannot be assessed

N0: No regional lymph node metastasis

N1: Metastasis in ipsilateral peribronchial and/or ipsilateral hilar lymph nodes and intrapulmonary nodes, including involvement by direct extension

N2: Metastasis in ipsilateral mediastinal and/or subcarinal lymph node(s)

N3: Metastasis in contralateral mediastinal, contralateral hilar, ipsilateral or contralateral scalene, or supraclavicular lymph node(s)

M – Distant metastasis

M0: No distant metastasis

M1: Distant metastasis

   M1a: Separate tumor nodule(s) in a contralateral lobe; tumor with pleural nodules or malignant pleural or pericardial effusion[c]

   M1b: Distant metastasis

   [a] The uncommon superficial spreading tumor of any size with its invasive component limited to the bronchial wall, which may extend proximal to the main bronchus, is also classified as T1a.
   [b] T2 tumors with these features are classified T2a if 5 cm or less or if size cannot be determined, and T2b if greater than 5 cm but not larger than 7 cm.
   [c] Most pleural (pericardial) effusions with lung cancer are due to tumor. In a few patients, however, multiple microscopic examinations of pleural (pericardial) fluid are negative for tumor, and the fluid is nonbloody and is not an exudate. Where these elements and clinical judgment dictate that the effusion is not related to the tumor, the effusion should be excluded as a staging element and the patient should be classified as M0.
   Reprinted with permission *courtesy of* the International Association for the Study of Lung Cancer. Copyright 2009 IASLC.

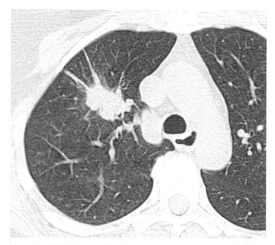

Fig. 1. NSCLC manifesting as a spiculated nodule. Axial contrast-enhanced CT shows an irregular, spiculated nodule. The solid component of the nodule measured 3 cm (T1), including the spicules in the measurement, which increased the size to 5.5 cm (T2). Note that there can be considerable variability in measurements if the lesion is irregular; this can potentially alter management.

appropriately undergo sublobar resection rather than lobectomy for curative resection.[27]

Regional Lymph Nodes

The N descriptor, which specifies the presence and location of nodal metastatic disease, has a significant effect on prognosis (see **Table 1**). Accordingly, a consistent and standardized description of the N descriptors is required to ensure uniformity in designating the clinical and

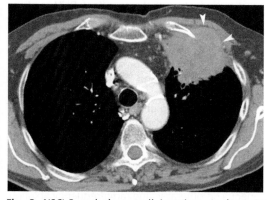

Fig. 2. NSCLC and chest wall invasion. A chest CT shows a large left upper lobe lung mass with invasion into the chest wall (*arrowheads*). CT is useful in determining frank chest wall invasion (T3), although limited locoregional invasion of the pleura is difficult to differentiate from abutment. Note chest wall invasion does not preclude resection.

pathologic extent of nodal metastases. In this regard, lymph node maps are used, in which the node stations are numbered according to anatomic structures.[28,29] For the 7th TNM edition, a standardized, internationally accepted nodal map with 7 node zones, created by unifying the previously used Mountain/Dressler-American Thoracic Society (MD-ATS) node map and the Japanese Naruke map, is used[30,31]; this was necessary because discordance between the 2 maps was high. Watanabe and colleagues[32] reported a discordance of 31.5% with 34% of patients considered to have N2 according to the MD-ATS map, having N1 by the Naruke map. The resulting International Association for the Study of Lung Cancer (IASLC) nodal map (**Fig. 4**) is used with the understanding that the designated oncologic midline of the superior mediastinum corresponds with the left lateral border of the trachea, such that all nodes anterior to the trachea are grouped with right paratracheal nodes (stations 2, 4). The oncologic midline and anatomic midline coincide at the carina.[30,33]

Accurate determination of the N descriptors is important because surgical resection and potential use of adjuvant therapy are dependent on this. Importantly, ipsilateral peribronchial or hilar (N1) nodes are usually resectable, whereas mediastinal nodes have a major influence on resectability. Specifically, ipsilateral mediastinal (including subcarinal) nodal metastasis (N2) can be resectable (usually after induction chemotherapy), whereas contralateral mediastinal and scalene or supraclavicular disease (N3) is unresectable. To potentially improve future patient management, data are currently being collected based on grouping of nodal stations together in 6 zones within the current N1 and N2 patient subsets for further evaluation.[34]

Nodal staging with CT relies on a threshold of greater than 1 cm in short-axis diameter as the indicator of metastatic disease. However, size is not a reliable indicator of nodal metastasis. The limitation of using size as a discriminator for nodal disease is underscored by a study that examined 2891 resected hilar and mediastinal nodes obtained from 256 patients with NSCLC. Seventy-seven percent of the 139 patients with no nodal metastases had at least one node greater than 1 cm in diameter and 12% of the 127 patients with nodal metastases had no nodes greater than 1 cm.[35] A meta-analysis of CT accuracy for nodal staging in 3438 patients showed a sensitivity of 57%, specificity of 82%, positive predictive value of 56%, and a negative predictive value of 83%.[36] Additional factors besides nodal size, such as histologic type (adenocarcinoma

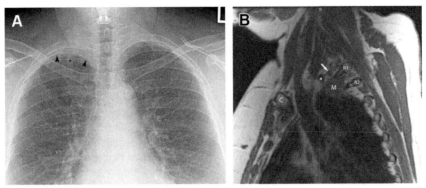

Fig. 3. A 57-year-old woman with a superior sulcus NSCLC presenting with right-hand numbness. (*A*) Posteroanterior chest radiograph shows a small nodular opacity in the right upper lobe (*asterisk*) and apical soft tissue (*arrowheads*) in the right lung apex. There are no findings of rib or vertebral body invasion. (*B*) Sagittal T1-weighted MRI shows the superior sulcus tumor (M) extending posteriorly into the T1/T2 vertebral space and involving the T1 nerve root. The C8 nerve root is preserved (*arrow*). Note that limited involvement of the brachial plexus does not preclude surgical resection. The patient underwent right upper lobe lobectomy and en-bloc resection of the superior sulcus and adjacent chest wall. C, clavicle; R1, first rib; R2, second rib; *, subclavian artery.

histology) and tumor size and location (larger size, central location), are associated with a higher risk of occult nodal disease and should be considered in the decision as to whether to perform invasive nodal sampling.[37,38]

FDG PET and FDG PET/CT have improved sensitivity and specificity for detecting mediastinal nodal metastasis compared with CT (**Fig. 5**). A meta-analysis incorporating 833 patients showed an overall sensitivity of 83% and specificity of 92% for FDG PET in detecting mediastinal nodal metastases compared with overall sensitivity and specificity of 59% and 78%, respectively, on CT.[39] Nevertheless, another study reported low sensitivity and accuracy of PET/CT for N staging based on nodal sampling.[40] From 1001 nodal specimens including mediastinal, hilar, and intrapulmonary stations, FDG PET/CT had a specificity of 94.5%, sensitivity of only 45% and accuracy of 85%. Furthermore, size of the node affected sensitivity: the sensitivity of PET/CT was 85% for nodes 1 cm or greater short axis, but 32% for nodes less than 1 cm.[40] de Langen and colleagues[41] have shown that nodal sampling may not be necessary for nodes measuring 10 to 15 mm on CT, as long as they are negative on FDG PET. However, mediastinal lymph nodes 16 mm or larger, even if negative on FDG PET, have a 21% posttest probability of metastatic involvement, necessitating preoperative pathologic staging.

Attempts to improve the detection of nodal metastasis on FDG PET have included measuring the SUVmax of the primary tumor to predict the likelihood of microscopic nodal metastatic disease and using a threshold SUVmax for FDG uptake to distinguish inflammatory disease from nodal

metastases.[42–46] In a study of 265 patients with NSCLC, Miyasaka and colleagues[42] reported that the SUVmax of the primary tumor was a significant predictor of pathologic nodal involvement. Of patients with primary tumors having SUVmax greater than 10, 41% had pN1-N2 disease, whereas only 12.7% of patients with tumor SUVmax less than 10 had pN1-N2 disease. However, there is significant variability in the definition of the SUV threshold among studies that preclude universal applicability.[42–46] Pertaining to false positive findings in nodal stations on FDG PET or FDG PET/CT due to infectious or inflammatory causes (**Fig. 6**), including endemic fungal infections, no FDG uptake threshold for nodal metastatic disease has been validated. This finding may partly be due to factors that can affect SUV such as time to imaging after FDG injection, scanner type, image reconstruction algorithm, and patient body weight. In fact, visual assessment of FDG uptake is considered superior to SUV in differentiating inflammatory and infectious causes from nodal metastasis.[47]

An understanding of the limitations of FDG PET and FDG PET/CT in the evaluation of the N descriptors is especially important because of the increasing utilization of nonsurgical definitive management options for early-stage NSCLC, including stereotactic body radiation therapy (SBRT), percutaneous cryotherapy, and radiofrequency ablation. Although studies have shown that the predominant pattern of recurrence following SBRT is distant metastatic disease, regional nodal metastases occur and may reflect pre-existing metastatic disease, not detected by FDG PET, before initiation of therapy.[48] Therefore, for patients with

#1 (Left/Right) Low cervical, supraclavicular and sternal notch nodes
Upper border: lower margin of cricoid cartilage
Lower border: clavicles bilaterally and, in the midline, the upper border of the manubrium, 1R designates right-sided nodes, 1L, left-sided nodes in this region.
#1 and #R1 limited by the midline of the trachea.

#2 (Left/Right) Upper paratracheal nodes
2R: Upper border: apex of the right lung and pleural space and, in the midline, the upper border of the manubrium
Lower border: intersection of caudal margin of innominate vein with the trachea
2L: Upper border: apex of the left lung and pleural space and, in the midline, the upper border of the manubrium
Lower border: superior border of the aortic arch
As for #4, in #2 the oncologic midline is along the left lateral border of the trachea.

#3 Pre-vascular and retrotracheal nodes
3a: Prevascular - On the right
upper border: apex of chest
lower border: level of carina
anterior border: posterior aspect of sternum
posterior border: anterior border of superior vena cava
3a: Prevascular - On the left
upper border: apex of chest
lower border: level of carina
anterior border: posterior aspect of sternum
posterior border: left carotid artery
3p: Retrotracheal
upper border: apex of chest
lower border: carina

#4 (Left/Right) Lower paratracheal nodes
4R: includes right paratracheal nodes, and pretracheal nodes extending to the left lateral border of trachea
upper border: intersection of caudal margin of innominate vein with the trachea
lower border: lower border of azygos vein
4L: includes nodes to the left of the left lateral border of the trachea, medial to the ligamentum arteriosum
upper border: upper margin of the aortic arch
lower border: upper rim of the left main pulmonary artery

MG57591 0409

#5 Subaortic (aorto-pulmonary window)
Subaortic lymph nodes lateral to the ligamentum arteriosum
upper border: the lower border of the aortic arch
lower border: upper rim of the left main pulmonary artery

#6 Para-aortic nodes ascending aorta or phrenic
Lymph nodes anterior and lateral to the ascending aorta and aortic arch
upper border: a line tangential to upper border of aortic arch
lower border: the lower border of the aortic arch

#7 Subcarinal nodes
upper border: the carina of the trachea
lower border: the upper border of the lower lobe bronchus on the left; the lower border of the bronchus intermedius on right

#8 (Left/Right) Para-esophageal nodes (below carina)
Nodes lying adjacent to the wall of the esophagus and to the right or left of the midline, excluding subcarinal nodes
upper border: the upper border of the lower lobe bronchus on the left; the lower border of the bronchus intermedius on right
lower border: the diaphragm

#9 (Left/Right) Pulmonary ligament nodes
Nodes lying within the pulmonary ligament
upper border: the inferior pulmonary vein
lower border: the diaphragm

#10 (Left/Right) Hilar nodes
Includes nodes immediately adjacent to the mainstem bronchus and hilar vessels including the proximal portions of the pulmonary veins and main pulmonary artery
upper border: the lower rim of the azygos vein on the right; upper rim of the pulmonary artery on the left
lower border: interlobar region bilaterally

#11 Interlobar nodes
Between the origin of the lobar bronchi
*#11s: between the upper lobe bronchus and bronchus intermedius on the right
*#11i: between the middle and lower lobe bronchi on the right

#12 Lobar nodes
Adjacent to the lobar bronchi

#13 Segmental nodes
Adjacent to the segmental bronchi

#14 Sub-segmental nodes
Adjacent to the subsegmental bronchi

Supraclavicular zone

● 1 Low cervical, supraclavicular, and sternal notch nodes

SUPERIOR MEDIASTINAL NODES

Upper zone

● 2R Upper Paratracheal (right)
○ 2L Upper Paratracheal (left)
● 3a Prevascular
● 3p Retrotracheal
● 4R Lower Paratracheal (right)
○ 4L Lower Paratracheal (left)

AORTIC NODES

AP zone

● 5 Subaortic
● 6 Para-aortic (ascending aorta or phrenic)

INFERIOR MEDIASTINAL NODES

Subcarinal zone

○ 7 Subcarinal

Lower zone

● 8 Paraesophageal (below carina)
● 9 Pulmonary ligament

N1 NODES

Hilar/Interlobar zone

○ 10 Hilar
● 11 Interlobar

Peripheral zone

● 12 Lobar
○ 13 Segmental
○ 14 Subsegmental

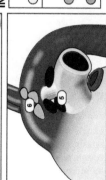

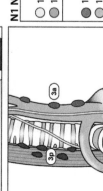

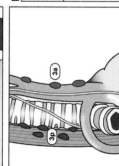

Fig. 4. IASLC nodal map. (Reprinted with permission *courtesy of* the International Association for the Study of Lung Cancer. Copyright 2009 IASLC).

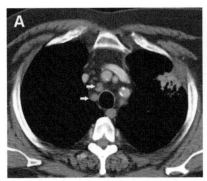
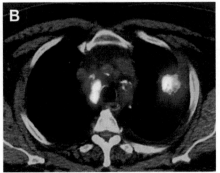

Fig. 5. A 63-year-old man with a left upper lobe NSCLC was evaluated for surgical resection. (*A*) Axial contrast-enhanced CT shows an irregular mass in the left upper lobe with small adjacent loculated pleural fluid and non-enlarged (short-axis diameters of <1 cm) contralateral right upper paratracheal nodes (*arrows*). (*B*) PET/CT shows increased FDG uptake in the left upper lobe mass and in the contralateral mediastinal nodes suspicious for N3 disease. Biopsy confirmed N3 nodal metastatic disease, and the patient was treated palliatively.

NSCLC undergoing SBRT or minimally invasive percutaneous ablative therapies, endobronchial ultrasound or endoscopic ultrasound should be strongly considered, especially when the likelihood of pN1 disease is high (high T designation, central tumors) and when CT and FDG PET findings are incongruent.[2,49]

Last, it is important to realize that the time interval between PET acquisition and surgical resection can affect the accuracy of nodal staging on PET. In this regard, Booth and colleagues[50] found that PET/CT had an accuracy of 94% for N2 disease when imaging was performed less than 9 weeks before resection, compared with 81% when imaging occurred ≥9 weeks before surgery.

Metastasis

Many patients with lung cancer have metastatic disease at presentation; common sites include the contralateral lung, pleura, liver, adrenal glands, brain, and bones.[1] The M1 descriptor describes these metastases and is divided into 2 subsets based on outcome data showing a modest but significant survival difference.[51] M1a includes one or more nodules in the contralateral lung, pleural effusion and nodules, and pericardial nodules, whereas M1b designates extrathoracic metastasis.[51,52]

The detection of metastases is important in determining whether the patient will be a candidate for surgical resection or receive palliative radiation and chemotherapy. CT is useful in determining the absence or presence of intrathoracic metastatic disease, including contralateral lung nodules, pleural and pericardial nodules, and effusions. For instance, the diagnosis of a malignant pleural effusion or pleural metastasis is important in patient management because these metastases preclude surgical resection. Pleural thickening and nodularity on CT suggest metastatic pleural disease, but these abnormalities may not be present in association with a malignant effusion.[53] This

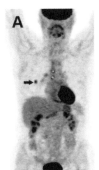
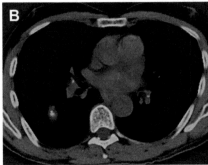
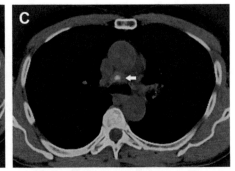

Fig. 6. A 65-year-old man with a poorly differentiated lung adenocarcinoma and increased FDG uptake in intrathoracic nodes suspicious for metastasis. (*A*) Whole-body PET coronal maximum intensity projection image shows increased FDG uptake in the right lower primary tumor (*arrow*), infrahilar and hilar lymph nodes, and mediastinal nodes (*asterisk*). (*B*) PET/CT fused axial image shows increased uptake of FDG in the right lower lobe nodule. (*C*) PET/CT shows increased FDG uptake in a right lower paratracheal node (*arrow*) suspicious for N2 disease. At surgical resection, anthracotic lymph nodes were found that were histologically negative for metastatic disease.

limitation is compounded by cytologic evaluation often being negative: mean sensitivity averages 72% (range, 49%–91%) when at least 2 pleural fluid specimens are analyzed.[53] FDG PET has an accuracy, sensitivity, and specificity for pleural malignancy of 92%, 100%, and 78%, respectively, and when FDG pleural uptake is increased and cytology is negative, pleural biopsy is necessitated in patients who are potential candidates for surgical resection.[54] False positive FDG uptake can be seen with talc pleurodesis and acute inflammatory conditions, including postsurgical sequelae.[55]

Although a nodule in the contralateral lung is potentially a metastasis (M1a), most additional pulmonary nodules (approximately 75%) seen on CT imaging in patients with potentially operable clinical stage I to IIIA lung cancer are benign.[56,57] Furthermore, an additional nodule can be a synchronous second primary lung cancer (incidence approximately 1.5%–2% per patient per year).[56] The American Joint Committee on Cancer criteria are confusing with regard to stage classification, but indicate that when a patient has simultaneous bilateral cancers in paired organs, the tumors are classified separately as independent tumors in different organs.[58] To clarify the staging ambiguity, the ACCP recommends that when 2 lung cancers are deemed to be synchronous primary cancers, they be classified with a TNM descriptor for each tumor.[56]

Although CT can be useful in detecting M1b disease, FDG PET and FDG PET/CT are more accurate (**Fig. 7**).[2] Nevertheless, the role of FDG PET/CT in the staging of patients with early-stage NSCLC is debated. A randomized controlled trial of patients primarily with T1-2N0 disease on conventional staging found that PET upstaged 22 of 91 patients as a result of N2 nodal disease and pleural metastases and would have changed management in 26% of patients.[59] However, occult distant metastases (M1b) were discovered in very few of these early-stage patients (<5%).[59] In more advanced NSCLC, FDG PET has been shown to detect extrathoracic metastatic disease in up to 24% of patients who were potentially eligible for curative resection.[7,60] The incidence of occult metastatic disease discovered with FDG PET is reported to increase with higher

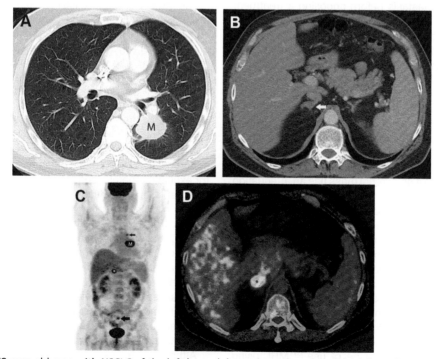

Fig. 7. A 58-year-old man with NSCLC of the left lower lobe and an adrenal nodule. (*A*) Axial contrast-enhanced chest CT shows a left lower lobe mass (M). (*B*) Axial contrast-enhanced abdominal CT shows a small low-attenuation right adrenal nodule (*arrow*). (*C*) Whole-body PET maximum intensity projection image shows increased FDG uptake in the left lung mass (M) and right adrenal (*asterisk*). Note increased FDG uptake in an ipsilateral mediastinal node (*small arrow*) and sacral bone suspicious for metastases (*large arrow*). (*D*) Axial PET/CT shows increased uptake of FDG in the right adrenal gland (*asterisk*) suspicious for a metastasis. Biopsy confirmed metastatic disease.

T and N descriptors.[60] Importantly, according to the American College of Surgeons Oncology Trial, the negative predictive value of FDG PET is 99% for M1 disease.[8]

Specific common sites for NSCLC metastases are now often evaluated by FDG PET/CT. In this regard, FDG PET/CT is more sensitive for osseous metastatic disease than bone scintigraphy with ^{99m}Technetium (Tc)-methylene diphosphonate (MDP). In fact, FDG PET/CT has almost entirely supplanted the use of ^{99m}Tc MDP in patients with NSCLC.[61–63] A meta-analysis reported overall sensitivity and specificity of 92% and 98%, respectively, for osseous metastases on PET/CT, compared with sensitivity of 86% and specificity of 88% for ^{99m}Tc MDP bone scintigraphy.[62] Results of ^{99m}Tc MDP and FDG PET/CT for bone involvement have been shown to be discordant in up to 20% of patients with lung cancer, primarily because ^{99m}Tc MDP cannot identify early metastatic bone marrow infiltration.[64] Although uptake of FDG in bone can occur on PET studies before radiologically evident bone destruction, inflammatory conditions can also cause focal uptake. For this reason, biopsy or correlation with anatomic imaging studies is mandated to confirm an osseous metastasis before choosing a treatment regimen, if it is the sole abnormality.

Adrenal gland metastases occur in up to 20% of patients with NSCLC.[65] Nevertheless, most adrenal nodules in patients with NSCLC are incidental adenomas.[66] CT and MRI are useful in the evaluation of adrenal masses, and CT and MRI features favoring malignancy include size greater than 3 cm, poorly defined margins, irregularly enhancing rim, invasion of adjacent structures, and high signal intensity on T2-weighted sequences.[67] A confident diagnosis of benignity can be made if an adrenal mass has an attenuation value less than 10 Hounsfield units (HU) on a noncontrast-enhanced CT. A meta-analysis of 10 studies to determine an optimal threshold for differentiating benign from malignant lesions yielded a sensitivity of 71% and a specificity of 98% for characterizing adrenal masses with a threshold of 10 HU.[68] Although the finding of low attenuation is useful to characterize an adenoma, up to 30% of adenomas do not contain sufficient lipid to demonstrate low attenuation on CT imaging.[69] In these cases, delayed contrast-enhanced CT has been shown to be of use.[70] MRI, using chemical shift analysis and dynamic gadolinium enhancement, can also be used to identify lipid-poor adenomas.[71–73] FDG PET-CT is also useful in detecting an adrenal metastasis and distinguishing benign from malignant adrenal masses detected on CT.[74] A meta-analysis of 21 studies

evaluating 1391 lesions (5 studies were specifically in patients with lung cancer) reported a combined sensitivity of 97% and specificity of 91% of FDG PET for characterizing adrenal masses as malignant.[74] In fact, FDG PET/CT has changed the imaging algorithm used to evaluate an indeterminate adrenal mass and is now often used as the definitive imaging modality rather than MRI, particularly when the adrenal mass is small. In patients with an FDG-avid adrenal nodule, biopsy is needed to confirm metastatic disease before treatment, if this finding will change therapeutic management.[2]

Central nervous system metastases are common and are detected in up to 18% of patients at presentation.[75,76] The standard of care for evaluating patients with lung cancer for potential brain lesions is MRI, which has exquisite soft tissue contrast resolution.[77,78] The detection of brain metastasis on CT or MRI in NSCLC patients with a negative clinical examination is reported to be 0% to 10% (**Fig. 8**).[2] To date, the use of routine MRI in staging patients with NSCLC and a negative clinical evaluation has not been studied adequately. However, Earnest and colleagues[79] have reported occult brain metastases in 6 of 27 (22%) patients with potentially resectable NSCLC (excluding early-stage lung cancer) on contrast-enhanced MRI. In addition, there is a substantial prevalence of early postoperative recurrence of tumor in the brain, particularly in patients with nonsquamous cell histology and stage of disease higher than T1N0, suggesting that undetected metastases were present at the time of surgical resection of the primary lung malignancy.[80,81] Consequently, there may be a limited role for imaging in the detection of occult brain metastases. In particular, imaging of the brain may be indicated for excluding metastases in patients with clinically resectable, locally advanced NSCLC with nonsquamous histology. Furthermore, the ACCP recommends that patients with clinical stage III or IV NSCLC have routine imaging of the brain with MRI (or CT if MRI is not available) even if the clinical evaluation is negative for brain metastases.[2] FDG PET and FDG PET/CT do not have a role in the assessment of metastatic brain disease. Normal brain cells are obligate glucose metabolizers; therefore, high uptake of FDG by normal brain tissue usually obscures metastatic lesions.

Although whole-body FDG PET/CT improves the accuracy of staging in patients with NSCLC, focal increased uptake of FDG in extrathoracic lesions unrelated to the primary NSCLC can mimic distant metastasis. Lardinois and colleagues[82] reported that in 350 patients with newly diagnosed NSCLC, 72 patients had

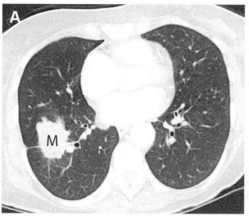
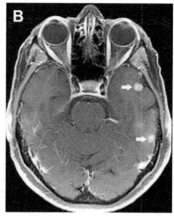

Fig. 8. A 72-year-old woman with a poorly differentiated adenocarcinoma presenting with hemoptysis. (*A*) Axial contrast-enhanced CT shows a right lower lobe mass (M). (*B*) Axial T1 contrast-enhanced MRI of the brain shows 2 small left temporal lobe metastases (*arrows*). Note that although the benefit of routine MRI in detecting occult brain metastasis is unclear, imaging of the brain may be indicated for the exclusion of brain metastases in patients with clinically resectable, locally advanced NSCLC with nonsquamous histology.

solitary extrathoracic FDG-avid lesions. Sixty-nine of these lesions were biopsied and 37 (54%) had a solitary metastasis, whereas 32 (46%) had lesions unrelated to the NSCLC. Accordingly, all extrathoracic FDG-avid lesions that potentially would alter patient management should be further imaged or biopsied to confirm the diagnosis of distant metastasis.

PEARLS AND PITFALLS
T Descriptor

Pearls

- CT accurately assesses most characteristics of the primary tumor (T descriptor), including size and location, but limited locoregional invasion can be difficult to diagnose.
- MRI is the optimal imaging modality to evaluate involvement of the brachial plexus, regional vessels, and spine in a patient with a superior sulcus tumor.
- FDG PET has poor intrinsic resolution and generally is not useful in evaluating the primary tumor.
- When margins of the tumor are obscured by postobstructive processes, FDG PET, PET/CT, and/or MRI can be helpful, particularly for radiation therapy planning.

Pitfalls

- Precise measurement of spiculated tumors is difficult and accordingly determination of the T descriptor can be inconsistent and inaccurate.

- Limited locoregional invasion of the pleura, chest wall, and mediastinum is difficult to differentiate from abutment.

N Descriptor

Pearls

- The IASLC lymph node map provides a standardized, internationally accepted map with 7 node zones and enables a consistent determination of the N descriptors.
- Accurate determination of the N descriptors is important because surgical resection and potential use of adjuvant therapy are dependent on this.
- Ipsilateral hilar (N1) node metastases are usually resectable; ipsilateral mediastinal nodes (N2) can be resectable (usually after induction chemotherapy), and contralateral mediastinal and scalene or supraclavicular adenopathy (N3) are unresectable.
- A CT threshold of greater than 1 cm in short-axis diameter is an unreliable indicator of nodal metastasis.
- FDG PET/CT has better sensitivity and specificity for mediastinal nodal staging compared with CT.
- PET/CT for nodal staging should be performed close to the anticipated resection date.

Pitfalls

- False positive FDG uptake by nodes due to infectious and/or inflammatory disease is common.

- The use of an SUV threshold in FDG PET/CT to distinguish nodal metastasis from infectious or inflammatory is not useful.
- SUVmax of the primary tumor to predict the likelihood of microscopic nodal metastatic disease is not universally applicable because of significant variability in the SUV threshold.

M Descriptor

Pearls

- The M1 descriptor is divided into M1a (one or more nodules in the contralateral lung, pleural effusion and nodules, and pericardial nodules) and M1b (extrathoracic metastasis).
- CT is useful in determining the absence or presence of M1a disease.
- Although a contralateral lung nodule on CT is potentially a metastasis (M1a), most are benign in patients with clinical stage I to IIIA NSCLC.
- FDG PET and FDG PET/CT are more sensitive for detection of distant extrathoracic metastases than CT alone.
- The incidence of occult metastatic disease discovered with FDG PET increases with higher T and N descriptors.
- Bone and adrenal metastases are optimally evaluated by FDG PET/CT, whereas MRI remains the imaging modality of choice in the detection of brain metastases.

Pitfalls

- False positive FDG uptake mimicking M1a pleural metastasis can be seen with talc pleurodesis.
- False positive FDG uptake in bone and adrenals can mimic metastatic disease, and biopsy or correlation with anatomic imaging studies is mandated to confirm M1b if this abnormality alters management.
- Single foci of extrathoracic FDG uptake in patients with newly diagnosed NSCLC mimicking a distant metastasis is often unrelated to the primary NSCLC, and biopsy is required to confirm metastatic disease before making treatment decisions.

CURRENT CONTROVERSIES

Many questions related to staging of lung cancer were unable to be addressed in the 7th edition of the TNM staging of NSCLC and it is hoped they will be clarified in the next revision.[33]

Staging of Contralateral Lung Nodules

In the 7th edition of TNM staging, nodules in the lung opposite the primary tumor constitute M1a disease, regardless of their multiplicity. However, in the absence of nodal metastatic disease, patients with lung cancer with a single metastatic nodule in the contralateral lung have a similar survival compared with patients with ipsilobar (T3) and ipsilateral (T4) lung nodules. De Leyn and colleagues[83] found that the 5-year survival rate in their series of patients with sequential resections for synchronous bilateral lung lesions was 38%, with no survival difference between patients with the same cancer histology versus different histologies in the bilateral tumors. The significantly higher survival of patients with a single contralateral lung nodule compared with patients having disseminated stage IV disease suggests that the single contralateral lung nodule should be assigned a descriptor that reflects its prognosis.[84]

Staging of Synchronous Primary Lung Cancers

The prognosis of synchronous primary lung cancers (SPLCs) if treated aggressively can be comparable with patients with single lung cancer of the same stage.[85] Therefore, it is important to identify patients with SPLCs. The Martini and Melamed criteria can be used to identify synchronous tumors. Clinical and pathologic criteria include the following: (1) different tumor histology; (2) tumors of different histologic subtypes; (3) tumors with similar histology that have a component of in situ carcinoma (implying separate occurrence); and (4) tumors with similar histology but without intervening locoregional nodal metastatic disease and without extrathoracic metastatic disease.[85,86]

Staging of Multilobar Primary Tumors

NSCLCs that invade the visceral pleura are classified as T2 in the 7th edition. Tumors that extend across a lung fissure to involve adjacent lobes are not categorized separately and therefore are considered by some to technically be categorized under the T2 descriptor. Early studies had conflicting results regarding the survival of these patients, but were also confounded by including pneumonectomy patients with increased morbidity.[87–89] More recently, Haam and colleagues[90] retrospectively evaluated 837 patients with T2 and T3 N0M0 disease, including 46 patients with direct translobar invasion, and found that 5-year survival of the invasion group was closer to T3 survival: 53% and 49%, respectively. The survival rate at 5 years in the T2 group was significantly different (68%). Joshi and colleagues[89] reported a reduction in survival for stage I tumors that cross a fissure compared with stage I tumors within a single lobe. Consequently, the categorization of primary tumors extending across a lung fissure deserves further investigation and validation.

Staging of Ground Glass Opacities

The measurement of part-ground glass, part-solid primary lung adenocarcinomas presents a dilemma. The solid part of the lesion corresponds on histology with the invasive component of the tumor; the solid portion of the tumor can be of varying sizes that can indicate different prognoses despite constancy of the overall dimensions that include the ground glass component and determine the T descriptor.[91,92]

Staging of Extrathoracic Nodal Disease

Lymph node metastases can occur in several nodal chains that are not addressed by the current TNM staging system. These lymph node metastases include internal mammary, axillary, intercostals, and diaphragmatic lymph nodes. In some practices, these are considered distant metastatic disease.[33]

FUTURE DIRECTIONS
Quantitative Imaging

An expanded role for CT in the evaluation of patients with NSCLC includes the assessment of quantitative imaging features in addition to the standard qualitative characteristics, such as size, spiculation, cavitation, and other morphologic features. An emerging technique referred to as texture analysis, in which objective measurements of heterogeneity based on the distribution of gray levels,[93] and a host of other characteristics reflecting variations in tumor morphology, heterogeneity, and texture, are being investigated (**Fig. 9**).[94] The term "radiomics" has been used to describe the extraction of advanced quantitative imaging features thought to be related to the underlying genotype and phenotype of tumors.[95] In NSCLC, quantitative imaging features have been used to distinguish between adenocarcinoma and squamous cell subtypes and suggest tumor characteristics such as stage, metabolism, hypoxia, angiogenesis, and prognosis.[96,97] Using a publicly available dataset consisting of 32 NSCLC patients, Kumar and colleagues[98] have identified 39 of 327 CT features that are reproducible, nonredundant, and informative. Recently, quantitative CT texture and spatial analysis techniques used to analyze mediastinal lymph nodes in 43 patients with primary lung malignancies showed a sensitivity of 81% and specificity of 80% for detecting nodal metastatic disease.[99]

Expanded Use of Magnetic Resonance in Staging

Recently, dynamic cine MR imaging used during quiet respiration has been reported to distinguish chest wall invasion from a tumor that is adjacent to but not invading the parietal pleura with a sensitivity of 100% and specificity of 70%.[100] Electrocardiogram-gated MR angiography has also been used to identify mediastinal and hilar invasion by NSCLC and is reported to have a sensitivity of 90%, specificity of 87%, and accuracy of 88%.[4]

MRI shows increasing utility in the detection of nodal disease and has been reported to have a sensitivity of 90.1%, specificity of 93.1%, and accuracy of 92.2% on a per-patient basis.[101,102] Recommended MR sequences for this purpose include cardiac- or respiratory-triggered short tau inversion recovery turbo spin-echo.[101,102] Metastatic lymph nodes have high signal intensity on these sequences, whereas normal nodes have low signal intensity. Other findings, such as eccentric cortical thickening or obliterated fatty hilum on T2 black-blood turbo spin-echo, also indicate nodal disease.[103] Diffusion-weighted imaging (DWI) has also been evaluated in the detection of lymph node involvement. One study has reported that DWI is more accurate that PET for nodal staging; nevertheless, DWI is limited for nodal detection and localization by intrinsically low spatial resolution.[104] A prospective study of 203 patients with NSCLC who underwent whole-body MRI with DWI imaging reported a sensitivity of 68%, specificity of 92%, and accuracy of 88% in detecting distant (M1b) metastatic disease. The authors concluded that MRI has an accuracy equivalent to that of PET/CT and can be used for assessment of M1b in patients with NSCLC.[105]

8th Edition TNM Staging for Lung Cancer

Although the 7th edition of TNM staging for lung cancer was based on evidence from the retrospective review of more than 100,000 international lung cancer cases, it is still entirely founded on anatomic data. The IASLC has been and is currently enrolling patients worldwide in a prospective database to prepare for the 8th edition of the TNM classification system, due in 2015. The goal is to focus on specific subsets of the T, N, and M descriptors. If validated, future editions may include additional parameters such as tumor histology, tumor markers, molecular genetic factors, and demographic data in the staging system.[106]

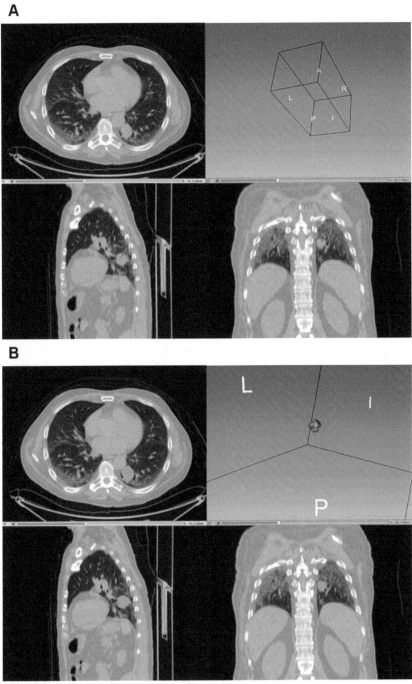

Fig. 9. Segmentation and quantitative analysis in a 58-year-old man with NSCLC of the left lower lobe. (*A*) Chest CT images show visual identification of the malignancy in the axial, sagittal, and coronal planes. (*B*) Images obtained after segmentation of the malignancy show appropriate selection of the nodule in the axial, sagittal, and coronal planes and, in the top right corner, the 3-dimensional image produced from these images that will be analyzed by the texture analysis software.

REFERENCES

1. Reck M, Heigener DF, Mok T, et al. Management of non-small-cell lung cancer: recent developments. Lancet 2013;382(9893):709–19.
2. Silvestri GA, Gonzalez AV, Jantz MA, et al. Methods for staging non-small cell lung cancer: diagnosis and management of lung cancer, 3rd ed: American College of Chest Physicians evidence-based clinical practice guidelines. Chest 2013;143(Suppl 5): e211S–50S.
3. Farjah F, Flum DR, Ramsey SD, et al. Multi-modality mediastinal staging for lung cancer among Medicare beneficiaries. J Thorac Oncol 2009; 4(3):355–63.
4. Ohno Y, Adachi S, Motoyama A, et al. Multiphase ECG-triggered 3D contrast-enhanced MR angiography: utility for evaluation of hilar and mediastinal invasion of bronchogenic carcinoma. J Magn Reson Imaging 2001;13(2):215–24.
5. Hollings N, Shaw P. Diagnostic imaging of lung cancer. Eur Respir J 2002;19(4):722–42.
6. Koyama H, Ohno Y, Seki S, et al. Magnetic resonance imaging for lung cancer. J Thorac Imaging 2013;28(3):138–50.
7. van Tinteren H, Hoekstra OS, Smit EF, et al. Effectiveness of positron emission tomography in the preoperative assessment of patients with suspected non-small-cell lung cancer: the PLUS multicentre randomised trial. Lancet 2002; 359(9315):1388–93.
8. Reed CE, Harpole DH, Posther KE, et al. Results of the American College of Surgeons Oncology Group Z0050 trial: the utility of positron emission tomography in staging potentially operable non-small cell lung cancer. J Thorac Cardiovasc Surg 2003;126(6):1943–51.
9. Antoch G, Stattaus J, Nemat AT, et al. Non-small cell lung cancer: dual-modality PET/CT in preoperative staging. Radiology 2003;229(2):526–33.
10. Weder W, Schmid RA, Bruchhaus H, et al. Detection of extrathoracic metastases by positron emission tomography in lung cancer. Ann Thorac Surg 1998;66:886–93.
11. Goldstraw P, Crowley J, Chansky K, et al. The IASLC Lung Cancer Staging Project: proposals for the revision of the TNM stage groupings in the forthcoming (seventh) edition of the TNM Classification of malignant tumours. J Thorac Oncol 2007;2(8):706–14.
12. Shepherd FA, Crowley J, Van Houtte P, et al. The International Association for the Study of Lung Cancer lung cancer staging project: proposals regarding the clinical staging of small cell lung cancer in the forthcoming (seventh) edition of the tumor, node, metastasis classification for lung cancer. J Thorac Oncol 2007;2(12):1067–77.
13. Jett JR, Schild SE, Kesler KA, et al. Treatment of small cell lung cancer: diagnosis and management of lung cancer, 3rd ed: American College of Chest Physicians evidence-based clinical practice guidelines. Chest 2013;143(Suppl 5):e400S–19S.
14. Rami-Porta R, Ball D, Crowley J, et al. The IASLC Lung Cancer Staging Project: proposals for the revision of the T descriptors in the forthcoming (seventh) edition of the TNM classification for lung cancer. J Thorac Oncol 2007;2(7):593–602.
15. Erasmus JJ, Gladish GW, Broemeling L, et al. Interobserver and intraobserver variability in measurement of non-small-cell carcinoma lung lesions: implications for assessment of tumor response. J Clin Oncol 2003;21(13):2574–82.
16. Wang J, Wu N, Zheng QF, et al. Application of the 2007 lung cancer staging system by International Association for the Study of Lung Cancer. Beijing Da Xue Xue Bao 2009;41(4):442–6 [in Chinese].
17. Ridge CA, Huang J, Cardoza S, et al. Comparison of multiplanar reformatted CT lung tumor measurements to axial tumor measurement alone: impact on maximal tumor dimension and T stage. AJR Am J Roentgenol 2013;201(5):959–63.
18. Ohno Y, Koyama H, Dinkel J, et al. Lung cancer. In: Kauczor H, editor. MRI of the Lung. Heidelberg (Germany): Springer-Verlag Berlin; 2009. p. 179–216.
19. Qi LP, Zhang XP, Tang L, et al. Using diffusion-weighted MR imaging for tumor detection in the collapsed lung: a preliminary study. Eur Radiol 2009;19(2):333–41.
20. Ratto GB, Piacenza G, Frola C, et al. Chest wall involvement by lung cancer: computed tomographic detection and results of operation. Ann Thorac Surg 1991;51:182–8.
21. Padovani B, Mouroux J, Seksik L, et al. Chest wall invasion by bronchogenic carcinoma: evaluation with MR imaging. Radiology 1993;187(1):33–8.
22. Freundlich IM, Chasen MH, Varma DG. Magnetic resonance imaging of pulmonary apical tumors. J Thorac Imaging 1996;11(3):210–22.
23. Bruzzi JF, Komaki R, Walsh GL, et al. Imaging of non-small cell lung cancer of the superior sulcus: part 1: anatomy, clinical manifestations, and management. Radiographics 2008;28(2):551–60 [quiz: 620].
24. Bruzzi JF, Komaki R, Walsh GL, et al. Imaging of non-small cell lung cancer of the superior sulcus: part 2: initial staging and assessment of resectability and therapeutic response. Radiographics 2008;28(2):561–72.
25. Dartevelle P, Macchiarini P. Surgical management of superior sulcus tumors. Oncologist 1999;4(5):398–407.
26. Bilsky MH, Vitaz TW, Boland PJ, et al. Surgical treatment of superior sulcus tumors with spinal and brachial plexus involvement. J Neurosurg 2002;97(Suppl 3):301–9.

27. Uehara H, Tsutani Y, Okumura S, et al. Prognostic role of positron emission tomography and high-resolution computed tomography in clinical stage IA lung adenocarcinoma. Ann Thorac Surg 2013; 96(6):1958–65.

28. Mountain CF, Dresler CM. Regional lymph node classification for lung cancer staging. Chest 1997;111:1718–23.

29. Naruke T, Suemasu K, Ishikawa S. Lymph node mapping and curability at various levels of metastasis in resected lung cancer. J Thorac Cardiovasc Surg 1978;76(6):832–9.

30. Goldstraw P. New staging system: how does it affect our practice? J Clin Oncol 2013;31(8):984–91.

31. Rusch VW, Asamura H, Watanabe H, et al. The IASLC lung cancer staging project: a proposal for a new international lymph node map in the forthcoming seventh edition of the TNM classification for lung cancer. J Thorac Oncol 2009;4(5):568–77.

32. Watanabe S, Ladas G, Goldstraw P. Inter-observer variability in systematic nodal dissection: comparison of European and Japanese nodal designation. Ann Thorac Surg 2002;73(1):245–8 [discussion: 248–9].

33. El-Sherief AH, Lau CT, Wu CC, et al. International association for the study of lung Cancer (IASLC) lymph node map: radiologic review with CT illustration. Radiographics 2014;34(6):1680–91.

34. Rusch VW, Crowley J, Giroux DJ, et al. The IASLC Lung Cancer Staging Project: proposals for the revision of the N descriptors in the forthcoming seventh edition of the TNM classification for lung cancer. J Thorac Oncol 2007;2(7):603–12.

35. Prenzel KL, Monig SP, Sinning JM, et al. Lymph node size and metastatic infiltration in non-small cell lung cancer. Chest 2003;123(2):463–7.

36. Toloza EM, Harpole L, McCrory DC. Noninvasive staging of non-small cell lung cancer: a review of the current evidence. Chest 2003;123(Suppl 1): 137S–46S.

37. Herth FJ, Eberhardt R, Krasnik M, et al. Endobronchial ultrasound-guided transbronchial needle aspiration of lymph nodes in the radiologically and positron emission tomography-normal mediastinum in patients with lung cancer. Chest 2008; 133(4):887–91.

38. Veeramachaneni NK, Battafarano RJ, Meyers BF, et al. Risk factors for occult nodal metastasis in clinical T1N0 lung cancer: a negative impact on survival. Eur J Cardiothorac Surg 2008;33(3):466–9.

39. Birim O, Kappetein AP, Stijnen T, et al. Meta-analysis of positron emission tomographic and computed tomographic imaging in detecting mediastinal lymph node metastases in nonsmall cell lung cancer. Ann Thorac Surg 2005;79(1):375–82.

40. Bille A, Pelosi E, Skanjeti A, et al. Preoperative intrathoracic lymph node staging in patients with non-small-cell lung cancer: accuracy of integrated positron emission tomography and computed tomography. Eur J Cardiothorac Surg 2009;36(3): 440–5.

41. de Langen AJ, Raijmakers P, Riphagen I, et al. The size of mediastinal lymph nodes and its relation with metastatic involvement: a meta-analysis. Eur J Cardiothorac Surg 2006;29(1):26–9.

42. Miyasaka Y, Suzuki K, Takamochi K, et al. The maximum standardized uptake value of fluoro-deoxyglucose positron emission tomography of the primary tumour is a good predictor of pathological nodal involvement in clinical N0 non-small-cell lung cancer. Eur J Cardiothorac Surg 2013;44(1): 83–7.

43. Park HK, Jeon K, Koh WJ, et al. Occult nodal metastasis in patients with non-small cell lung cancer at clinical stage IA by PET/CT. Respirology 2010;15(8):1179–84.

44. Trister AD, Pryma DA, Xanthopoulos E, et al. Prognostic value of primary tumor FDG uptake for occult mediastinal lymph node involvement in clinically N2/N3 node-negative non-small cell lung cancer. Am J Clin Oncol 2014;37(2):135–9.

45. Maeda R, Isowa N, Onuma H, et al. The maximum standardized 18F-fluorodeoxyglucose uptake on positron emission tomography predicts lymph node metastasis and invasiveness in clinical stage IA non-small cell lung cancer. Interact Cardiovasc Thorac Surg 2009;9(1):79–82.

46. Lee PC, Port JL, Korst RJ, et al. Risk factors for occult mediastinal metastases in clinical stage I non-small cell lung cancer. Ann Thorac Surg 2007;84(1):177–81.

47. Hellwig D, Groschel A, Graeter TP, et al. Diagnostic performance and prognostic impact of FDG-PET in suspected recurrence of surgically treated non-small cell lung cancer. Eur J Nucl Med Mol Imaging 2006;33(1):13–21.

48. Bradley J, Thorstad WL, Mutic S, et al. Impact of FDG-PET on radiation therapy volume delineation in non-small-cell lung cancer. Int J Radiat Oncol Biol Phys 2004;59(1):78–86.

49. Perigaud C, Bridji B, Roussel JC, et al. Prospective preoperative mediastinal lymph node staging by integrated positron emission tomography-computerised tomography in patients with non-small-cell lung cancer. Eur J Cardiothorac Surg 2009;36(4):731–6.

50. Booth K, Hanna GG, McGonigle N, et al. The mediastinal staging accuracy of 18F-Fluorodeoxyglycose positron emission tomography/computed tomography in non-small cell lung cancer with variable time intervals to surgery. Ulster Med J 2013; 82(2):75–81.

51. Postmus PE, Brambilla E, Chansky K, et al. The IASLC Lung Cancer Staging Project: proposals

for revision of the M descriptors in the forthcoming (seventh) edition of the TNM classification of lung cancer. J Thorac Oncol 2007;2(8):686–93.

52. Rami-Porta R, Bolejack V, Goldstraw P. The new tumor, node, and metastasis staging system. Semin Respir Crit Care Med 2011;32(1):44–51.

53. Rivera MP, Mehta AC, Wahidi MM. Establishing the diagnosis of lung cancer: diagnosis and management of lung cancer, 3rd ed: American College of Chest Physicians evidence-based clinical practice guidelines. Chest 2013;143(Suppl 5):e142S–65S.

54. Erasmus JJ, McAdams HP, Rossi SE, et al. FDG PET of pleural effusions in patients with non-small cell lung cancer. AJR Am J Roentgenol 2000; 175(1):245–9.

55. Schaffler GJ, Wolf G, Schoellnast H, et al. Non-small cell lung cancer: evaluation of pleural abnormalities on CT scans with 18F FDG PET. Radiology 2004;231(3):858–65.

56. Detterbeck FC, Postmus PE, Tanoue LT. The stage classification of lung cancer: diagnosis and management of lung cancer, 3rd ed: American College of Chest Physicians evidence-based clinical practice guidelines. Chest 2013;143(Suppl 5):e191S–210S.

57. Gould MK, Donington J, Lynch WR, et al. Evaluation of individuals with pulmonary nodules: when is it lung cancer? Diagnosis and management of lung cancer, 3rd ed: American College of Chest Physicians evidence-based clinical practice guidelines. Chest 2013;143(Suppl 5):e93S–120S.

58. American Joint Committee on Cancer. AJCC Cancer staging manual. 7th edition. New York: Springer; 2009.

59. Viney RC, Boyer MJ, King MT, et al. Randomized controlled trial of the role of positron emission tomography in the management of stage I and II non-small-cell lung cancer. J Clin Oncol 2004; 22(12):2357–62.

60. MacManus MP, Hicks RJ, Matthews JP, et al. High rate of detection of unsuspected distant metastases by PET in apparent stage III non-small-cell lung cancer: implications for radical radiation therapy. Int J Radiat Oncol Biol Phys 2001;50(2):287–93.

61. Min JW, Um SW, Yim JJ, et al. The role of whole-body FDG PET/CT, Tc 99m MDP bone scintigraphy, and serum alkaline phosphatase in detecting bone metastasis in patients with newly diagnosed lung cancer. J Korean Med Sci 2009;24(2):275–80.

62. Qu X, Huang X, Yan W, et al. A meta-analysis of ^{18}FDG-PET-CT, ^{18}FDG-PET, MRI and bone scintigraphy for diagnosis of bone metastases in patients with lung cancer. Eur J Radiol 2012;81(5):1007–15.

63. Liu N, Ma L, Zhou W, et al. Bone metastasis in patients with non-small cell lung cancer: the diagnostic role of F-18 FDG PET/CT. Eur J Radiol 2010;74(1):231–5.

64. Ak I, Sivrikoz MC, Entok E, et al. Discordant findings in patients with non-small-cell lung cancer: absolutely normal bone scans versus disseminated bone metastases on positron-emission tomography/computed tomography. Eur J Cardiothorac Surg 2010;37(4):792–6.

65. Oliver TW Jr, Bernardino ME, Miller JI, et al. Isolated adrenal masses in nonsmall-cell bronchogenic carcinoma. Radiology 1984;153(1):217–8.

66. Sahdev A, Reznek RH. The indeterminate adrenal mass in patients with cancer. Cancer Imaging 2007;7(Spec No A):S100–9.

67. Mayo-Smith WW, Boland GW, Noto RB, et al. State-of-the-art adrenal imaging. Radiographics 2001; 21(4):995–1012.

68. Boland GW, Lee MJ, Gazelle GS, et al. Characterization of adrenal masses using unenhanced CT: an analysis of the CT literature. AJR Am J Roentgenol 1998;171:201–4.

69. Pena CS, Boland GW, Hahn PF, et al. Characterization of indeterminate (lipid-poor) adrenal masses: use of washout characteristics at contrast-enhanced CT. Radiology 2000;217(3):798–802.

70. Boland GW, Hahn PF, Pena C, et al. Adrenal masses: characterization with delayed contrast-enhanced CT. Radiology 1997;202(3):693–6.

71. Boland GW, Lee MJ. Magnetic resonance imaging of the adrenal gland. Crit Rev Diagn Imaging 1995; 36:115–74.

72. Outwater EK, Siegelman ES, Huang AB, et al. Adrenal masses: correlation between CT attenuation value and chemical shift ratio at MR imaging with in-phase and opposed-phase sequences. Radiology 1996;200(3):749–52.

73. Schwartz LH, Ginsberg MS, Burt ME, et al. MRI as an alternative to CT-guided biopsy of adrenal masses in patients with lung cancer. Ann Thorac Surg 1998;65(1):193–7.

74. Boland GW, Dwamena BA, Jagtiani Sangwaiya M, et al. Characterization of adrenal masses by using FDG PET: a systematic review and meta-analysis of diagnostic test performance. Radiology 2011; 259(1):117–26.

75. Hooper RG, Tenholder MF, Underwood GH, et al. Computed tomographic scanning of the brain in initial staging of bronchogenic carcinoma. Chest 1984;85(6):774–6.

76. Mintz BJ, Tuhrim S, Alexander S, et al. Intracranial metastases in the initial staging of bronchogenic carcinoma. Chest 1984;86(6):850–3.

77. Posther KE, McCall LM, Harpole DH Jr, et al. Yield of brain 18F-FDG PET in evaluating patients with potentially operable non-small cell lung cancer. J Nucl Med 2006;47(10):1607–11.

78. Ettinger DS, Akerley W, Bepler G, et al. Non-small cell lung cancer. J Natl Compr Canc Netw 2010; 8(7):740–801.

79. Earnest FT, Ryu JH, Miller GM, et al. Suspected non-small cell lung cancer: incidence of occult

brain and skeletal metastases and effectiveness of imaging for detection–pilot study. Radiology 1999; 211(1):137–45.

80. Yokoi K, Kamiya N, Matsuguma H, et al. Detection of brain metastasis in potentially operable non-small cell lung cancer. A comparison of CT and MRI. Chest 1999;115:714–9.

81. Robnett TJ, Machtay M, Stevenson JP, et al. Factors affecting the risk of brain metastases after definitive chemoradiation for locally advanced non-small-cell lung carcinoma. J Clin Oncol 2001; 19(5):1344–9.

82. Lardinois D, Weder W, Roudas M, et al. Etiology of solitary extrapulmonary positron emission tomography and computed tomography findings in patients with lung cancer. J Clin Oncol 2005; 23(28):6846–53.

83. De Leyn P, Moons J, Vansteenkiste J, et al. Survival after resection of synchronous bilateral lung cancer. Eur J Cardiothorac Surg 2008;34(6):1215–22.

84. Boiselle PM, Erasmus JJ, Ko JP, et al. Expert opinion: lung cancer staging. J Thorac Imaging 2011;26(2):85.

85. Finley DJ, Yoshizawa A, Travis W, et al. Predictors of outcomes after surgical treatment of synchronous primary lung cancers. J Thorac Oncol 2010; 5(2):197–205.

86. Martini N, Melamed MR. Multiple primary lung cancers. J Thorac Cardiovasc Surg 1975;70(4):606–12.

87. Okada M, Tsubota N, Yoshimura M, et al. How should interlobar pleural invasion be classified? Prognosis of resected T3 non-small cell lung cancer. Ann Thorac Surg 1999;68(6):2049–52.

88. Miura H, Taira O, Uchida O, et al. Invasion beyond interlobar pleura in non-small cell lung cancer. Chest 1998;114(5):1301–4.

89. Joshi V, McShane J, Page R, et al. Clinical upstaging of non-small cell lung cancer that extends across the fissure: implications for non-small cell lung cancer staging. Ann Thorac Surg 2011; 91(2):350–3.

90. Haam SJ, Park IK, Paik HC, et al. T-stage of non-small cell lung cancer directly invading an adjacent lobe. Eur J Cardiothorac Surg 2012;42(5):807–10 [discussion: 810–1].

91. Borczuk AC, Qian F, Kazeros A, et al. Invasive size is an independent predictor of survival in pulmonary adenocarcinoma. Am J Surg Pathol 2009; 33(3):462–9.

92. Sakao Y, Miyamoto H, Sakuraba M, et al. Prognostic significance of a histologic subtype in small adenocarcinoma of the lung: the impact of non-bronchioloalveolar carcinoma components. Ann Thorac Surg 2007;83(1):209–14.

93. Ravanelli M, Farina D, Morassi M, et al. Texture analysis of advanced non-small cell lung cancer (NSCLC) on contrast-enhanced computed tomography: prediction of the response to the first-line chemotherapy. Eur Radiol 2013;23(12):3450–5.

94. Davnall F, Yip CS, Ljungqvist G, et al. Assessment of tumor heterogeneity: an emerging imaging tool for clinical practice? Insights Imaging 2012;3(6):573–89.

95. Lambin P, Rios-Velazquez E, Leijenaar R, et al. Radiomics: extracting more information from medical images using advanced feature analysis. Eur J Cancer 2012;48(4):441–6.

96. Ganeshan B, Abaleke S, Young RC, et al. Texture analysis of non-small cell lung cancer on unenhanced computed tomography: initial evidence for a relationship with tumour glucose metabolism and stage. Cancer Imaging 2010;10:137–43.

97. Balagurunathan Y, Kumar V, Gu Y, et al. Test-retest reproducibility analysis of lung CT image features. J Digit Imaging 2014;27(6):805–23.

98. Kumar V, Gu Y, Basu S, et al. Radiomics: the process and the challenges. Magn Reson Imaging 2012;30(9):1234–48.

99. Bayanati H, E Thornhill R, Souza CA, et al. Quantitative CT texture and shape analysis: can it differentiate benign and malignant mediastinal lymph nodes in patients with primary lung cancer? Eur Radiol 2014;25(2):480–7.

100. Sakai S, Murayama S, Murakami J, et al. Bronchogenic carcinoma invasion of the chest wall: evaluation with dynamic cine MRI during breathing. J Comput Assist Tomogr 1997;21:595–600.

101. Ohno Y, Koyama H, Nogami M, et al. STIR turbo SE MR imaging vs coregistered FDG-PET/CT: quantitative and qualitative assessment of N-stage in non-small-cell lung cancer patients. J Magn Reson Imaging 2007;26(4):1071–80.

102. Ohno Y, Hatabu H, Takenaka D, et al. Metastases in mediastinal and hilar lymph nodes in patients with non-small cell lung cancer: quantitative and qualitative assessment with STIR turbo spin-echo MR imaging. Radiology 2004;231(3):872–9.

103. Yi CA, Shin KM, Lee KS, et al. Non-small cell lung cancer staging: efficacy comparison of integrated PET/CT versus 3.0-T whole-body MR imaging. Radiology 2008;248(2):632–42.

104. Nomori H, Mori T, Ikeda K, et al. Diffusion-weighted magnetic resonance imaging can be used in place of positron emission tomography for N staging of non-small cell lung cancer with fewer false-positive results. J Thorac Cardiovasc Surg 2008; 135(4):816–22.

105. Ohno Y, Koyama H, Onishi Y, et al. Non-small cell lung cancer: whole-body MR examination for M-stage assessment–utility for whole-body diffusion-weighted imaging compared with integrated FDG PET/CT. Radiology 2008;248(2):643–54.

106. Cogen A, Dockx Y, Cheung KJ, et al. TNM-classification for lung cancer: from the 7th to the 8th edition. Acta Chir Belg 2011;111(6):389–92.

Imaging Infection

Loren Ketai, MD[a],*, Kirk Jordan, MD[b], Katrina H. Busby, MD[c]

KEYWORDS

- Thoracic imaging • Infection • Chest radiography • Computed tomography

KEY POINTS

- Among immunocompetent hosts, the combination of clinical and radiographic findings performs better than radiographic findings alone in the detection and follow-up of pneumonia.
- Computed tomography (CT) findings are most useful in evaluating pleural disease and pulmonary necrosis. Recognition of CT patterns of micronodules can help differentiate infection from noninfectious acute disease.
- In immunocompromised hosts who do not have AIDS, identification of radiologic patterns of invasive fungal disease are key to its early diagnosis and treatment.
- Despite the declining incidence of *Pneumocystis jiroveci* pneumonia (PJP) among patients with human immunodeficiency virus (HIV), recognition of its CT pattern remains important, because PJP may be the presenting illness in patients previously undiagnosed with AIDS. The possibility of immune reconstitution inflammatory syndrome should be considered when new thoracic radiologic findings develop in a patient initiating treatment of HIV.

NORMAL HOSTS

Chest radiography (CR) is sufficiently accurate to diagnose community-acquired pneumonia (CAP) in most immunocompetent patients. Interobserver agreement of 80% to 90% has been reported, but accuracy is diminished in patients with chronic obstructive pulmonary disease (COPD), atelectasis, or congestive heart failure.[1–3] Patients with these confounding conditions who receive a clinical diagnosis of lower respiratory tract infection may have similar rates of septicemia and mortality regardless of whether CR confirms the diagnosis of pneumonia.[2]

In most cases, CR performed at the time of pneumonia diagnosis has clinical utility. For instance, the number of lobes involved and the presence of pleural disease are predictors of disease severity and need for intensive care unit (ICU) admission.[4] The benefit of follow-up CR is less certain. Speed of radiographic improvement is related to patient age as well as initial pneumonia extent and is often outpaced by clinical improvement (**Fig. 1**). After a week of treatment, more than 50% of patients hospitalized with CAP experience resolution of symptoms, whereas only 25% show radiologic resolution (see **Fig. 1**).[5] CR performed within 4 weeks of initiating treatment rarely detects progression of infection in patients clinically responding to therapy.[6]

The accuracy of CR for the detection of hospital-acquired pneumonia is less than that for CAP, and lower still for ventilator-acquired pneumonia (VAP) because of confounding opacities caused by atelectasis and pleural effusions. Among patients receiving mechanical ventilation, approximately 60% to 70% of focal parenchymal opacities that contain air bronchograms represent VAP. However, air bronchograms are not helpful in identifying pneumonia in the setting of diffuse

Disclosures: None.
[a] Department of Radiology, University of New Mexico Health Science Center, MSC10 5530, 1 University of New Mexico, Albuquerque, NM 87131-0001, USA; [b] Department of Radiology, University of Texas Southwestern, 5323 Harry Hines Boulevard, Dallas, TX 75390-8548, USA; [c] Division of Pulmonary, Critical Care and Sleep Medicine, University of New Mexico Health Science Center, MSC10 5550, 1 University of New Mexico, Albuquerque, NM 87131-0001, USA
* Corresponding author.
E-mail address: lketai@salud.unm.edu

Clin Chest Med 36 (2015) 197–217
http://dx.doi.org/10.1016/j.ccm.2015.02.005
0272-5231/15/$ – see front matter © 2015 Elsevier Inc. All rights reserved.

chestmed.theclinics.com

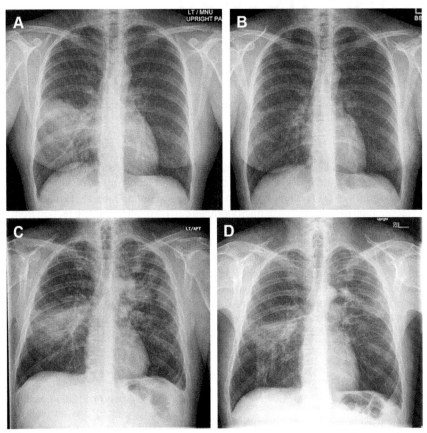

Fig. 1. Resolution of CAP. (*A, B*) Two posteroanterior (PA) radiographs 2 weeks apart show nearly complete radiographic resolution of CAP in a 27-year-old woman without comorbidities. (*C, D*) Two PA radiographs 2 months apart show minimal improvement in legionella pneumonia. Legionella characteristically shows slow radiographic resolution, in part because of its predilection for hosts with comorbidities.

parenchymal opacities seen with acute respiratory distress syndrome.[7,8] Given these limitations, CR was not chosen as a component of newly proposed criteria for the diagnosis of VAP.[9]

Computed tomography (CT) also has its limitations in the ICU because it cannot reliably differentiate diffuse alveolar damage caused by systemic disease from that caused by diffuse pneumonia.[10] Given its ability to resolve overlying structures and its superior contrast resolution compared with radiography, it can be helpful in differentiating atelectasis or cardiogenic edema from pneumonia and identifying radiographically occult infectious bronchiolitis (discussed later).

Complications of Pneumonia

After pneumonia is diagnosed, additional imaging is often performed if there are clinical or radiographic findings that suggest the presence of pleural disease, lung necrosis, or lymphadenopathy. Presence of parapneumonic effusion

is clinically relevant and is the sole imaging finding included in the Pneumonia Severity Index.[11] In most cases, cross-sectional imaging is not necessary if CR shows only very small effusions. An occasional patient can present with a small effusion that rapidly expands over days despite minimal apparent parenchymal infection. This scenario has been termed explosive pleuritis, and is associated with *Streptococcus pyogenes* infections (**Fig. 2**).[12]

Ultrasonography is widely used to assess effusions for pleural drainage, often at the bedside, and may show septations within pleural fluid collections that are not visible on contrast-enhanced CT scanning.[13] These septations are often fibrinous strands rather than dense adhesions between visceral and parietal pleura and are not reliable in predicting efficacy of catheter drainage.[14]

CT scanning is superior to ultrasonography in providing a global assessment of multiloculated pleural fluid, including paramediastinal collections

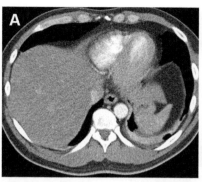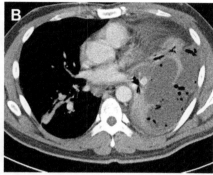

Fig. 2. Explosive pleuritis. (*A*) CT shows a small effusion and adjacent atelectasis in a patient with fever and pleuritic pain. (*B*) CT performed 3 days later shows multiloculated empyema.

that do not have good ultrasonographic windows. On CT scans performed with intravenous contrast (optimally using a delay of 45–60 seconds) the pleura enhances in most noninfected parapneumonic effusions and in 85% to 100% of empyemas (**Fig. 3**).[13,15] Absence of parietal pleural enhancement on CT argues strongly against the presence of an empyema.

CR can suggest the presence of lung necrosis by depicting focal lucency within an area of consolidation. Lucencies scattered within lobar consolidation early in the course of pneumonia often represent underlying centrilobular emphysema rather than cavitation but development later in the disease course favors developing lung necrosis (**Fig. 4**). CT imaging in this instance may show geographic areas of nonenhancing lung parenchyma, some of which progress to discrete abscesses. CT can also be used to differentiate large abscesses from empyemas (**Table 1**).

Other manifestations of lung necrosis are less common. Occasionally focal alveolar or bronchiolar necrosis allows air to dissect into the pulmonary parenchyma and create pneumatoceles; thin-walled air cysts that may give rise to pneumothoraces. In rare cases, necrosis may extend into the pulmonary vasculature, producing in situ thrombosis of a pulmonary artery or destruction of the arterial wall and leading to formation of a pseudoaneurysm. Both complications often require surgical resection but some cases of pulmonary artery pseudoaneurysm may be amenable to transcatheter embolization (**Fig. 5**).[16]

In addition to pleural effusion and lung parenchymal necrosis, CR of pneumonia occasionally reveals hilar or mediastinal lymphadenopathy. Lymphadenopathy that is apparent on CR suggests an underlying neoplasm, sarcoidosis, or a short list of infectious agents that include primary tuberculosis, endemic fungal infections, tularemia, and anthrax. However, the detection of enlarged lymph nodes on chest CT is nonspecific and can be found in about half of patients with either bacteremic pneumococcal pneumonia or an empyema.[17]

Differentiation of Pneumonia from Noninfectious Diseases

Among normal hosts with suspected pneumonia the radiologic pattern helps determine which noninfectious diseases might also be considered

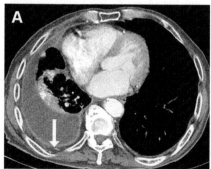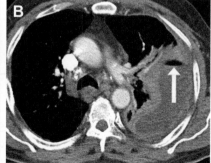

Fig. 3. Empyemas. (*A*) CT shows right-sided empyema with thickened high-attenuation extrapleural fat (*arrow*), which is a slightly more specific finding for empyema than contrast enhancement alone. (*B*) CT shows focal gas (*arrow*) within uninstrumented pleural fluid in the left hemithorax, which is diagnostic of empyema.

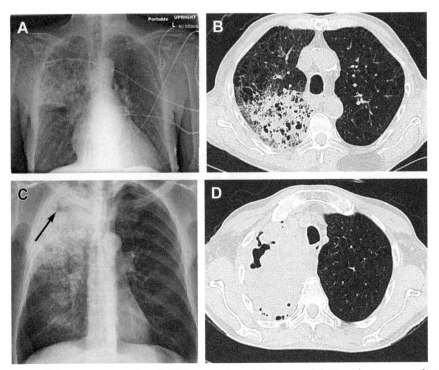

Fig. 4. Lobar consolidation. (*A, B*) CR and CT images show lobar consolidation that appears heterogenous because of underlying centrilobular emphysema. (*C, D*) CR and CT images in patient with lobar pneumonia show larger, irregular lucencies (*arrow*) caused by necrosis.

in the differential diagnosis. A linear interstitial pattern is dominated by Kerley lines, subpleural edema (thickening the fissures), and pleural effusions. The CT equivalent of this pattern is smooth thickening of the interlobular septa. These septa are 1 to 2 cm in length and represent the divisions between secondary lobules, which are the smallest unit of lung surrounded by connective tissue (**Fig. 6**). Infectious agents rarely cause this pattern, with the notable exception of the North American hantaviruses and occasionally rickettsial diseases.[18]

Reticulonodular or nodular patterns are the most common interstitial appearance of pneumonia on CR. In the setting of lower respiratory tract infections, this appearance is often caused by bronchial wall thickening and small nodules. These inflammatory nodules are centered on the bronchioles in the center of the secondary lobule. CT shows that these bronchioles do not extend to the pleura and accordingly nodules that form around them (centrilobular nodules) spare the pleural surfaces. Nodules that are ground glass in attenuation (not sufficiently opaque to obscure pulmonary vasculature) usually range from 1 to 5 mm in diameter. When they are the predominant finding, they more commonly represent noninfectious than infectious diseases (**Table 2**).[19]

If bronchioles connecting centrilobular nodules are thickened or filled with secretions they may also become visible on CT. The resulting pattern of centrilobular nodules connected by branching

Table 1
CT findings of abscess versus empyema

Structure	Abscess	Empyema
Wall inner contour	Irregular	Smooth
Wall thickness	Varying thickness	Uniform thickness
Shape	Round	Lenticular
Adjacent bronchi/vessels	Truncated	Deviated

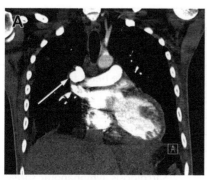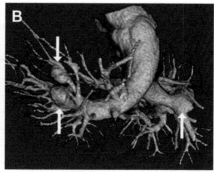

Fig. 5. Pseudoaneurysms caused by staphylococcal sepsis. (*A*) Coronal CT image shows a focal right upper lobe pseudoaneurysm (*arrow*). (*B*) Multiple additional pseudoaneurysms (*arrows*) seen on volume-rendered imaging.

structures is termed a tree-in-bud (TIB) pattern. This subset of centrilobular nodules has strong association with infection or, in acutely ill patients, aspiration (**Figs. 7** and **8**).[20] Centrilobular nodules with soft tissue attenuation (sufficiently opaque to obscure vasculature) can accompany TIB opacities. These nodules vary in size but are slightly larger (4–10 mm) than ground-glass nodules and, when seen in the setting of infection, probably represent filling of centrally located acini.

By distinguishing centrilobular nodules from nodules with either a random or perilymphatic distribution, CT can narrow the differential diagnosis. Randomly distributed nodules are often caused by blood-borne dissemination of disease (eg, miliary tuberculosis or metastases); pathogenic material reaching small capillaries in all portions of the secondary lobules. Unlike centrilobular nodules, random nodules can touch pleural surfaces, including the fissures. A third micronodular pattern, the perilymphatic distribution, in which nodules show a predilection for interlobular septa and pleural surfaces, is almost always noninfectious (**Fig. 9**).

Rather than causing reticulonodular opacities, most pneumonias fill airspaces, creating a bronchopneumonia or lobar pneumonia pattern. On CR, bronchopneumonias appear as patchy opacities that may be accompanied by bronchial wall thickening. CT often shows bronchiolitis affecting the center of the pulmonary lobule accompanied by other portions of the lung parenchyma in which inflammation has progressed to involve the entire lobule. The resulting opacities are sharply

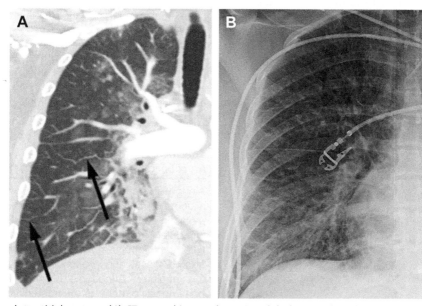

Fig. 6. Linear interstitial pattern. (*A*) CT coronal image shows interlobular septal thickening (*arrows*). (*B*) Magnified image from PA chest radiograph shows the corresponding Kerley B lines in the lung periphery.

Table 2
Radiologic patterns shared by infectious and noninfectious disease

CT Pattern	Infection	Noninfectious Disease
Linear interstitial	Rare	Congestive heart failure, drug reaction
Nodules		
Centrilobular GG	Common	HP, respiratory bronchiolitis
Centrilobular ST	Common	Adenocarcinoma,[a] PLCH[a]
TIB	Common	Aspiration
Random	Uncommon	Metastases
Perilymphatic	Rare	Sarcoidosis, lymphangitic spread of cancer

Abbreviations: GG, ground glass; HP, hypersensitivity pneumonitis; PLCH, pulmonary Langerhans cell histiocytosis; ST, soft tissue; TIB, tree in bud.
  [a] If chronic.

marginated by interlobular septa (**Fig. 10**). Opacities that are sufficiently transparent to allow visualization of underlying vasculature are termed ground-glass opacity (GGO), and those dense enough to obscure vessels are termed consolidation. In addition to bronchopneumonia, a lobular pattern of GGO or consolidation may be caused by drug toxicity, chronic infiltrative lung diseases, pulmonary hemorrhage, or pulmonary edema.[21] The presence of a TIB configuration combined with lobular opacities on CT favors pneumonia rather than these other diagnoses.

Lobar pneumonias characteristically begin in the lung periphery and then spread centrally. Consolidation is confluent rather than patchy and often sufficient to form air bronchograms. In an acutely ill patient, opacification of an entire lobe without volume loss almost always indicates pneumonia rather than atelectasis. When less than a lobe is affected, volume loss may be subtle on chest CR, making differentiation between pneumonia and atelectasis more difficult. CT more clearly shows the displacement and crowding of fissures and bronchi seen with atelectasis. Contrast enhancement pattern may also help differentiate atelectasis from pneumonia. On contrast-enhanced CT, areas of passive atelectasis enhance markedly.[22] Some pneumonias and areas of obstructive atelectasis enhance to a lesser degree, increasing the contrast between pulmonary vasculature and surrounding lung parenchyma (**Fig. 11**).[23] Low attenuation of lung parenchyma in conjunction with air-filled bronchi favors pneumonia. The presence of airless bronchi suggests obstructive atelectasis.

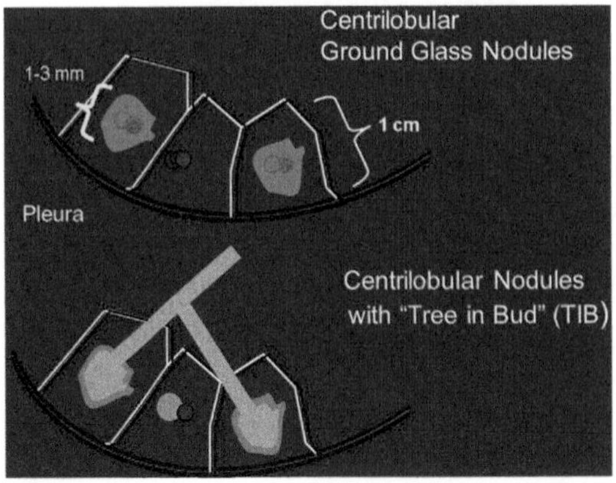

Both pulmonary infarcts and early lobar/segmental pneumonia arise in the periphery of the lung and may appear similar on CR. On CT, an infarct may appear as triangular opacity, with its base against the pleura and its truncated apex pointing centrally, but these findings are nonspecific (**Fig. 12**). Absence of air bronchograms and the presence of central ground glass are more specific signs of pulmonary infarct.[24]

Specific Diagnosis: Mycoplasma, Viruses, and Mycobacterium

Along with pneumococcus, *Mycoplasma* remains a common cause of CAP.[25] Mycoplasma pneumonia in adults commonly presents with a reticulonodular radiographic pattern that correlates with centrilobular nodules, peribronchovascular ground glass, and bronchial wall thickening on CT imaging.[26] Although a bronchiolitis bronchopneumonia pattern is characteristic of mycoplasma infection in adults, similar findings may be caused by *Chlamydia* and bacterial infections

Fig. 7. Centrilobular ground-glass nodules and TIB nodules.

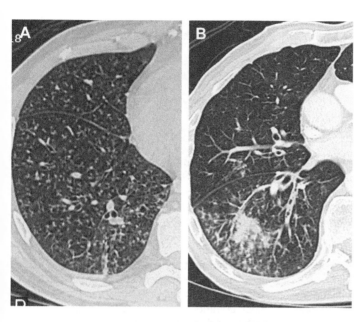

Fig. 8. CT of TIB pattern from 2 different causes. (*A*) CT shows diffuse TIB pattern caused by mycoplasma infection. (*B*) CT shows TIB pattern in the dependent lung in a patient with acute aspiration. Nodules in both images largely spare the subpleural lung.

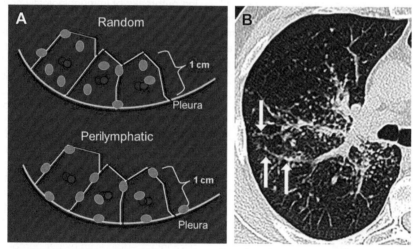

Fig. 9. Perilymphatic and random nodules. (*A*) Random and perilymphatic nodules. (*B*) CT of patient with sarcoidosis showing perilymphatic nodules (*arrows*) along the bronchovascular bundles and interlobular septa.

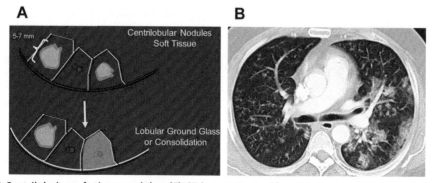

Fig. 10. (*A*) Centrilobular soft tissue nodules. (*B*) CT in a patient with respiratory syncytial virus infection shows lobules with varying degrees of opacification in the right lung. TIB pattern is visible on the right.

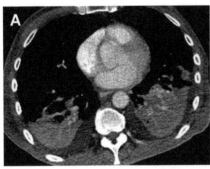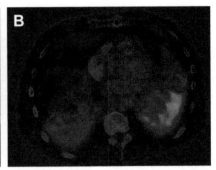

Fig. 11. Pneumonia versus atelectasis. (*A*) Contrast-enhanced CT showing low attenuation in the left lower lobe consolidation relative to that in the right lower lobe. (*B*) PET/CT confirms asymmetrically increased metabolic activity on the left, consistent with pneumonia.

(particularly *Haemophilus influenzae*) and by viruses.[27]

Recent diagnostic tests, particularly polymerase chain reactions, have allowed more frequent identification of viral pathogens, which are probably present in 15% to 35% of lower respiratory tract infections among immunocompetent adults.[28,29] These viruses may be the sole causative organism but frequently occur as coinfections. On CT images, many viruses are as likely to appear as

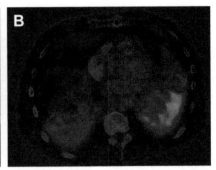

Fig. 12. Pulmonary infarct. CT shows a wedge-shaped opacity with ground-glass center and surrounding consolidation consistent with a pulmonary infarct. Central feeding vessel is a confirmatory sign, but is an uncommon finding.

pneumonia as they are to appear as bronchiolitis/bronchitis. However, some viruses, such as respiratory syncytial virus (RSV) and parainfluenza, most commonly present with an airway centric pattern of disease.[29] Adenoviruses are more likely to cause confluent consolidation, particularly during outbreaks of immunologically novel strains.[30]

Compared with its diagnostic role in bacterial and viral infections, CT abnormalities can be more specific for diagnosis of mycobacterial disease, and can serve as an adjunct to interferon gamma release assays.[31] Upper lobe predominance of centrilobular nodules is a common early manifestation of tuberculosis when presenting as what was traditionally termed reactivation tuberculosis (**Fig. 13**). Centrilobular nodules, lobular opacities, and thick-walled cavities suggest active infection, whereas parenchymal bands, bronchiectasis, and calcified adenopathy are typical of inactive disease. Cavitation and macronodules, particularly those created by aggregation of micronodules (galaxy sign), are associated with production of smear-positive sputum.[32,33]

Nontuberculous mycobacteria (NTM) infections can appear as a classic form that mimics reactivation tuberculosis, in a bronchiectatic form, or as hypersensitivity pneumonitis.[34] Centrilobular nodules are common to all 3 forms but the bronchiectatic form has the most distinctive radiologic pattern. It manifests as centrilobular nodules with or without TIB configuration accompanied by cylindrical bronchiectasis and localized areas of volume loss. Bronchiectasis characteristically occurs in the middle and lingular lobes, but positive cultures are most commonly obtained in patients with involvement of all lobes (**Fig. 14**).[35]

NON-AIDS IMMUNOCOMPROMISED HOSTS

Imaging of infections in immunocompromised hosts relies heavily on CT scanning to detect and

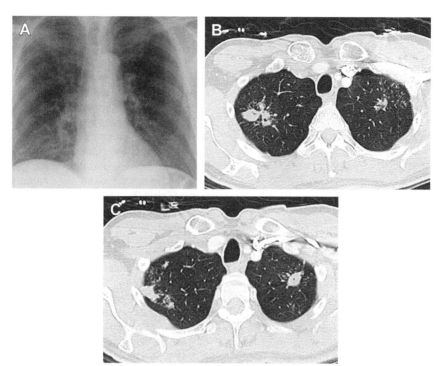

Fig. 13. Early tuberculosis. (*A*) Subtle upper lung nodules on present on CR. (*B, C*) CT shows centrilobular nodules accompanied by macronodules (5–10 mm in diameter) containing small areas of cavitation; a finding uncommon in mycoplasma and viral infection.

characterize lower respiratory tract infections. Among neutropenic patients with fever for more than 48 to 72 hours, up to half of those with a normal chest radiograph can be found to have pneumonia on CT scanning.[36] Earlier diagnosis is relevant because early identification of opportunistic infections, specifically invasive fungi, can improve survival.[37]

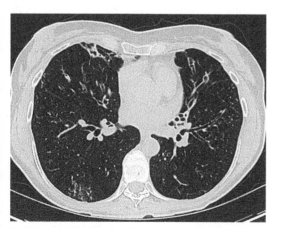

Fig. 14. CT of patient with nonclassic NTM infection. Bronchiectasis is most evident in the right middle lobe and lingua. Centrilobular nodules are scattered throughout all lobes.

Fungal Infections

Invasive mold pulmonary infections are responsible for more than 10% of pulmonary infections after hematopoietic stem cell transplantation (HCT), and are most likely to be seen in the first month of transplant, when profound prolonged neutropenia is present. These infections are less common among solid organ transplant recipients and are usually seen within the first 6 months after transplantation, when therapeutic immunosuppression is highest (**Fig. 15**).[38]

Aspergillus is the most common invasive fungal infection and, on CT, often presents with findings related to angioinvasion. More than 90% of these patients show 1 or more nodules on CT, which are usually larger than 1 cm in diameter. Masslike consolidation, sometimes peripheral and wedge shaped, can also occur (**Fig. 16**).

Nodules that show the halo sign are seen in more than half of the patients with invasive aspergillosis, and are much more common among patients with HCT and hematologic malignancy than among patients with solid organ transplants.[39] The sign describes a solid nodule surrounded by peripheral GGO. GGO in this setting is thought to represent hemorrhage caused by thrombosis from the fungal angioinvasion.

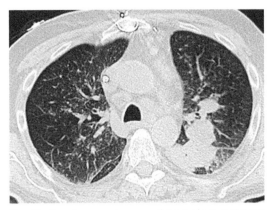

Fig. 15. *Cryptococcus* in a renal transplant recipient. CT shows multiple masses in the left lung and scattered micronodules. Cerebrospinal fluid infection was also present.

Prevalence of the halo sign is similar in aspergillus, Zygomycetes, and candida infections (**Fig. 17**). The reversed halo sign (focal area of GGO surrounded by a rim of consolidation) is much less common and has been associated with Zygomycetes infection.[40] Both halo sign and the reversed halo sign appear early in the course of infection (**Fig. 18**). Because results of cultures from biopsies for suspected fungal pneumonia may yield a diagnosis in less than 50% of cases,[41] characteristic CT patterns (sometimes combined with serum or bronchoalveolar lavage markers such as galactomannan) can be used as the basis for empiric antifungal therapy.[42,43]

Later in the course of infection, when neutropenia is resolving, necrotic material is digested, causing cavitation that can be eccentric, giving rise to the crescent sign. The crescent sign usually occurs 2 to 3 weeks after initiation of treatment and usually indicates a good prognosis. Although the halo and crescent signs suggest invasive fungal disease, they can also be seen in bacterial infections (eg, *Pseudomonas aeruginosa*) and in noninfectious diseases in immunocompetent hosts (**Table 3**).

Infections with other fungi may also occur in immunocompromised patients. Mucormycosis (zygomycosis) appears similar to aspergillosis on imaging, but is more likely to directly cross fissures or invade the chest wall and pulmonary arteries (**Fig. 19**).[44] Patients with diabetes are at higher risk of mucormycosis pneumonia, which often coexists with sinus infection. Fusarium rarely causes a halo sign, whereas candida pneumonia closely mimics aspergillus infections, except for a greater likelihood to cause randomly distributed nodules.[45]

Infections with the fungus *Pneumocystis jiroveci* in immunocompromised patients without AIDS have become uncommon since the routine administration of trimethoprim/sulfamethoxazole (TMP/SMX) prophylaxis. The typical CT features of *P jiroveci* pneumonia (PJP) include upper lobe, perihilar and scattered GGO, and septal thickening interspersed with normal lung parenchyma. Parenchymal cysts of various sizes may also be present, but are less common than in PJP infections among patients with AIDS (discussed later). Progression to consolidation may be more common in patients who do not have AIDS because of more vigorous immune response.[46] The mosaic (patchwork) pattern of GGO can also be seen with cytomegalovirus (CMV) pneumonia; however, PJP is more likely to have an upper lobe predominance and a mosaic pattern with sharp demarcation, and is less likely to cause micronodules.[47]

Viral Infections

Viral pneumonias are most common among those non–AIDS immunocompromised patients who have received HCTs. CMV is the most common, occurring in up to 35% of allogeneic HCT recipients. CMV pneumonia also occurs in up to 55% of lung transplants but is much less common in other solid organ transplants. Incidence among patients with both HCT and lung transplants is markedly diminished by prophylaxis. When CMV pneumonia does occur, CT usually shows it to be

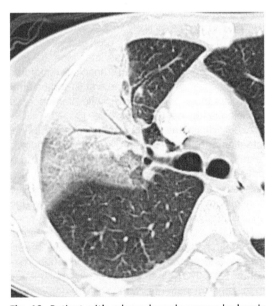

Fig. 16. Patient with relapsed myelogenous leukemia after HCT. CT shows a wedge-shaped consolidation and adjacent GGO caused by invasive aspergillus infection.

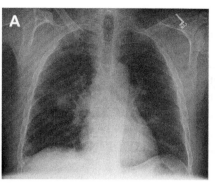
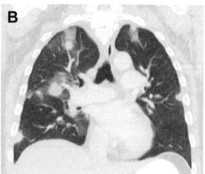

Fig. 17. Angioinvasive aspergillus. (*A*) CR in a patient with angioinvasive aspergillus reveals multiple nodules. (*B*) CT scan in the same patient shows that most of the nodules are surrounded by GGO, consistent with the halo sign.

bilateral, and most patients have a combination of GGO and/or consolidation (90%) and pulmonary nodules (50%).[48] Unlike fungal infections, in CMV pneumonia, the nodules are all smaller than 1 cm (**Fig. 20**). Radiologic findings cannot readily distinguish CMV from other respiratory viruses.[49]

Bacterial and Mycobacterial Infections

Nosocomial bacterial pneumonias are most common within the first month after solid organ transplantation, in the first 100 days of HCT, and

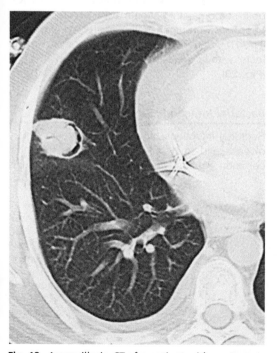

Fig. 18. Aspergillosis. CT of a patient with acute myelogenous leukemia and neutropenia 2 weeks after treatment initiation shows an eccentric cavity in the middle lobe nodule consistent with the crescent sign. (*Courtesy of* E. Marom, MD, MD Anderson, Houston, TX.)

in patients undergoing chemotherapy when neutrophil counts are less than 500/mL. These pneumonias most commonly appear as bronchopneumonias. Some bacterial pathogens, such as *Pseudomonas* or *Staphylococcus aureus*, can present with nodular or masslike lesions. Nocardia infection can cause multiple nodules or masses in patients with depressed cellular immunity following solid organ transplants (or in patients with AIDS; discussed later).

Although the risk of reactivation tuberculosis in transplant recipients is much higher than in the general population, in developed countries, tuberculosis is still uncommon after solid organ transplant or HCT. Infection tends to occur several months after organ transplant and is associated with chronic graft-versus-host disease in HCT recipients.[50] Most literature on immunocompromised patients with NTM infections has addressed those patients with human immunodeficiency virus (HIV)–AIDS (discussed later). Among non-AIDS immunocompromised patients, both classic and bronchiectatic patterns occur, but may show more numerous cavities and larger opacities (>2 cm) than are seen in immunocompetent patients.[51]

PATIENTS WITH AIDS
Detection of Infections in AIDS

CR is useful in assessing patients infected with HIV and with suspected bacterial pneumonia. If acute fever and productive cough are caused by bacterial pneumonia, CR is commonly abnormal.[52–54] In contrast, bacterial pneumonia is rarely the cause of an abnormal chest radiograph in the absence of symptoms, and in asymptomatic patients an alternative diagnosis, such as tuberculosis, should be considered.[52]

The utility of CR is more limited in the setting of suspected PJP or tuberculosis. CR may be normal

Table 3
Causes of radiologic signs in immunosuppressed and normal hosts

Sign	Immunosuppressed Hosts	Normal Hosts
Halo sign	Early invasive fungal infection	Hemorrhagic metastases
Reversed halo sign	Early invasive fungal infection	Pulmonary infarct, cryptogenic organizing pneumonia
Crescent sign	Resolving invasive fungi	Aspergilloma (colonization of preexisting cavity)

or near normal at initial presentation in 2% to 39 % of patients with PJP and in 10% to 20% of patients with tuberculosis, most commonly those with advanced AIDS (**Fig. 21**).[55–57] CT imaging is useful in these settings and in evaluating patients with AIDS suspected of having bacterial pyogenic airway infections (discussed later). CT imaging has also become important in detecting noninfectious diseases occurring with increased incidence in this population, including HIV-associated cardiomyopathy, ischemic cardiomyopathy, pulmonary hypertension, lung cancer, and COPD.[58,59]

Radiologic Patterns

In patients with AIDS, the combination of focal consolidation and history of fever less than 1 week is 94% specific for bacterial pneumonia. Sensitivity is much less; about half of bacterial pneumonias have a radiographic pattern other than focal consolidation.[60] Twenty percent of bacterial pneumonias, most commonly *H influenzae* infections, cause bilateral alveolar and interstitial opacities that mimic PJP.[61]

Centrilobular micronodules seen on CT in individuals infected with HIV, often with a TIB pattern, commonly represent bacterial infection.

Mycobacteria, viruses, and fungal infections can have a similar appearance.[62] Lymphocytic interstitial pneumonia (LIP) is uncommon in adults but can occasionally cause GGO or TIB centrilobular nodules.[63] Unlike many infections, LIP does not show a predilection for patients with diminished CD4 lymphocyte counts and runs an indolent waxing and waning course (**Fig. 22**).[64]

As in immunocompetent hosts, miliary nodules in patients with HIV infection usually represent hematogenous spread of infection or malignancy. In addition to tuberculosis and NTM, disseminated endemic fungal infections can cause this pattern, usually in patients with CD4 counts less than 100 cells/mm^3. Perilymphatic nodules usually indicate noninfectious disease such as Kaposi sarcoma. In patients with HIV undergoing treatment with highly active antiretroviral therapy (HAART), sarcoidosis can also occur and manifests with a perilymphatic pattern on imaging (**Fig. 23**).

Bacterial Infection

Bacterial infections, specifically pyogenic airway disease and bacterial pneumonia, are the most common pulmonary infections in individuals

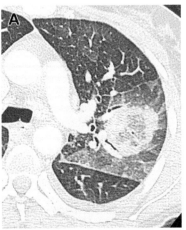 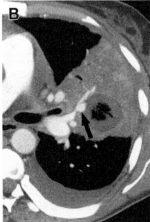

Fig. 19. Mucormycosis. (*A*) Initial CT shows a ring of consolidation surrounding a central area of GGO consistent with the reversed halo sign in a patient with neutropenic fever following induction chemotherapy for acute myelogenous leukemia. (*B*) Follow-up CT shows interval development of a pseudoaneurysm (*arrow*). (*Courtesy of* E. Marom, MD, MD Anderson, Houston, TX.)

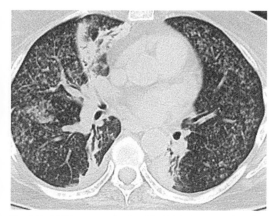

Fig. 20. CT from a patient with CMV pneumonia after HCT. Diffuse micronodules are present bilaterally, most of which spare the pleural surfaces, which is atypical for PJP.

infected with HIV.[65,66] Even mildly immunocompromised patients with CD4 counts lower than 500 cell/mm^3 are at an increased risk for developing bacterial CAP. *Streptococcus pneumoniae* and *H influenzae* are the most common pathogens. *H influenzae* infection occurs less frequently overall and is observed more commonly in patients with CD4 counts less than 100 cells/mm^3.[61]

Radiographic findings of bacterial pneumonias in patients with AIDS are similar to those in normal hosts, but progress more rapidly, and are more commonly complicated by cavity and abscess formation and by bacteremia (**Fig. 24**).[65] Bacterial pneumonia is the most common cause of cavitary lung disease, often caused by *P aeruginosa* or *Staphylococcus*. Occasionally, cavitary disease can be caused by less common pathogens such *Nocardia*, or in severely immunocompromised patients with AIDS by *Rhodococcus equi*.[67,68]

Recurrent bronchitis and bronchiolitis is common in patients with AIDS and manifests on CR as bronchial wall thickening and reticulonodular opacities that can mimic the perihilar opacities of PJP. CT findings include bronchial dilatation and wall thickening as well as nodules with TIB pattern (**Fig. 25**).

Pneumocystis jiroveci Pneumonia

PJP has become much less common among patients infected with HIV after widespread adoption of prophylactic use of TMP/SMX and HAART.[45,55] Despite its decline in frequency, PJP remains the most common cause of life-threatening infection in patients with AIDS and is the most common presenting illness in patients previously undiagnosed with AIDS. In 85% to 90% of patients it occurs at CD4 counts less than 200 cells/mm^3.

The classic CR pattern of PJP is a bilateral perihilar or diffuse symmetric interstitial opacity, which may have a granular, reticular, or ground-glass appearance (**Fig. 26**). As mentioned earlier, on CT scans PJP often appears as bilateral patchy or geographic GGOs with a central perihilar predominance. GGOs are sometimes interleaved by smooth interlobular septal thickening. CMV infection can have a similar appearance, but occurs in patients with more severe immunosuppression (CD4 counts <100 cells/mm^3) and more commonly causes retinitis or enteritis rather than pneumonia. Cystic lung disease occurs in 10% to 34% of PJP cases. These cysts have a predilection for the upper lobes and a subpleural location, the latter accounting for an increased incidence of pneumothoraces (**Fig. 27**). Cysts may decrease in size or resolve with treatment, but CT scans frequently show residual cysts and fibrosis.[69] A small percentage of PJP infections cause nodules; however, TIB micronodules, enlarged lymph nodes, and pleural effusions are uncommon and suggest an alternative diagnosis.[45,55]

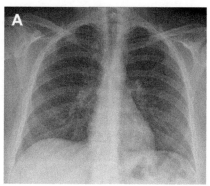
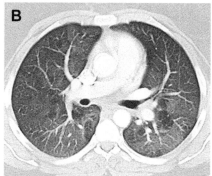

Fig. 21. PJP. (*A*) CR from a patient with PJP appears normal. (*B*) CT shows widespread GGO with some areas showing geographic margination.

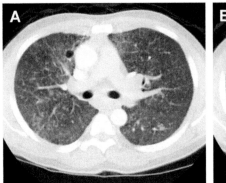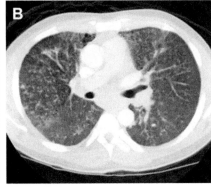

Fig. 22. (*A, B*) LIP. CT images in an adult patient with AIDS and LIP shows widespread micronodules, some with TIB pattern and others with ground-glass attenuation. An air cyst is also present in the right upper lobe, which is typical of LIP.

Mycobacterial Infections

The risk of developing active tuberculosis is increased up to 50 times in patients infected with HIV. Tuberculosis occurs in patients infected with HIV at all levels of immunosuppression, but the risk increases with decreasing CD4 counts, as does the likelihood of progression to miliary/disseminated disease.[70] The radiographic appearance of pulmonary tuberculosis in patients infected with HIV depends on the degree of immunosuppression.[71,72] In patients with CD4 counts greater than 200 cell/mm^3, radiographic findings are similar to the reactivation pattern seen in immunocompetent patients.

In more severely immunocompromised patients (CD4 counts <200 cells/mm^3), the radiographic findings of tuberculosis resemble those of primary-type tuberculosis regardless of whether the infection is newly acquired or reactivated. CR shows consolidation and lymphadenopathy, either alone and/or in combination (**Fig. 28**). From 60% to 75% of patients infected with HIV with pulmonary tuberculosis show enlarged lymph nodes on CT imaging, some of which show low-attenuation centers and peripheral rim enhancement following intravenous contrast. Enlarged neck/supraclavicular lymph nodes may also be present, and may be

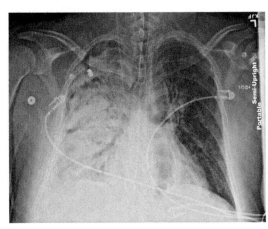

Fig. 23. Kaposi sarcoma. CT image shows nodular thickening of interlobular septa and perilymphatic macronodules, a pattern that is unlikely to represent infection.

Fig. 24. CAP in AIDS. CR of right lung CAP with extensive necrosis in a patient with AIDS.

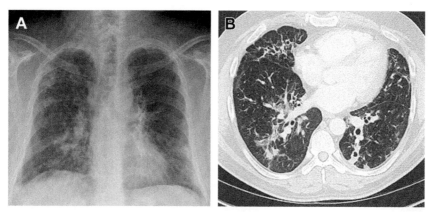

Fig. 25. Pyogenic airway disease. (*A*) CR from patient with pyogenic airway disease shows basilar bronchiectasis confirmed on CT (*B*).

more readily accessible for biopsy. Pleural effusions, when present, are often loculated and tend to be large. With advanced immunosuppression, the likelihood of disseminated tuberculosis increases. Seventy percent of patients with CD4 counts less than 100 cells/mm[3] show extrathoracic disease and approximately one-half of patients infected with HIV with extrathoracic involvement have a miliary pattern in the lungs (**Fig. 29**).[69]

NTM, almost always the *Mycobacterium avium* complex (MAC) species, are the most common opportunistic bacterial infection in patients with AIDS. HAART therapy and the institution of macrolide prophylaxis in patients the CD4 counts less than 50 cells/mm[3] have diminished the incidence to 1% per year.[73] CR is frequently normal with disseminated MAC and localized pulmonary disease is less common than with tuberculosis. When present, CT abnormalities are most commonly confined to mediastinal and hilar adenopathy (typically low attenuation on CT). Multifocal patchy consolidation, ill-defined nodules (some of

which may cavitate), and findings of infectious bronchiolitis may also be present.[37]

Patients with opportunistic infections and other HIV-related diseases, such as Kaposi sarcoma, who initiate HAART may develop paradoxic worsening of clinical and radiologic findings as their cell-mediated immunity is partially restored.[74] This heightened inflammatory response that occurs as CD4 counts increase and HIV viral load diminishes is referred to as immune reconstitution inflammatory syndrome (IRIS).[75] In the setting of NTM infection, IRIS characteristically causes lymphadenopathy with a low-attenuation center, whereas in the setting of PJP it may present as GGOs that progress over days to weeks.[76] IRIS manifestations of tuberculosis often commence within 2 to 3 weeks of initiating HAART. Patients may develop new or worsening lymphadenopathy, pulmonary opacity, and pleural effusions (**Fig. 30**). The diagnosis of IRIS requires exclusion of new infections; drug toxicity; and, in the setting of tuberculosis, noncompliance with therapy or the presence a multidrug-resistant organism.[77]

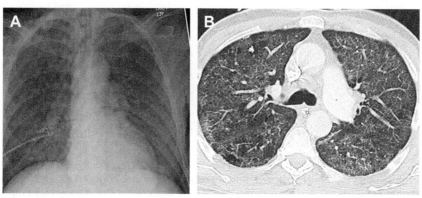

Fig. 26. PJP. (*A*) CR shows perihilar GGO and reticular opacity. (*B*) CT image shows widespread GGO and scattered areas of septal thickening.

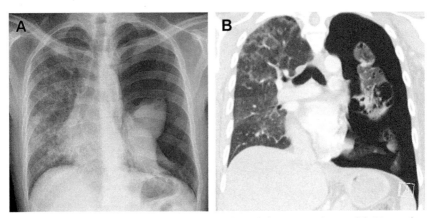

Fig. 27. PJP and pneumothorax. (*A*) PA radiograph shows a large left pneumothorax. (*B*) CT reveals numerous underlying cysts in the left lung. GGO in the right lung is consistent with PJP.

Fungal Infections

Three of the endemic fungi (*Cryptococcus neoformans*, *Histoplasma capsulatum*, and *Coccidioides immitis*), exploit the defect in cell-mediated immunity in severely affected (CD4 counts <100 cell/mm^3) patients with AIDS. In contrast, *Aspergillus* and Mucorales species, which are killed by phagocytes, are less pathogenic in patients with AIDS. *C neoformans*, the most common cause of fungal infection among patients with AIDS, can cause a wide range of imaging findings, including reticular opacities, consolidation, single or multiple nodules (including miliary nodules), lymphadenopathy, and pleural effusions. Histoplasma pneumonia frequently becomes disseminated in patients with AIDS.[78] At presentation, up to 50% of patients with disseminated disease have a normal chest radiograph but later develop diffuse opacities concurrent with development of respiratory symptoms (**Fig. 31**).

Aspergillosis is uncommon in patients infected with HIV and most frequently occurs in patients with advanced immunosuppression (ie, CD4 counts frequently <50 cells/mm^3) who are also neutropenic or have received corticosteroids.[79] The most common imaging finding is a thick-walled cavitary lesion; airway involvement similar to that in non–AIDS immunocompromised patients can occur (**Fig. 32**).

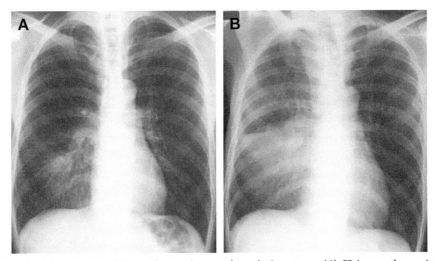

Fig. 28. Tuberculosis in an HIV-positive patient; primary tuberculosis pattern. (*A*) CR image shows right hilar adenopathy and right middle lobe parenchymal opacity. (*B*) CR 1 month later shows progressive right middle lobe consolidation as well as right hilar and right paratracheal lymphadenopathy. Effusions are commonly present in this pattern but are not seen on this radiograph.

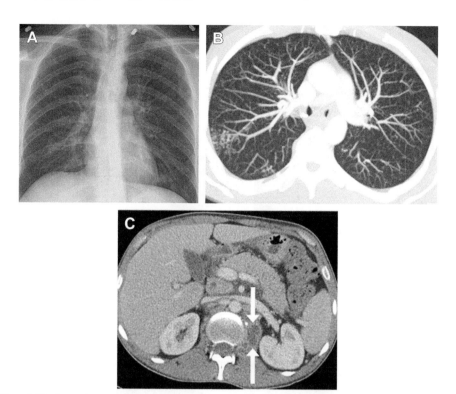

Fig. 29. CR and CT of a patient with disseminated tuberculosis. (*A*) Micronodules are difficult to detect on CR. (*B*) Maximum intensity projection image from CT shows widespread micronodules. (*C*) Abdominal CT shows a tuberculous psoas abscess (*arrows*) consistent with extrapulmonary spread of disease.

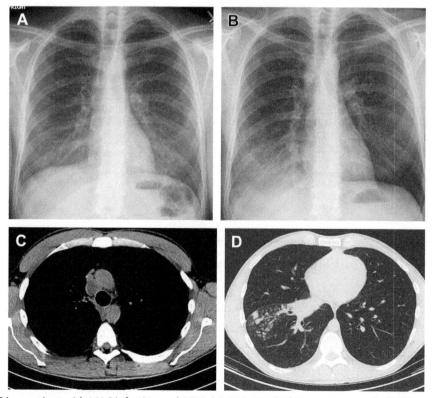

Fig. 30. IRIS in a patient with MAC infection and AIDS. (*A*) CR image before starting HAART is normal. (*B*) Several months later, CR image shows right paratracheal widening, left lung cavity, and right lower lobe opacity. (*C, D*) CT images show low-attenuation right paratracheal adenopathy (*C*) and consolidation and bronchiolitis in the right lower lobe (*D*).

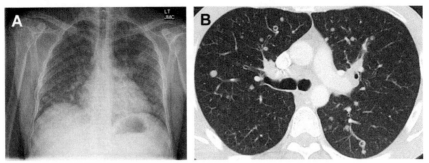

Fig. 31. Disseminated histoplasmosis in an patient with AIDS. (*A*) CR and (*B*) CT images show numerous small nodules, some of which are cavitary.

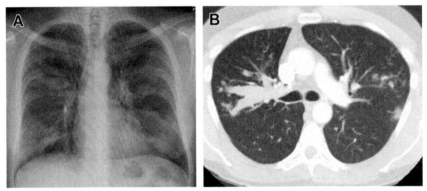

Fig. 32. Invasive airway disease in a patient with AIDS. (*A*) CR image shows perihilar tubular opacities. (*B*) CT image shows a large bronchocele in the right upper lobe and airway centric nodules in the left upper lobe.

Table 4
Examples of radiologic patterns and associated pathogens, depending on the type of immunosuppression

Finding	AIDS	HCT
Macronodules	TB, *Cryptococcus*, *Nocardia*	*Aspergillus*, mucormycosis
Predominant GGO	PJP	CMV
Centrilobular Nodules		
TIB	Bacteria, TB	Viruses; eg, RSV, parainfluenza
GGO nodules	Uncommon, LIP	Uncommon
Perilymphatic nodules	Kaposi sarcoma, sarcoidosis	Rare

Abbreviations: CMV, cytomegalovirus; LIP, lymphocytic interstitial pneumonitis; PJP, *Pneumocystis jiroveci* pneumonia; TB, tuberculosis.

SUMMARY

CR remains the initial means of assessing suspected lower respiratory tract infection. CT is most useful in assessing complications of infection, particularly pleural disease and the sequelae of lung necrosis. In immune-competent patients with micronodular opacities on CR, CT can also differentiate between airway-centered infections, such as mycoplasma, and blood-borne disseminated disease, such as miliary tuberculosis. Occasionally CT suggests that parenchymal opacities are caused by unsuspected noninfectious disease.

CT should be used early in suspected respiratory infection in immunocompromised patients to confirm diagnosis and help identify potential pathogens. In severely immunocompromised patients who do not have AIDS, the presence of large nodules and visualization of the halo sign are most suggestive of fungal infection.[39] Other findings are helpful in identifying a specific organism only if combined with clinical setting (eg, the combination of GGO and micronodules can suggest CMV infection after HCT) (**Table 4**). CT remains useful in assessing patients with HIV-AIDS because prophylactic TMP/SMX and HAART have shifted the relative frequency of opportunistic infections and made bacterial airway disease and atypical PJP infections more common.

REFERENCES

1. Boersma WG, Daniels JM, Lowenbery A, et al. Reliability of radiographic findings and the relation to etiologic agents in community acquired pneumonia. Respir Med 2006;100(5):916–32.

2. Basi SK, Marrie TJ, Huang JQ, et al. Patients admitted to the hospital with suspected pneumonia and normal chest radiographs: epidemiologic, microbiology and outcomes. AM J Med 2004; 117(5):305–11.

3. Hopstaken RM, Witbraad T, van Engelshoven JM, et al. Inter-observer variation in the interpretation of chest radiographs for pneumonia in community acquired lower respiratory tract infections. Clin Radiol 2004;59(8):743–52.

4. Woodhead W, Blasi F, Ewig S, et al. Guidelines for the management of adult lower respiratory tract infections. Eur Respir J 2005;26:1138–80.

5. Bruns AH, Oosterheert JJ, Prokop M, et al. Patterns of resolution of chest radiograph abnormalities in adults hospitalized with severe community-acquired pneumonia. Clin Infect Dis 2007;45: 983–91.

6. Bruns AH, Oosterheert JJ, El Moussaoui R, et al. Pneumonia recovery; discrepancies in perspectives

of the radiologist, physician and patient. J Gen Intern Med 2009;25(3):203–6.

7. Wunderink R, Wokknberg LS, Zeiss J, et al. The radiologic diagnosis of autopsy proven ventilator-associated pneumonia. Chest 1992;101:458–63.

8. Fàbregas N, Ewig S, Torres A, et al. Clinical diagnosis of ventilator associated pneumonia revisited: comparative validation using immediate post-mortem lung biopsies. Thorax 1999;54(10):867–73.

9. Magill SS, Klompas M, Balk R, et al. Developing a new, national approach to surveillance for ventilator-associated events. Crit Care Med 2013; 41(11):2467–75.

10. Desai SR, Wells AU, Suntharalingam G, et al. Acute respiratory distress syndrome caused by pulmonary and extrapulmonary injury: a comparative CT study. Radiology 2001;218(3):689–93.

11. Aujesky D, Fine MJ. The pneumonia severity index: a decade after the initial derivation and validation. Clin Infect Dis 2008;47:S133–9.

12. Johnson JL. Pleurisy, fever, and rapidly progressive pleural effusion in a healthy, 29-year-old physician. Chest 2001;119:1266–9.

13. Kearney SE, Davies CW, Davies RJ, et al. Computed tomography and ultrasound in parapneumonic effusions and empyema. Clin Radiol 2000;55(7):542–7.

14. Heffner JE, Klein JS, Hampson C. Diagnostic utility and clinical application of chest imaging for pleural space infections. Chest 2010;137:467–79.

15. Arenas-Jimenez J, Alonso-Charterina S, Sanchez-Paya J, et al. Evaluation of CT findings for diagnosis of pleural effusions. Eur Radiol 2000;10(4):681–90.

16. Mody GN, Lau CL, Bhalla S, et al. Mycotic pulmonary artery pseudoaneurysm. J Thorac Imaging 2005;20(4):310–2.

17. Stein DL, Haramati LB, Spindola-Franco H, et al. Intrathoracic lymphadenopathy in hospitalized patients with pneumococcal pneumonia. Chest 2005; 127(4):1271–5.

18. Boroja M, Barrie JR, Raymond GS. Radiographic findings in 20 patients with hantavirus pulmonary syndrome correlated with clinical outcome. AJR Am J Roentgenol 2002;178(1):159–63.

19. Raoof S, Amchentsev A, Vlahos I, et al. Pictorial essay: multinodular disease. A high resolution CT scan diagnostic algorithm. Chest 2006;129(3):805–15.

20. Rossi SE, Franquet T, Volpacchio M, et al. Tree in bud pattern at thin-section CT of the lungs: radiologic-pathologic overview. Radiographics 2005;25(3):789–801.

21. Shah RM, Miller W. Widespread ground glass opacity of the lung in consecutive patients undergoing CT: does lobular distribution assist diagnosis? AJR Am J Roentgenol 2003;180(4):965–8.

22. Eisenhuber E, Schaefer-Prokop CM, Prosch H, et al. Bedside chest radiography. Respir Care 2012;57(3): 427–43.

23. Shah RM, Friedman AC. CT angiogram sign: incidence and significance in lobar consolidations evaluated by contrast-enhanced CT. AJR Am J Roentgenol 1998;170(3):719–21.

24. Revel MP, Triki R, Chatellier G, et al. Is it possible to recognize pulmonary infarction on multisection CT images? Radiology 2007;244(3):875–82.

25. Nambu A, Saito A, Tsutomu A, et al. Comparison with findings of *Mycoplasma pneumoniae* and *Streptococcus pneumoniae* at thin-section CT. Radiology 2006;238(1):330–8.

26. Miyashita N, Kawai Y, Yamaguchi T. Clinical potential of diagnostic methods for the rapid diagnosis of *Mycoplasma pneumoniae* pneumonia in adults. Eur J Clin Microbiol Infect Dis 2011;30(3):439–46.

27. Okada F, Ando Y, Tanoue S, et al. Radiographic findings in acute *Haemophilus influenzae* pulmonary infection. Br J Radiol 2012;85(1010):121–6.

28. Choi SH, Hong SB, Ko GB, et al. Viral infection in patients with severe pneumonia requiring intensive care unit admission. Am J Respir Crit Care Med 2012;186:325–32.

29. Miller WT Jr, Mickus TJ, Barbosa E Jr, et al. CT of viral lower respiratory tract infections in adults: comparison among viral organisms and between viral and bacterial infections. AJR Am J Roentgenol 2011;197(5):1088–95.

30. Lewis PF, Schmidt MA, Lu X, et al. A community-based outbreak of severe respiratory illness caused by human Adenovirus serotype 14. J Infect Dis 2009;199:1427–34.

31. Lee SW, Jang YS, Park CM, et al. The role of chest CT scanning in TB outbreak investigation. Chest 2010;137(5):1057–64.

32. Ors F, Deniz O, Bozlar U, et al. High resolution CT findings in patients with pulmonary tuberculosis: correlation with degree of smear positivity. J Thorac Imaging 2007;22(2):154–9.

33. Yeh JJ, Yua JK, Tenga WB. High-resolution CT for identify patients with smear-positive active pulmonary tuberculosis. Eur J Radiol 2012;81:195–201.

34. Martinez S, McAdams HP, Batchu CS. The many faces of pulmonary nontuberculous mycobacterial infection. AJR Am J Roentgenol 2007;189(1):177–86.

35. Koh WJ, Lee KS, Kwon OJ, et al. Bilateral bronchiectasis and bronchiolitis at thin section CT: diagnostic implications in nontuberculous mycobacterial pulmonary infection. Radiology 2005;225(1):282–8.

36. Godet C, Elsendoorn A, Roblot F. Benefit of CT scanning for assessing pulmonary disease in the immune-depressed patient. Diagn Interv Imaging 2012;93:425–30.

37. Caillot D, Casasnovas O, Bernard A, et al. Improved management of invasive pulmonary aspergillosis in neutropenic patients using early thoracic computed tomographic scan and surgery. J Clin Oncol 1997; 15:139–47.

38. Ahuja J, Kanne JP. Thoracic infections in immunocompromised thoracic infections in immunocompromised patients. Radiol Clin North Am 2014;52(1): 121–36.

39. Marom EM, Kontoyiannis DP. Imaging studies for diagnosing invasive fungal pneumonia in immunocompromised patients. Curr Opin Infect Dis 2011; 24:309–14.

40. Wahba H, Truong T, Lei X, et al. Reversed halo sign in invasive pulmonary fungal infections. Clin Infect Dis 2008;46:1733–7.

41. Kallenberg MH, Gill RR, Factor RE, et al. Diagnostic efficacy and safety of computed tomography-guided transthoracic needle biopsy in patients with hematologic malignancies. Acad Radiol 2009;16: 1408–15.

42. Letourneaua A, Issaa NC, Badena L. Pneumonia in the immunocompromised host. Curr Opin Pulm Med 2014;20:272–9.

43. Greene RE, Schlamm HT, Oestmann JW, et al. Imaging findings in acute invasive pulmonary aspergillosis: clinical significance of the halo sign. Clin Infect Dis 2007;44:373–9.

44. McAdams HP, Rosado de Christenson M, Strollo DC, et al. Pulmonary mucormycosis: radiologic findings in 32 cases. AJR Am J Roentgenol 1997;168:1541–8.

45. Althoff Souza C, Muller NL, Marchiori E, et al. Pulmonary invasive aspergillosis and candidiasis in immunocompromised patients: a comparative study of the high-resolution CT findings. J Thorac Imaging 2006;21:184–9.

46. Kanne JP, Yandow DR, Meyer CA. *Pneumocystis jiroveci* pneumonia: high-resolution CT findings in patients with and without HIV infection. AJR Am J Roentgenol 2012;198:W555–61.

47. Vogel MN, Brodoefel H, Hierl T, et al. Differences and similarities of cytomegalovirus and pneumocystis pneumonia in HIV-negative immunocompromised patients – thin-section CT-morphology in the early phase of the disease. Br J Radiol 2006;80(955): 516–23.

48. Franquet T, Lee KS, Muller NL. Thin-section CT findings in 32 immunocompromised patients with cytomegalovirus pneumonia who do not have AIDS. AJR Am J Roentgenol 2003;181:1059–63.

49. Franquet T. Imaging of pulmonary viral pneumonia. Radiology 2011;260(1):18–39.

50. Kotloff RM, Ahya VN, Crawford SW. Pulmonary complications of solid organ and hematopoietic stem cell transplantation. Am J Respir Crit Care Med 2004; 170:22–48.

51. Lee Y, Song JW, Chae EJ, et al. CT findings of pulmonary non-tuberculous mycobacterial infection in non-AIDS immunocompromised patients: a

case-controlled comparison with immunocompetent patients. Br J Radiol 2013;86:20120209.

52. Gold JA, Rom WA, Harkin TJ. Significance of abnormal chest radiograph findings in patients with HIV-1 infection without respiratory symptoms. Chest 2002;121:395–408.

53. Selwyn PA, Pumerantz AS, Durante A, et al. Clinical predictors of *Pneumocystis carinii* pneumonia, bacterial pneumonia, and tuberculosis in hospitalized patients with HIV infection. AIDS 1998;12: 885–93.

54. Boiselle PM, Tocino I, Hooley RJ, et al. Chest radiograph diagnosis of *Pneumocystis carinii* pneumonia, bacterial pneumonia and pulmonary tuberculosis in HIV-positive patients: accuracy, distinguishing features, and mimics. J Thorac Imaging 1997;12: 47–53.

55. Boiselle PM, Crans CA, Kaplan MA. The changing face of *Pneumocystis carinii* pneumonia in AIDS patients. AJR Am J Roentgenol 1999;172:1301–9.

56. Gruden JF, Huang L, Turner J, et al. High-resolution CT in the evaluation of clinically suspected *Pneumocystis carinii* pneumonia in AIDS patients with normal, equivocal, or nonspecific radiographic findings. AJR Am J Roentgenol 1997;169:967–75.

57. Greenberg SD, Frager D, Suster B, et al. Active pulmonary tuberculosis in patients with AIDS; spectrum of radiographic findings (including a normal appearance). Radiology 1994;193:115–9.

58. Lichtenberger JP, Sharma A, Zachary KC, et al. What a differential a virus makes: a practical approach to thoracic imaging findings in the context of HIV infection—part 1, pulmonary findings. AJR Am J Roentgenol 2012;198:1295–304.

59. Chou S, Prabhu S, Crothers K, et al. Thoracic diseases associated with HIV infection in the era of antiretroviral therapy: clinical and imaging findings. Radiographics 2014;34:895–911.

60. Benito N, Moreno A, Miro JM, et al. Pulmonary infections in HIV-infected patients: an update in the 21st century. Eur Respir J 2012;39(3):730–45.

61. Cordero E, Pachon J, Rivero A, et al. *Haemophilus influenzae* pneumonia in human immunodeficiency virus-infected patients. Clin Infect Dis 2000;30: 461–5.

62. Jasmer RM, Edinburgh KJ, Thompson A, et al. Clinical and radiographic predictors of pulmonary nodules in HIV-infected patients. Chest 2000;117: 1023–30.

63. Edinburgh KJ, Jasmer RM, Huang L. Multiple pulmonary nodules in AIDS: usefulness of CT in distinguishing among potential causes. Radiology 2000; 214:427–32.

64. Lichtenberger JP, Sharma A, Zachary KC, et al. What a differential a virus makes: a practical approach to thoracic imaging findings in the context of HIV infection—part 2, extrapulmonary

findings, chronic lung disease, and immune reconstitution syndrome. AJR Am J Roentgenol 2012; 198:1305–12.

65. Brecher CW, Aviram G, Boiselle PM. CT and radiography of bacterial respiratory infections in AIDS patients. AJR Am J Roentgenol 2003;180:1203–9.

66. Crothers K, Thompson B, Burkhardt K, et al. HIV-associated lung infections and complications in the era of combination antiretroviral therapy. Proc Am Thorac Soc 2011;8:275–81.

67. Aviram G, Fishman JE, Sagar M. Cavitary lung disease in AIDS: etiologies and correlation with immune status. AIDS Patient Care STDS 2001;15:353–61.

68. Kanne JP, Yandow DR, Mohammed TH, et al. CT findings of pulmonary nocardiosis. AJR Am J Roentgenol 2011;197:W266–72.

69. Hardak E, Brook O, Yigla M. Radiological features of *Pneumocystis jirovecii* pneumonia in immunocompromised patients with and without AIDS. Lung 2010;188(2):159–63.

70. Kim JY, Jeong YJ, Kim K, et al. Miliary tuberculosis: a comparison of CT findings in HIV seropositive and HIV-seronegative patients. Br J Radiol 2010;83:206–11.

71. Saurborn DP, Fishman JE, Boiselle PM. The imaging spectrum of pulmonary tuberculosis in AIDS. J Thorac Imaging 2002;17(1):28–33.

72. Geng E, Kreiswirth B, Burzynski J, et al. Clinical and radiographic correlates to primary and reactivation tuberculosis: a molecular epidemiology study. JAMA 2005;293:2740–5.

73. Karakousis PC, Moore RD, Chaisson RE. *Mycobacterium avium* complex in patients with HIV infection in the era of highly active antiretroviral therapy. Lancet Infect Dis 2004;4:557–65.

74. French MA, Price P, Stone SF. Immune restoration disease after antiretroviral therapy. AIDS 2004;18: 1615–27.

75. Wittram C, Fogg J, Farber H. Immune restoration syndrome manifested by pulmonary sarcoidosis. AJR Am J Roentgenol 2001;177:1427.

76. Fishman JE, Saraf-Lavi E, Narita M, et al. Pulmonary tuberculosis in AIDS patients: transient chest radiographic worsening after initiation of antiretroviral therapy. AJR Am J Roentgenol 2000; 174:43–9.

77. Berman EJ, Iyer RS, Addrizzo-Harris D, et al. Immune-reconstitution syndrome related to atypical mycobacterial infection in aids. J Thorac Imaging 2008;23:182–7.

78. Heller HM, Wu CW, Pierce VM, et al. Case 31-2013: a 29-year-old man with abdominal pain, fever, and weight loss. N Engl J Med 2013;369:1453–61.

79. Mylonakis E, Barlam TF, Flanigan T, et al. Pulmonary aspergillosis and invasive disease in AIDS; review of 342 cases. Chest 1998;114:251–62.

Intensive Care Unit Imaging

Matthew R. Bentz, MD[a],*, Steven L. Primack, MD[b]

KEYWORDS

- ICU • Imaging • Chest radiograph • Pulmonary edema • Atelectasis

KEY POINTS

- Imaging plays a crucial role in caring for the critically ill.
- The radiograph is essential for evaluating the positioning of ICU support and monitoring equipment, and in evaluating for complications of these devices.
- The chest radiograph is useful in diagnosing and evaluating the progression of atelectasis, aspiration, pulmonary edema, pneumonia, and pleural fluid collections.
- CT can be useful when the clinical and radiologic presentations are discrepant, the patient is not responding to therapy, or in further defining a radiographic abnormality.

INTRODUCTION

The chest radiograph is a crucial tool in the care of the critically ill. It serves to diagnose and monitor a variety of cardiopulmonary disorders. Additionally, it is used to evaluate a broad range of thoracic medical devices, ensuring proper positioning and surveying for complications. Daily rounds and prompt communication between radiologist and intensivist can help to improve diagnostic accuracy and manage potential complications.

Indications for Portable Chest Radiography

Posteroanterior and lateral upright radiographs are standard practice for chest radiography. Indications for portable anteroposterior (AP) chest radiography include critically ill patients, trauma patients, those with cardiopulmonary symptoms following surgery, and after line or tube placement, according to the American College of Radiology practice guidelines (revised 2011).[1] There are no absolute guidelines dictating the frequency of chest radiography for intensive care unit (ICU) patients. Several studies assessing the benefit of

daily chest radiography in the ICU have been performed, with varied findings.[2–5] Two recent meta-analyses found that eliminating routine daily radiographs in ICU patients did not lead to any negative outcomes compared with a restrictive strategy, which only ordered radiographs based on clinical indications.[6,7] The American College of Radiology recommends chest radiography for patients with clinical changes, and not as a matter of routine.[8] Chest radiographs also should be obtained immediately after the placement of endotracheal tubes, enteric tubes, vascular catheters, and chest tubes.[8] Follow-up is warranted if tube or catheter position is suspected to have changed, or is otherwise clinically indicated.

Technical Factors

Inherent challenges exist in ICU chest radiography, all of which limit diagnostic accuracy. Many patients are debilitated and not readily able to cooperate with the examination, precluding optimal upright posteroanterior positioning. Radiographs are usually obtained in a semi upright or supine AP position. Lateral radiographs are

Disclosure statement: Neither author has any financial interests or potential conflicts of interest to disclose.
[a] Department of Radiology, Oregon Health and Science University, 3181 Southwest Sam Jackson Park Road, L340, Portland, OR 97239, USA; [b] Division of Pulmonary Medicine, Department of Radiology, Oregon Health and Science University, 3181 Southwest Sam Jackson Park Road, L340, Portland, OR 97239, USA
* Corresponding author.
E-mail address: bentzm@ohsu.edu

Clin Chest Med 36 (2015) 219–234
http://dx.doi.org/10.1016/j.ccm.2015.02.006
0272-5231/15/$ – see front matter © 2015 Elsevier Inc. All rights reserved.

usually impractical. Decubitus views may be obtained to evaluate for pleural effusions. External monitoring devices, overlying tubes, and electro-cardiographic leads can obscure underlying disease, mimic pathology, and create ambiguity as to the positioning of other support equipment.

MONITORING AND SUPPORT DEVICES

Evaluation of support equipment and monitoring devices is of utmost importance in imaging of patients in the ICU. Early recognition of malpositioning reduces the likelihood of potentially serious complications. Radiologists often review the position of all support equipment as their initial step in appraisal of the radiograph. For this reason, and to underline its importance, evaluation of monitoring and support devices is discussed first.

Endotracheal and Tracheostomy Tubes

Endotracheal tubes are used in patients requiring short-term respiratory support with mechanical ventilation. With the patient's head in a neutral position, the endotracheal tube tip should be located 4 ± 1 cm above the carina. Neck flexion results in inferior movement of the tube by up to 2 cm, whereas neck extension can cause 2 cm superior migration, hence the colloquial saying "the hose goes with the nose."

A malpositioned endotracheal tube is not an uncommon finding. Intubation of the main bronchi can occur when endotracheal tube position is too low, resulting in subsegmental atelectasis, segmental collapse, or complete collapse of the contralateral lung. The ipsilateral lung may be overventilated, increasing the risk of pneumothorax. Main bronchus intubation is most frequently right-sided, because of a more direct angle of the trachea and right main bronchus (**Fig. 1**). If the endotracheal tube is too high, there may be inadvertent extubation or damage to the larynx. Esophageal intubation is a severe complication compromising ventilation and introducing excessive amounts of air into the gastrointestinal tract, but is typically clinically apparent. Aspiration has been reported to occur in up to 8% of intubations.[9]

The endotracheal balloon cuff should not be inflated beyond the normal diameter of the trachea (**Fig. 2**), and inflation to 1.5 times the normal tracheal diameter frequently causes tracheal damage.[10] Overinflation can rarely lead to acute rupture or can lead to the chronic complication of tracheal stenosis (**Fig. 3**).

Tracheostomy tubes are placed when long-term intubation is necessary. The tracheostomy tube tip should be at approximately the T3 level. Position is

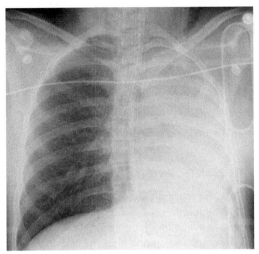

Fig. 1. Right main bronchus intubation. AP chest radiograph in this trauma patient demonstrates the endotracheal tube tip in the right main bronchus. Associated collapse of the left upper and lower lobes is present, with leftward shift of the mediastinum.

maintained with neck flexion and extension. Tracheostomy tube diameter should be approximately two-thirds that of the trachea and as with the endotracheal tube, the cuff should not distend the tracheal wall. Mediastinal air can be seen after uncomplicated tube placement.

Enteric Tubes

Enteric tubes are used for feeding, medication administration, and suction. For feeding, ideal tip position is in the gastric antrum or more distally to reduce aspiration risk. If the enteric tube is

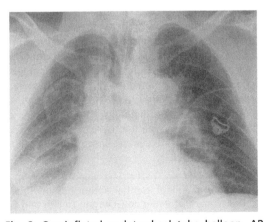

Fig. 2. Overinflated endotracheal tube balloon. AP chest radiograph shows an endotracheal tube cuff that is inflated sufficiently to cause widening of the trachea. The cuff should fill, but not expand, the tracheal lumen.

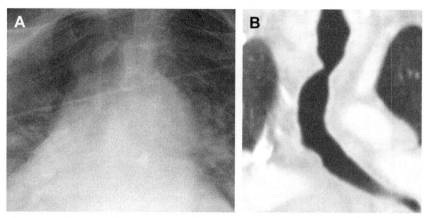

Fig. 3. Tracheal stenosis. (*A*) Magnified AP view of the trachea in a patient with a history of prolonged intubation shows focal tracheal stenosis. (*B*) Corresponding coronal CT image of the trachea in the same patient shows the area of narrowing in more detail.

used exclusively for suction or medication administration, placement within the stomach is adequate. The proximal sidehole of a nasogastric tube should extend beyond the gastroesophageal junction to decrease aspiration risk.

Radiography is important in detecting aberrant tube location, and preventing potentially lethal complications. Tubes can coil within the pharynx or esophagus, creating a high risk of aspiration if nutrition is administered. Pharyngeal and esophageal perforations are extremely rare complications. Enteric tubes occasionally terminate in the trachea or bronchi where ectopic feeding can result in direct bronchopulmonary injury and pneumonia (**Fig. 4**). Pneumothorax, pulmonary laceration, and pulmonary contusion may be seen if the lung parenchyma is punctured. If an enteric tube

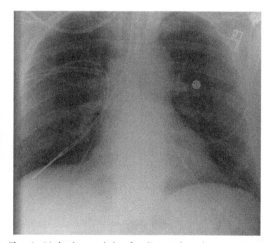

Fig. 4. Right lower lobe feeding tube placement. AP chest radiograph demonstrates an aberrant enteric tube terminating in the right lower lobe.

has been placed in the airway and extends to the periphery or into the pleura, it is essential to obtain a follow-up radiograph because pneumothorax may only be apparent postremoval (**Fig. 5**).

Venous Catheters

The central venous catheter tip should be located within the superior vena cava (SVC), beyond venous valves, to reduce the risk of thrombosis. Positioning of the catheter tip in the lower SVC or at the cavoatrial junction has been shown in one study to result in reduction of thrombosis around the catheter tip.[11] When catheter position is too caudal, it may enter the right atrium. Right atrial positioning increases risk of dysrhythmia and of the very rare complication of cardiac perforation. Thus, catheters should ideally terminate within the lower SVC or at the cavoatrial junction.

Aberrant positioning of venous catheters is quite common. Usually, the aberrantly located catheter is intravenous or within the right atrium. Peripherally inserted catheters can coil in the veins of the upper extremity, course cephalad within the internal jugular vein, traverse midline into the contralateral brachiocephalic vein, or enter the azygos vein (**Fig. 6**). Catheter location within a persistent left-sided SVC, an anomalous vein occurring in 0.3% of the population,[12] occasionally occurs (**Fig. 7**). Positioning within a left SVC is acceptable; however, a left SVC catheter that is too deep enters the coronary sinus, which increases the risk of arrhythmia. Additionally, a left SVC catheter may mimic an intra-arterial location on an AP chest radiograph.

Occasionally, arteries are inadvertently accessed, most often the subclavian artery or common carotid artery (**Fig. 8**). Arterial

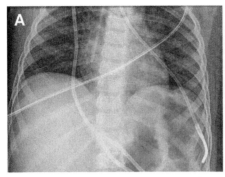
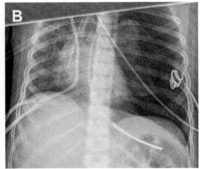

Fig. 5. Left lower lobe feeding tube placement. AP chest radiograph (*A*) demonstrates an aberrant enteric tube terminating in the left lower lobe. Tubes terminating in the costophrenic sulcus may overlie the gastric bubble. Follow-up AP chest radiograph (*B*) after tube removal shows a large left pneumothorax.

catheterization is usually clinically apparent with pulsatile flow of bright red oxygenated blood from the catheter. However, intra-arterial placement may not be clinically apparent in patients with severe heart failure, sepsis, or hypotension. On the AP chest radiograph, subclavian artery placement should be suspected if the catheter course projects above the clavicle. If uncertainty remains after radiographic analysis, determination of wave form (arterial vs venous) can confirm location.

When the catheter tip is directed at and abuts the venous wall, the catheter should be repositioned or withdrawn to reduce the risk of vessel perforation. Vascular perforation causes hematoma in the surrounding soft tissues. Fluid and medications can accumulate in adjacent soft tissues or pleural space if extravascular catheter position (**Figs. 9** and **10**) is unnoticed. The chest radiograph should also be used to evaluate for hemothorax and pneumothorax following line placement. Pneumothorax occurs uncommonly with peripherally inserted central catheter placement and is most frequently seen when the subclavian vein is accessed.

Pulmonary Artery Catheters

Pulmonary artery catheters, or Swan-Ganz catheters, are used to measure pulmonary artery pressure, pulmonary capillary wedge pressure, and cardiac output. The catheter tip should be within the right main pulmonary artery, left main pulmonary artery, or the proximal interlobar pulmonary artery. If the catheter extends beyond the pulmonary hilum on the chest radiograph, the catheter should be retracted.[13] Distal catheter location increases the risk of arterial occlusion and rupture. Pulmonary artery occlusion and subsequent pulmonary infarct can also be secondary to pericatheter thrombus. Pulmonary artery catheters are subject to the same complications as central venous catheters, namely dysrhythmia, cardiac perforation, pneumothorax, and hemothorax.

Chest Tubes

Approximately 10% of chest tubes are malpositioned.[8] Chest tube sideholes, radiographically evident as interruptions of the tube's radiopaque line, should be located within the pleural space.

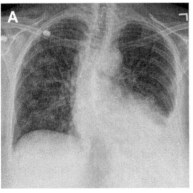
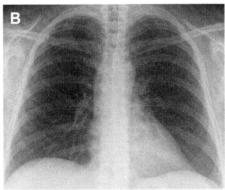

Fig. 6. Peripherally inserted central catheter (PICC) terminating in the azygos vein. (*A*) AP radiograph shows a left upper extremity PICC terminating in the azygos vein. (*B*) AP radiograph in another patient with a right upper extremity PICC terminating in the azygos vein.

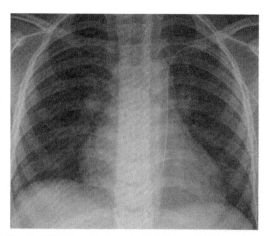

Fig. 7. PICC terminating in left-sided SVC. AP chest radiograph shows a left PICC traveling lateral to the descending aorta within a persistent left SVC. Note the rightward deviation inferiorly, as the left SVC drains into the right atrium via the coronary sinus.

Improper chest tube location may manifest as a poorly functioning or nonfunctioning tube. When a chest tube is inserted into the pulmonary parenchyma, pulmonary contusion may be seen, resulting in a new opacity adjacent to the chest tube. Location in the pulmonary fissures may or may not affect tube function. An inappropriately positioned chest tube can injure the heart, major blood vessels, diaphragm, and upper abdominal organs. Critical assessment of support equipment is

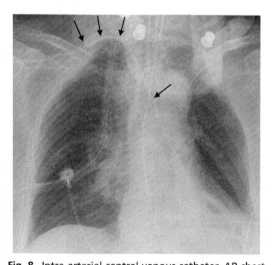

Fig. 8. Intra-arterial central venous catheter. AP chest radiograph of a trauma patient demonstrates a right subclavian approach central venous catheter (*arrows*) with an aberrant course. The catheter travels above the clavicle, and crosses midline. Both features are concerning for intra-arterial placement of a subclavian catheter, as was proved in this case.

essential, because appropriate placement can mimic aberrant placement and vice versa. The following example illustrates this point, with a sub-diaphragmatic chest tube mimicking placement in the posterior costophrenic sulcus (**Fig. 11**).

PULMONARY PARENCHYMAL ABNORMALITIES

Atelectasis, aspiration, pneumonia, hydrostatic pulmonary edema, and noncardiogenic pulmonary edema all present as opacities on chest radiography and computed tomography (CT). Although it is often difficult, and sometimes impossible, to distinguish between these entities, certain radiographic features can aid in their diagnoses.

Atelectasis

Atelectasis, a decrease in lung volume, is the most common cause of pulmonary opacities in the ICU population. It is frequently found after general anesthesia and thoracic or upper abdominal surgery, occurring in up to 64% of patients in one surgical investigation.[14] The most common location is the left lower lobe (66%), followed by the right lower lobe (22%), and right upper lobe (11%).[15] Atelectasis is usually subsegmental. Atelectasis can mimic pneumonia, particularly when signs of volume loss, such as crowding of air bronchograms, fissural deviation, mediastinal shift, and diaphragmatic elevation, are absent. Flat, platelike opacities are characteristic of discoid atelectasis (**Fig. 12**). Complete lung collapse, lobar collapse, or segmental collapse can also be seen (**Fig. 13**). Atelectasis is categorized according to mechanism as obstructive, compressive, cicatricial, and adhesive. Adhesive atelectasis is common in premature neonates secondary to insufficient production of surfactant and is not discussed further.

Obstructive atelectasis is the most common type of atelectasis. Impaired mucociliary function, increased secretions, and altered consciousness are all predisposing factors. When only the distal, small airways are obstructed, crowded air bronchograms are seen. Air bronchograms are absent if the obstruction is more proximal, in larger airways. Mucous plugging is a common cause of acute segmental, lobar, and complete lung collapse (**Fig. 14**). The absence of air bronchograms in patients with acute lobar collapse favors mucoid impaction as the cause, and predicts a higher rate of therapeutic success with bronchoscopy (79%–89% in favorable patients).[16]

Compressive atelectasis is volume loss secondary to mass effect exerted on the lung. In the ICU population, pleural fluid is usually the cause. Cicatricial atelectasis is volume loss secondary to

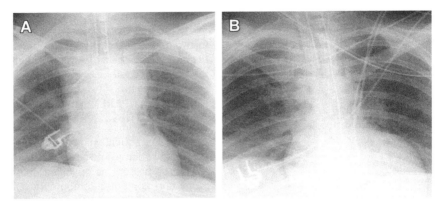

Fig. 9. Mediastinal hematoma following catheter placement. (*A*) AP chest radiograph shows new widening of the mediastinum after left subclavian central venous catheter placement. More importantly, the right upper mediastinum is more dense than on the radiograph from the day prior (*B*), consistent with mediastinal hematoma.

pulmonary fibrosis and can be seen in those with underlying pulmonary disease or as an associated finding with acute respiratory distress syndrome (ARDS).

On CT, atelectasis can often be identified by signs of volume loss, such as crowding of vessels and airways. On contrast-enhanced CT, atelectasis results in relatively high attenuation of the lung parenchyma, a useful feature distinguishing it from relatively lower attenuating consolidative processes, such as pneumonia. This is discussed further in the section on pneumonia (see **Fig. 19**).

Aspiration

Intubation, diminished cough reflex, sedation, and enteric tube feeds all increase aspiration risk. Aspiration can occur in mechanically ventilated patients despite adequate inflation of the endotracheal tube cuff. Clinically, aspiration events may

go unnoticed or may be severe, causing respiratory distress. Aspiration can result in airway obstruction, chemical pneumonitis, or infectious pneumonia, depending on the volume and type of aspirate. Small amounts of aspirated saliva may result in no radiographic abnormality, whereas aspiration of large amounts of food substance increases the likelihood of aspiration pneumonia.

Patchy, ill-defined ground-glass, consolidative, and nodular opacities are the most frequently encountered radiographic manifestations of aspiration (**Fig. 15**). Opacities typically appear rapidly, and are most commonly located in the dependent regions of the lungs: the posterior segment of the upper lobes and the superior and posterior basal segments of the lower lobes.[17] Opacities may increase in conspicuity over the first 1 to 2 days in aspiration pneumonitis, but should resolve relatively rapidly thereafter (**Fig. 16**). If opacities

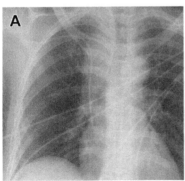
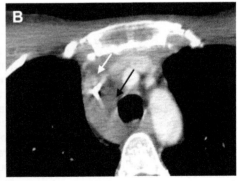

Fig. 10. Extravascular catheter placement. (*A*) AP chest radiograph demonstrates an apparent right subclavian approach central venous catheter. Hyperdensity and widening of the mediastinum were new compared with the prior radiograph, and were concerning for mediastinal hematoma. The course of the catheter on the radiograph was not aberrant, but the new mediastinal hematoma appropriately prompted further investigation. (*B*) CT showed that the attempted subclavian line was extravascular, traveling posterior to, but not within, the superior vena cava (*white arrow*). CT confirmed a mediastinal hematoma (*black arrow*).

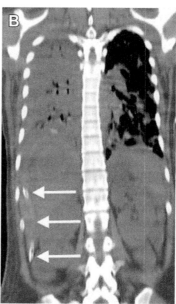

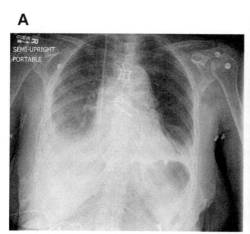

Fig. 11. Chest tube in the abdominal cavity. (*A*) An AP chest radiograph was obtained following chest tube placement. The position of the tip was more inferior than expected and sanguineous output was obtained from the chest tube. This prompted a CT for localization of the tube. (*B*) CT showed the tube (*white arrows*) looping underneath the diaphragm and terminating in the upper abdomen.

persist or increase over several days, aspiration pneumonia is likely present (**Fig. 17**).

Patchy, dependent ground-glass and consolidative opacities are also seen on CT. "Tree-in-bud" opacities[18] result from filling and inflammation of the distal airways. When tree-in-bud opacities are present in a dependent distribution, they are highly suggestive of aspiration (see **Figs. 16** and **17**).

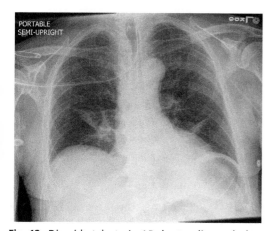

Fig. 12. Discoid atelectasis. AP chest radiograph demonstrates low lung volumes and linear opacities in the lung bases, greater on the right, consistent with discoid atelectasis.

Pneumonia

Pneumonia is another cause of pulmonary opacities in ICU patients. Aspiration and mechanical ventilation[19] are two important risk factors for pneumonia in the ICU population. Ventilator-associated pneumonia occurs in 9% to 24% of patients ventilated for more than 48 hours.[20] Most pneumonias in the ICU are caused by mixed anaerobic or, in the ventilated patient, aerobic gram-negative bacteria, such as *Pseudomonas aeruginosa*.[21]

Pneumonia may present as a focal consolidation on the chest radiograph. However, it is often multifocal (**Fig. 18**). Pneumonia can be difficult to differentiate from other causes of pulmonary opacities, such as atelectasis, aspiration, and pulmonary edema. Typically, radiographic findings of pneumonia change more slowly than these other ARDS entities. In addition, air bronchograms may be seen, and can be differentiated from those seen in atelectasis by noting the absence of volume loss and crowding of bronchi. On contrast-enhanced CT, pneumonia can often be discriminated from atelectasis by its lack of enhancement, whereas atelectasis enhances (**Fig. 19**).

When ARDS is present, the diagnostic accuracy of CT and chest radiography for the detection of pneumonia is diminished.[22,23] The presence of underlying consolidation in ARDS limits the ability

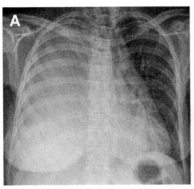
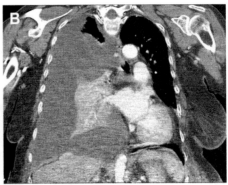

Fig. 13. Right lung collapse. (*A*) AP chest radiograph demonstrates opacification of the right hemithorax, silhouetting of the right hemidiaphragm, and mediastinal shift to the left. These findings were suggestive of a unilateral large pleural effusion. Because this was a new finding, CT was performed for further investigation. (*B*) This coronal CT image shows a large pleural effusion with complete collapse of the right lower lobe and only minimal aeration of the right upper lobe.

to diagnose or exclude concurrent pneumonia. The incidence of pneumonia in patients with diffuse lung injury at autopsy has been reported to be 58%.[24]

Pulmonary Edema

Pulmonary edema can be classified as either hydrostatic pulmonary edema or noncardiogenic pulmonary edema, also referred to as increased permeability edema. These entities can be difficult to distinguish radiographically, and may coexist,

further increasing the challenge of differentiating the two.

Noncardiogenic Pulmonary Edema

Noncardiogenic pulmonary edema is caused by primary pulmonary pathologies, such as pneumonia, aspiration, and pulmonary contusion.[24,25] Extrathoracic causes of increased permeability include drug toxicity, systemic inflammatory response syndrome, sepsis, shock, and extrathoracic trauma. Neurogenic pulmonary edema demonstrates radiographic features of hydrostasis and capillary leak.[26] Diffuse alveolar damage (DAD) results from injury to the alveolar capillaries and epithelium. The degree of DAD varies from

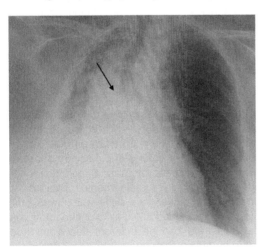

Fig. 14. Atelectasis, mucous plug. AP chest radiograph demonstrates opacification of the right mid and lower lung, with silhouetting of the right hemidiaphragm and shift of the mediastinum to the right. The shift of the mediastinum indicates volume loss/atelectasis, and evaluation of the right main bronchus is notable for an abrupt cutoff (*arrow*), suggesting mucous plugging. Bronchoscopy revealed viscous secretions in the right bronchus, with markedly improved aeration seen on the postprocedure radiograph.

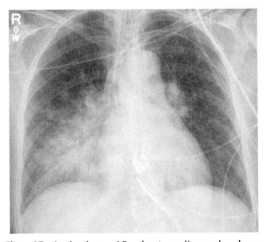

Fig. 15. Aspiration. AP chest radiograph shows nodular consolidation with air bronchograms in the right lower lobe. Of note, the enteric tube tip is pointed superiorly within the distal esophagus. These findings are highly suggestive of aspiration into the right lung.

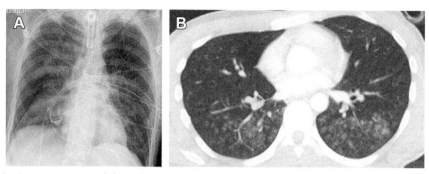

Fig. 16. Aspiration pneumonitis. (*A*) AP chest radiograph obtained after an acute event in a patient on long-term mechanical ventilation. An appropriately positioned tracheostomy tube is noted. Right lower lobe atelectasis is present, with subtle nodularity throughout the lower lobes. (*B*) Corresponding CT shows bilateral dependent "tree in bud" nodularity, indicating aspiration. This resolved on subsequent imaging, consistent with aspiration pneumonitis.

severe in cases of ARDS, to relatively nonexistent, as in many cases of heroin-induced pulmonary edema.[26] When DAD is minimal, radiographic abnormalities are likely to be relatively transient.

Respiratory symptoms may precede radiographic abnormalities in noncardiogenic pulmonary edema, and the initial radiograph is often normal. Within the first 24 hours, patchy, bilateral ground-glass and consolidative opacities typically appear. These opacities frequently coalesce, forming diffuse pulmonary opacification (**Fig. 20**A) that lasts for days to months depending on the cause, degree of DAD, complications, such as aspiration and pneumonia, and treatment. Radiographic features typically associated with hydrostatic pulmonary edema, including septal lines, pleural fluid, and widening of the vascular pedicle, may also be seen with noncardiogenic pulmonary edema. Aberle and colleagues[27] found that a patchy, peripheral distribution is much more commonly seen in noncardiogenic (50%) than

cardiogenic (13%) pulmonary edema, although this is not commonly sufficient to differentiate between the two entities in clinical practice. Radiographic change is typically slow and monitoring of noncardiogenic edema requires the comparison of multiple chest radiographs.

ARDS was originally described by Ashbaugh and colleagues[28] in 1967, with multiple subsequent definitions. The 1994 American-European Consensus Conference (AECC) presented a specific definition of a clinical syndrome characterized by hypoxemia resistant to oxygen therapy, the absence of clinically apparent left atrial hypertension, and bilateral pulmonary opacification on the chest radiograph.[29] In 2011, a panel of experts met to address some of the limitations of the AECC definition of ARDS. Using data from more than 4000 patients with ARDS, the panel revised the definition such that different levels of severity are well defined, reproducible, and reflective of patient mortality. The "Berlin Definition" created

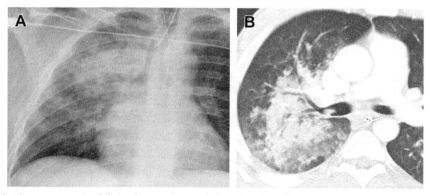

Fig. 17. Aspiration pneumonia. (*A*) AP chest radiograph in an intubated ICU patient shows nodular consolidation in the right upper lobe. (*B*) Corresponding CT demonstrates nodular consolidation and foreign material within the right upper lobe bronchus. The consolidation persisted on the following radiograph, consistent with aspiration pneumonia.

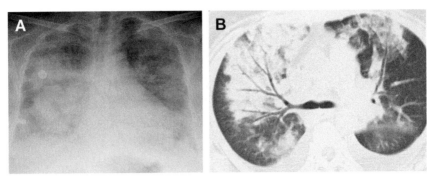

Fig. 18. Bacterial pneumonia. (A) AP chest radiograph shows bilateral, multifocal consolidation. (B) Axial CT image of the right upper lobe shows the consolidation and demonstrates air bronchograms. Note the absence of airway crowding that is seen in atelectasis. Findings are consistent with a bacterial pneumonia, *Staphylococcus aureus* in this case.

by the ARDS definition task force was released in 2012, and defined ARDS as respiratory failure (1) within 1 week of a known clinical insult or new or worsening respiratory symptoms; (2) with bilateral opacities on lung imaging, with the opacities not fully explained by atelectasis, effusions, or nodules; (3) not attributable solely to cardiac failure or volume overload; and (4) with an arterial partial pressure of oxygen to fraction of inspired oxygen (Pao_2/Fio_2) ratio of less than 300 mm Hg. The levels of severity were defined as mild, with Pao_2/Fio_2 between 200 and 300 mm Hg; moderate, with Pao_2/Fio_2 between 100 and 200 mm Hg; and severe as having Pao_2/Fio_2 less than 100 mm Hg.[30]

Acute lung injury (ALI) was a term used by the AECC. Under the new Berlin definition, ALI has been replaced with the term "mild ARDS," and ALI should no longer be used in this setting.[29,30] The incidence of ARDS/ALI has not been well-defined. A study conducted in the United States by Rubenfeld and colleagues[31] determined the age-adjusted incidence of ALI to be 86.2 per 100,000 person-years with an in-hospital mortality rate of 38.5%.

Pulmonary opacities on CT are often more heterogeneous than on the chest radiograph. Goodman and colleagues[32] found that asymmetric ground-glass and consolidative opacities predominate when ARDS is secondary to pulmonary disease. When ARDS is caused by extrapulmonary causes, a relatively symmetric ground-glass distribution predominates (see **Fig. 20**B). CT patterns in ARDS may be described as typical or atypical. In the typical pattern, dense consolidation involves the posterior lungs, in a dependent distribution (see **Fig. 20**C). This can change with position (supine vs prone), reflective of the contribution of atelectasis in ARDS. Ground-glass opacities are seen in a nondependent distribution. In the atypical pattern, dense consolidation is seen in nondependent locations. The atypical distribution of consolidation is more likely to be found when ARDS is incited by pulmonary disease.[33] Air bronchograms are frequently seen in both forms. "Crazy paving" is the term for ground-glass opacities with superimposed interlobular septal

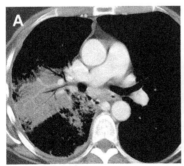
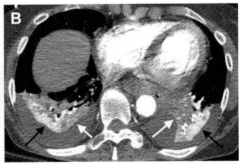

Fig. 19. CT of pneumonia, atelectasis, and effusion. (A) Axial CT of the lungs in soft tissue window demonstrates consolidation in the right lung with decreased enhancement, consistent with pneumonia. In contrast, atelectasis demonstrates volume loss and homogeneous enhancement. (B) An axial CT image in another patient demonstrates bilateral lower lobe pneumonia (*white arrows*), which shows decreased enhancement compared with areas of adjacent atelectasis (*black arrows*). Small layering bilateral pleural effusions are present.

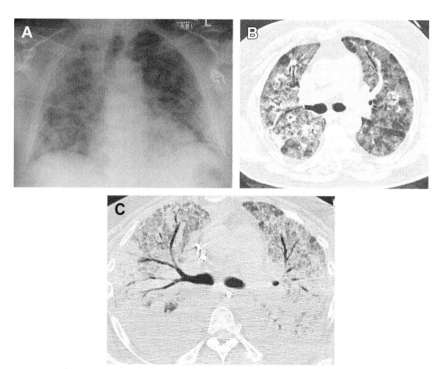

Fig. 20. ARDS. (*A*) AP chest radiograph shows low lung volumes and diffuse bilateral pulmonary opacities. (*B*) Axial CT image at the level of the carina in the same patient shows ground-glass and consolidative opacities without pleural effusions. The patient was intubated shortly after imaging. (*C*) Axial CT image from another patient shows dense bilateral consolidation with air bronchograms and diffuse ground-glass opacity. This patient had ARDS secondary to H1N1 infection.

thickening. This pattern may be seen in ARDS; however, crazy paving is not a pattern specific for ARDS.[34]

DAD can be categorized into exudative, proliferative, and fibrotic phases on pathologic findings, although varying degrees of these phases may be occurring at any one time. The early exudative phase cannot be reliably identified using CT.[35] However, in the proliferative and fibrotic phases, traction bronchiectasis and bronchiolectasis may be seen.[35] Ichikado and colleagues[36] found that the presence of

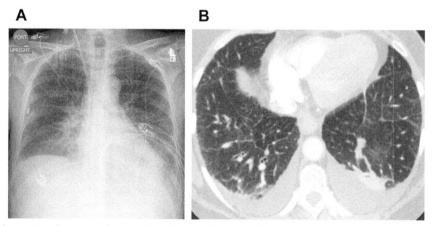

Fig. 21. Hydrostatic pulmonary edema. (*A*) AP chest radiograph of a patient who received large volumes of intravenous fluid during resuscitation shows classic findings of hydrostatic pulmonary edema: pulmonary vascular indistinctness, diffuse ground-glass opacification with lower lobe predominance, and septal thickening. Blunting of the costophrenic angles indicates bilateral pleural effusions. (*B*) Axial CT image through the lower lobes of a patient with hydrostatic pulmonary edema, demonstrating smooth interlobular septal thickening, ground opacities, and small bilateral pleural effusions.

extensive fibroproliferative change early in the clinical course of ARDS is predictive of poor prognosis.

Survivors of ARDS often show marked improvement over the first 6 months with normal spirometric findings, although diffusion capacity often remains low after 1 year.[37] Anterior reticular opacities are the most frequent finding on follow-up CT in survivors of ARDS.[38]

Hydrostatic Pulmonary Edema

Hydrostatic pulmonary edema may be caused by cardiac disease, renal failure, or overhydration. The radiographic findings may not be temporally synchronous with clinical disease. Characteristic radiographic findings of hydrostatic pulmonary edema include pulmonary vascular indistinctness, bilateral ground-glass opacities, and interlobular septal thickening. Indistinctness of the pulmonary vessels may be subtle, but is often the most useful radiographic finding in diagnosing pulmonary edema (**Fig. 21**) in the ICU. Consolidative opacities are present in more advanced cases. Distribution is gravity dependent, and abnormalities are most notable at the lung bases. However, this gradient may be absent in the supine ICU patient. Pleural fluid and a widened vascular pedicle are also characteristically seen. Pleural effusions may be bilateral or unilateral. When unilateral, right-sided pleural effusions are more common. Radiographic

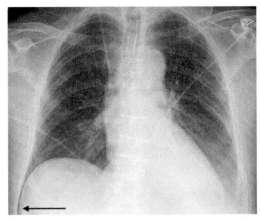

Fig. 23. Pneumothorax, "deep sulcus sign." AP chest radiograph in a supine trauma patient demonstrating lucent deep lateral costophrenic sulcus (*arrow*) and lucency of the right lower hemithorax, characteristic of basilar pneumothorax.

changes of hydrostatic pulmonary edema typically occur much more rapidly than those of noncardiogenic pulmonary edema.

Renal failure may present with similar findings and characteristic perihilar opacities, sometimes referred to as "batwing edema." Aggressive hydration is often seen in settings of trauma and postoperative patients, and may coincide with noncardiogenic pulmonary edema.

CT findings of hydrostatic pulmonary edema include smooth interlobular septal thickening, ground-glass and consolidative opacities, and pleural fluid (see **Fig. 21**B). When underlying pulmonary disease, such as emphysema, is present, hydrostatic pulmonary edema may have an atypical appearance and mimic other pathology, such

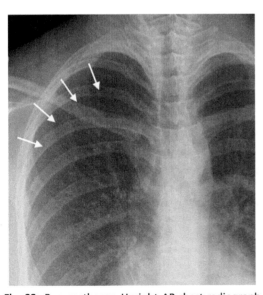

Fig. 22. Pneumothorax. Upright AP chest radiograph showing a moderate right apical pneumothorax. A thin line of visceral pleura is visible (*arrows*), with no pulmonary vessels visible beyond the line. Concentric retraction of the collapsed right lung toward the right hilum is present.

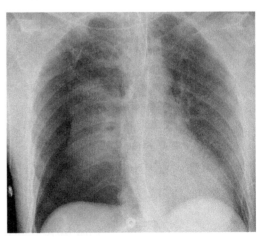

Fig. 24. Tension pneumothorax. Semi upright AP chest radiograph demonstrates a large right pneumothorax following central line placement. Note the shift of the mediastinum away from the pneumothorax, indicative of tension physiology.

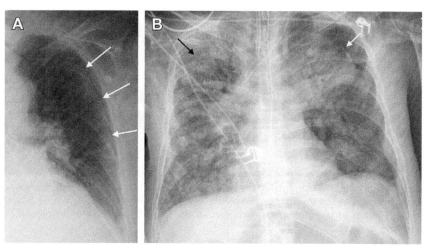

Fig. 25. Skin fold versus pneumothorax. (*A*) AP radiograph shows a skin fold (*arrows*) masquerading as a left pneumothorax. A skin fold demonstrates a gradient of density, contrasted to the thin visceral pleural line seen in pneumothorax. In this case, additional skin folds are also present over the superior mediastinum and left hilar region. Although subtle, pulmonary vessels are visible peripheral to the skin fold. (*B*) AP radiograph of an ICU patient with ARDS demonstrates a left pneumothorax (*white arrow*) and a right skin fold (*black arrow*).

as aspiration pneumonitis or pneumonia. Mitral regurgitation can present as asymmetric pulmonary edema of the right upper lobe.

PNEUMOTHORAX, PNEUMOMEDIASTINUM, AND PLEURAL FLUID

Pleural space abnormalities include pnuemothorax and pleural fluid, and are extremely common in the ICU setting. Pneumomediastinum is less commonly encountered but is important to recognize because it may indicate underlying tracheobronchial injury or alveolar rupture in a mechanically ventilated patient.

Pneumothorax

Underlying pulmonary disease, trauma, and iatrogenic causes may all result in pneumothorax (**Fig. 22**). The classic sign of a thin curvilinear pleural line, bordered by lung on one side and pleural air on the other, is often absent in the supine ICU patient. Detection often requires a high degree of suspicion. In the ventilated patient, a small pneumothorax can rapidly progress to tension, and recognition is critical.

When supine, pleural air initially accumulates in the anteromedial recess, the least dependent location in the hemithorax. Abnormal lucency at the lung base or projecting over the upper abdomen is suggestive of pneumothorax. A lucent deep sulcus may be visualized in the medial or lateral hemithorax (**Fig. 23**). In addition, the mediastinum may be unusually well outlined.[39,40] If pneumothorax is suspected, an upright or lateral decubitus radiograph should be obtained for confirmation.

Tension pneumothorax occurs when intrathoracic pressure is greater than atmospheric pressure. Radiographically, tension pneumothorax is most reliably diagnosed by inversion or flattening of the hemidiaphragm (**Fig. 24**). Mediastinal shift may also be seen but is less specific and frequently less pronounced in those with ARDS because of reduced lung compliance.

Skin folds can mimic pneumothoraces. There are important distinguishing features that should be recognized. A skin fold is seen as a soft

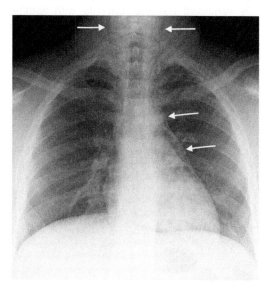

Fig. 26. Pneumomediastinum. AP chest radiograph of a 27-year-old man with asthma who presented with spontaneous pneumomediastinum. Linear and curvilinear lucencies (*arrows*) are present along the mediastinum and in the soft tissues at the base of the neck.

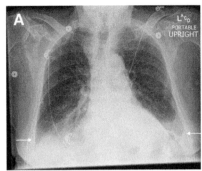
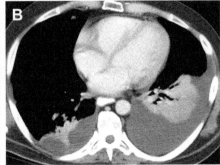

Fig. 27. Layering pleural fluid. (*A*) Upright AP chest radiograph shows blunting of the costophrenic angles bilaterally and a small amount of fluid tracking up the pleural space laterally (*arrows*), indicating bilateral pleural effusions. (*B*) Axial CT image in the same patient confirms moderate left and small right pleural effusions, with adjacent compressive atelectasis.

tissue–air interface, with radiopacity on one side and normal lung on the other. In pneumothorax, a pleural line is often bordered by air on both sides: normal lung and pleural air (**Fig. 25**). The diagnosis may be more complex if the lung is abnormally opaque, creating the illusion of a soft tissue–air interface. If pulmonary vessels extend peripheral to the interface, the opacity is a skin fold. If no pulmonary vessels are seen peripherally, a pneumothorax is present.

Pneumomediastinum

Pneumomediastinum is extraluminal air within the mediastinum. It can be seen in tracheobronchial injury, tracheostomy tube placement, mechanically ventilated patients, patients with asthma, and esophageal rupture (although this is a rare cause). Pneumomediastinum most commonly occurs via the Macklin effect. This is the process by which air from ruptured alveoli dissects along the bronchovascular interstitium to the mediastinum.[41,42] Pulmonary interstitial emphysema in the mechanically ventilated patient is a sign of alveolar rupture. Air may dissect cephalad into the subcutaneous tissues of the neck (**Fig. 26**) and caudad into the retroperitoneum.

Pleural Fluid

Pleural fluid is common in ICU patients, and is most frequently transudative. The supine radiograph is relatively insensitive in the detection of pleural fluid, and often underestimates the amount of pleural fluid. On the semi- or full upright radiograph, blunting of the costophrenic angles and silhouetting of the diaphragm are the classic findings of pleural effusion (**Fig. 27**). On the upright lateral radiograph, blunting of the costophrenic angle usually occurs when 200 mL of fluid is present but may be absent with as much as 500 mL.[43] Layering pleural fluid is more difficult to detect on the supine radiograph. The costophrenic angle is often not blunted, and the supine radiograph may only demonstrate hazy "veil-like" opacification caused by layering pleural fluid. The apex is the most dependent

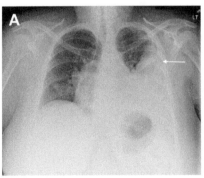
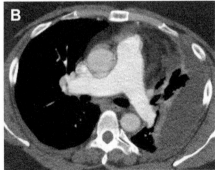

Fig. 28. Loculated pleural effusion. (*A*) Upright AP chest radiograph demonstrates a large left pleural effusion. The effusion tracks higher than expected along the lateral hemithorax (*arrow*), suggesting that it may not freely layer and may be loculated. (*B*) Axial CT image through the mid chest in the same patient demonstrates that the fluid is loculated along the lateral pleural space, and does not freely layer in the dependent pleural space.

location in the supine patient, and pleural effusion may manifest as an apical cap.[43]

Consolidation, atelectasis, and pleural fluid all cause opacities on the chest radiograph, and frequently coexist, particularly at the thoracic base. CT may be useful in demonstrating loculated pleural fluid collections, and in differentiating pleural fluid from pulmonary parenchymal disease and atelectasis (see **Fig. 19**; **Fig. 28**, respectively). CT also better characterizes loculated pleural fluid collections. Empyema is suggested when pleural fluid is bordered by enhancing, thick pleura. Hemothorax is suggested by relatively high attenuation of pleural fluid,[44] commonly 35 to 70 Hounsfield units.[39] Ultrasound is usually readily available and can also be very useful in demonstrating loculations and in guiding fluid sampling.

SUMMARY

Chest radiography is an integral component in the evaluation of the ICU patient. It is critical in ensuring the proper positioning of support and monitoring equipment, and in evaluating for potential complications of this equipment. The radiograph is useful in diagnosing and evaluating the progression of atelectasis, aspiration, pulmonary edema, pneumonia, and pleural fluid collections. CT can be useful when the clinical and radiologic presentations are discrepant, the patient is not responding to therapy, or in further defining the pattern and distribution of a radiographic abnormality. Daily rounds involving critical care physicians and radiologists can assist in more accurate and expedient diagnoses.

REFERENCES

1. ACR Practice Guideline for the Performance of Pediatric and Adult Portable (Mobile Unit) Chest Radiography. ACR Practice Guideline; Revised 2011. Available at: http://www.acr.org/Quality-Safety/Standards-Guidelines. Accessed February 17, 2015.
2. Hall JB, White SR, Karrison T. Efficacy of daily routine chest radiographs in intubated, mechanically ventilated patients. Crit Care Med 1990;19(5):689–93.
3. Krivopal M, Shlobin OA, Schwartzstein RM. Utility of daily routine portable chest radiographs in mechanically ventilated patients in the medical ICU. Chest 2003;123(5):1607–14.
4. Marik PE, Janower ML. The impact of routine chest radiography on ICU management decisions: an observational study. Am J Crit Care 1997;6(2):95–8.
5. Strain DS, Kinasewitz GT, Vereen LE, et al. Value of routine daily chest x-rays in the medical intensive care unit. Crit Care Med 1985;13(7):534–6.
6. Oba Y, Zaza T. Abandoning daily routine chest radiography in the intensive care unit: meta-analysis. Radiology 2010;255(2):386–95.
7. Ganapathy A, Adhikari N, Spiegelman J, et al. Routine chest x-rays in intensive care units: a systematic review and meta-analysis. Crit Care 2012;16(2):R68.
8. American College of Radiology. ACR Appropriateness Criteria: Routine Chest Radiographs in ICU Patients. 2011. Available at: https://acsearch.acr.org/docs/69452/Narrative/. Accessed October 28, 2014.
9. Wechsler RJ, Steiner RM, Kinori I. Monitoring the monitors: the radiology of thoracic catheters, wires, and tubes. Semin Roentgenol 1988;23:61–84.
10. Khan F, Reddy NC, Khan A. Cuff/trachea ratio as an indicator of tracheal damage. Chest 1976;70:431.
11. Cadman A, Lawrance JA, Fitzsimmons L, et al. To clot or not to clot? That is the question in central venous catheters. Clin Radiol 2004;59:349–55.
12. Collins J, Stern EJ. Monitoring and support devices: "tubes and lines.". In: Collins J, Stern EJ, editors. Chest radiology the essentials. Philadelphia: Lippincott Williams & Wilkins; 1999. p. 59–71.
13. Kazerooni EA, Gross BH. Lines, tubes, and devices. In: Kazerooni EA, Gross BH, editors. Cardiopulmonary imaging. Philadelphia: Lippincott Williams & Wilkins; 2004. p. 255–93.
14. Gale GD, Teasdale SJ, Sanders DE, et al. Pulmonary atelectasis and other respiratory complications after cardiopulmonary bypass and investigation of aetiological factors. Can Anaesth Soc J 1979;26(1):15–21.
15. Sheuland JE, Hireleman MR, Hoang KA, et al. Lobar collapse in the surgical intensive care unit. Br J Radiol 1983;56:531–4.
16. Kreider ME, Lipson DA. Bronchoscopy for atelectasis in the ICU. A case report and review of the literature. Chest 2003;124(7):344–50.
17. Franquet T, Giménez A, Rosón N, et al. Aspiration diseases: findings, pitfalls, and differential diagnosis. Radiographics 2000;20:673–85.
18. Rossi SE, Franquet T, Volpacchio M, et al. Tree-in-bud pattern at thin-section CT of the lungs: radiologic-pathologic overview. Radiographics 2005;25:789–801.
19. Cunnion KM, Weber DJ, Broadhead WE, et al. Risk factors for nososcomial pneumonia: comparing adult critical-care populations. Am J Respir Crit Care Med 1996;153(1):158–62.
20. Morehead RS, Pinto SJ. Ventilator-associated pneumonia. Arch Intern Med 2000;160:1926–36.
21. Winer-Muram HT, Jennings SG, Wunderink RG, et al. Ventilator-associated *Pseudomonas aeruginosa* pneumonia: radiographic findings. Radiology 1995;195:247–52.
22. Winer-Muram HT, Rubin SA, Ellis JV, et al. Pneumonia and ARDS in patients receiving mechanical ventilation: diagnostic accuracy of chest radiography. Radiology 1993;188:479–85.

23. Winer-Muram HT, Steiner RM, Gurney JW, et al. Ventilator-associated pneumonia in patients with adult respiratory distress syndrome: CT evaluation. Radiology 1998;208(1):193–9.

24. Andrews CP, Coalson JJ, Smith JD, et al. Diagnosis of nosocomial bacterial pneumonia in acute, diffuse lung injury. Chest 1981;80(3):254–8.

25. Miller PR, Croce MA, Bee TK, et al. ARDS after pulmonary contusion: accurate measurement of contusion volume identifies high-risk patients. J Trauma 2001;51(2):223–30.

26. Gluecker T, Capasso P, Schnyder P, et al. Clinical and radiologic features of pulmonary edema. Radiographics 1999;19:1507–31.

27. Aberle DR, Wiener-Kronish JP, Webb WR, et al. Hydrostatic versus increased permeability pulmonary edema: diagnosis based on radiographic criteria in critically ill patients. Radiology 1988;168:73–9.

28. Ashbaugh DG, Bigelow DB, Petty TL, et al. Acute respiratory distress in adults. Lancet 1967;2:319–23.

29. Bernard GR, Artigas A, Brigham KL, et al. The American-European Consensus Conference on ARDS: definitions, mechanisms, relevant outcomes, and clinical trial coordination. Am J Respir Crit Care Med 1994;149:818–24.

30. ARDS Definition Task Force. Acute respiratory distress syndrome: the Berlin definition. JAMA 2012;307(23):2526–33.

31. Rubenfeld GD, Caldwell E, Peabody E, et al. Incidence and outcomes of acute lung injury. N Engl J Med 2005;353(16):1685–93.

32. Goodman LR, Fumagalli R, Tagliabue P. Adult respiratory distress syndrome due to pulmonary and extrapulmonary causes: CT, clinical, and functional correlations. Radiology 1999;213:545–52.

33. Desai SR, Suntharalingam G, Rubens MB, et al. Acute respiratory distress syndrome caused by pulmonary and extrapulmonary injury: a comparative CT study. Radiology 2001;218:689–93.

34. Rossi SE, Erasmus JJ, Volpacchio M. "Crazy-Paving" pattern at thin-section CT of the lungs: radiologic-pathologic overview. Radiographics 2003;23:1508–19.

35. Ichikado K, Suga M, Gushima Y, et al. Hyperoxia-induced diffuse alveolar damage in pigs: correlation between thin-section CT and histopathologic findings. Radiology 2000;216:531–8.

36. Ichikado K, Suga M, Muranaka S, et al. Prediction of prognosis for acute respiratory distress syndrome with thin-section CT: validation in 44 cases. Radiology 2006;238(1):321–9.

37. Herridge MS, Cheung AM, Tansey CM, et al. One-year outcomes in survivors of the acute respiratory distress syndrome. N Engl J Med 2003;348(8):683–93.

38. Desai SR, Wells AU, Rubens MB, et al. Acute respiratory distress syndrome: CT abnormalities at long-term follow-up. Radiology 1999;210:29–35.

39. Rivas LA, Fishman JE, Múnera F, et al. Multislice CT in thoracic trauma. Radiol Clin North Am 2003;41: 599–616.

40. Tocino IM. Pneumothorax in the supine patient: radiographic anatomy. Radiographics 1985;5(4): 557–86.

41. Wintermark M, Schnyder P. The Macklin effect. Chest 2001;120(2):543–6.

42. Zylak CM, Standen JR, Barnes GR, et al. Pneumomediastinum revisited. Radiographics 2000;20: 1043–57.

43. Müller N. Imaging of the pleura. Radiology 1993; 186:297–309.

44. Kuhlman JE, Sinha NK. Complex disease of the pleural space: radiographic and CT evaluation. Radiographics 1997;17:63–79.

Pulmonary Vascular Diseases

Kristopher W. Cummings, MD[a], Sanjeev Bhalla, MD[b],*

KEYWORDS

- Acute pulmonary embolism • Chronic thromboembolic pulmonary hypertension
- Pulmonary arteriovenous malformation • Hereditary hemorrhagic telangiectasia
- Granulomatosis with polyangitis • Microscopic polyangitis

KEY POINTS

- Multidetector CT (MDCT) is the study of choice for the evaluation of acute pulmonary embolism (PE), simultaneously detecting thromboemboli and, in its absence, providing alternative explanations for presentation.
- MDCT plays a role in the detection and distribution characterization of disease in patients with chronic thromboembolic pulmonary hypertension (CTEPH), especially in cases of prior emboli or abnormal ventilation-perfusion (V/Q) scan.
- In patients with suspected pulmonary arteriovenous malformation (PAVM) or HHT who have abnormal bubble echocardiography, MDCT is the study of choice.
- Vasculitides can affect the large central pulmonary vessels or more commonly the small vessels of the lung, resulting in various parenchymal manifestations.

INTRODUCTION

Pulmonary vascular diseases encompass a large and diverse group of underlying pathologies ranging from venous thromboembolism to congenital malformations to inflammatory vasculitides. As a result, patients can present either acutely with dyspnea and chest pain or chronically with dyspnea on exertion, hypoxia, and right heart failure. Imaging, particularly with MDCT, plays a key role in the evaluation and management of patients with suspected pulmonary vascular disease.

ACUTE PULMONARY EMBOLISM

Venous thromboembolism is reportedly the third most common vascular disease after myocardial infarction and stroke, affecting approximately 600,000 people each year.[1] Because acute PE can be a challenging clinical diagnosis to make given the variability in patient presentation, CT pulmonary angiography (CTPA) is one of the most commonly ordered imaging studies performed for pulmonary vascular disease, especially in the emergency department.

The vast majority of PE arises from the deep venous system of the lower extremities, frequently in the setting of risk factors, such as recent surgery, prolonged immobilization, hypercoagulable disorders, and malignancy. No predisposing factor, however, is identified in up to 30% of cases,[2] and 50% of patients studied with deep venous thrombosis are found to have clinically silent PE.[3] For these reasons, clinical prediction criteria, such as the Wells score, and laboratory assays, like the D-dimer, are used to risk stratify for acute PE. The combination of the 2 can safely exclude the risk of acute PE.[4]

MDCT has emerged as the imaging study of choice for those patients with intermediate or high

Disclosures: None.
[a] Cardiothoracic Radiology, Mayo Clinic Arizona, 5777 E. Mayo Boulevard, Phoenix, AZ 85054, USA;
[b] Cardiothoracic Imaging, Mallinckrodt Institute of Radiology, Washington University School of Medicine in St Louis, 510 South Kingshighway Boulevard, Box 8131, St Louis, MO 63110, USA
* Corresponding author.
E-mail address: bhallas@mir.wustl.edu

Clin Chest Med 36 (2015) 235–248
http://dx.doi.org/10.1016/j.ccm.2015.02.007
0272-5231/15/$ – see front matter © 2015 Elsevier Inc. All rights reserved.

clinical risk for acute PE and those with abnormal D-dimer assays. In PIOPED II (Prospective Investigation of Pulmonary Embolism Diagnosis), which studied the accuracy of CTPA with V/Q and conventional pulmonary angiography, CTPA in patients with a high pretest probability was shown to have a sensitivity of 83% and specificity of 96% for the diagnosis.[5] The rapid evolution of MDCT technology has, however, likely resulted in greatly improved accuracy in comparison to the 4-, 8-, and 16-row scanners used in the PIOPED II study. In addition to its widespread availability and rapid assessment, another major advantage of MDCT over V/Q and conventional angiography is the ability to detect alternative causes for clinical symptoms in up to a third of cases, which is important given the widespread low positivity rates for acute PE, in many cases as low as 10%.[6]

Although techniques vary slightly among institutions and vendors, generally CTPA is performed with 80 to 100 mL of nonionic iodinated intravenous contrast administered at a rate of 4 mL/s from an upper extremity antecubital vein cannulated with an 18- or 20-gauge intravenous (IV). In the era of widespread advanced and even ultrafast MDCT, automated bolus tracking and test bolus techniques are widely used to time optimal contrast delivery to the pulmonary system during the time of imaging. Test bolus technique is useful in patients with very poor cardiac function who frequently have delayed opacification of the pulmonary arteries. Although caudal to cranial scanning is often used to reduce effect of respiratory motion at the lung bases where more emboli are seen and more diaphragmatic motion occurs, the availability of ultrafast MDCT usually obviates this modification. Thin collimation allowing for isovolumetric 1-mm slice reconstruction allows for detailed analysis and multiplanar reconstruction.

The hallmark finding of acute PE on MDCT is a low-attenuation filling defect in a contrast-filled pulmonary artery. MDCT findings of acute PE include (**Fig. 1**)[7,8]

- Complete arterial occlusion (vessel cutoff) without luminal enhancement with or without vessel dilatation
- Partial, central filling defect surrounded by contrast (rim or polo mint sign when viewed perpendicular to the vessel axis or railway sign when viewed longitudinal to the vessel axis)
- Peripheral filling defects forming acute angles with the vessel walls or at vessel branch points

To prevent obscuration of small segmental emboli by dense iodinated contrast, window and level values that enable visualization of right heart structures, such as trabeculations, or the pulmonary valve leaflets should be chosen.

Parenchymal findings that can be seen with acute PE include (**Fig. 2**)

- Pulmonary hemorrhage (ground-glass opacification)
- Infarct (peripheral consolidation with central ground-glass)
- Oligemia (vascular mosaic attenuation)
- Atelectasis
- Pleural effusion

The prognosis for patients with acute PE has been shown to correlate with circulatory effects and right ventricular dysfunction. Clinically, the term, massive PE, is applied to patients with evidence of hemodynamic compromise (systemic hypotension), whereas those patients with hemodynamic stability are labeled submassive. Cardiac findings that can be seen in the setting of acute PE include (**Fig. 3**)

- Right ventricle–to–left ventricle (RV:LV) diameter ratio greater than 1 (measured on axial image)
- Leftward interventricular septal bowing
- Inferior vena cava and/or azygous vein dilatation
- Reflux of contrast material into the inferior vena cava

Of the findings listed, RV:LV ratio best correlates with echocardiographic evidence of right heart strain with reported sensitivities of 80% or greater for RV:LV ratio greater than 1 but variable specificity.[9] CT findings of right heart dysfunction should be reported, because they may triage a patient to a more closely monitored nursing division. The CT findings of right heart dysfunction, however, are not used for determining whether thrombolysis is warranted. That decision is based on systemic symptoms and echocardiographic findings.

Artifacts that can limit assessment for acute PE include

- Flow artifacts (transient interruption of the contrast column)
- Respiratory or patient motion
- Image noise
- Partial volume averaging with adjacent structures

It is important to interrogate the pulmonary arteries on all contrast-enhanced CT scans, especially in oncologic populations, because PEs

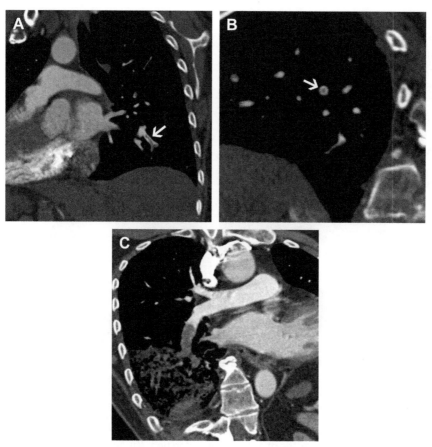

Fig. 1. Acute PE. (*A*) Oblique coronal and (*B*) oblique sagittal CT images demonstrate a linear central filling defect in a segmental right lower lobe pulmonary artery. When viewed longitudinal to the axis of the vessel, the defect produces the railway sign (*arrow, A*) as it is outlined on both sides by intravenous contrast. In cross-section to the vessel, the defect is central and produces a rim or polo mint sign (*arrow, B*). (*C*) Occlusive embolism in the right lower lobar pulmonary artery is seen in a different patient on an oblique coronal image. Note contrast column surrounding the proximal aspect of the embolus is concave indicative of an acute thrombus, and there is airspace opacification in the affected lung in keeping with hemorrhage.

have been reported as incidental findings in as many as 1.5% of patients imaged for other reasons.[10]

CHRONIC THROMBOEMBOLIC PULMONARY HYPERTENSION

Most acute PEs resolve with or without treatment and, in the absence of recurrent episodes of venous thromboembolism, leave no significant clinical sequela. A small subset (1%–4%), however, of patients with acute PE proceed to the development of CTEPH.[11,12] Nonspecific symptoms, such as exertional dyspnea, often predominate, mimicking more common pathologies, such as ischemic heart disease or interstitial lung disease. A confounding issue is the absence of a documented episode of prior PE in one-third to one-half of patients with an eventual diagnosis of

CTEPH, presumably due to misdiagnosed or previously asymptomatic emboli.[13]

A variety of mechanisms for the development of CTEPH have been postulated but the most widespread is the failure in or alteration of clot degradation pathways responsible for clearing thromboemboli, resulting in their endothelization and incorporation into the vessel wall. Vessel luminal narrowing and occlusion subsequently result in elevated pulmonary vascular resistance. There is histologic evidence, however, to support the development of a diffuse pulmonary arteriopathy similar to that seen in primary pulmonary hypertension, possibly induced by a previous thromboembolic event.[14] Patients with myeloproliferative disorders, chronic inflammatory conditions (such as inflammatory bowel disease and chronic osteomyelitis), ventriculoatrial shunts, and splenectomy are at a higher risk of developing CTEPH.[15]

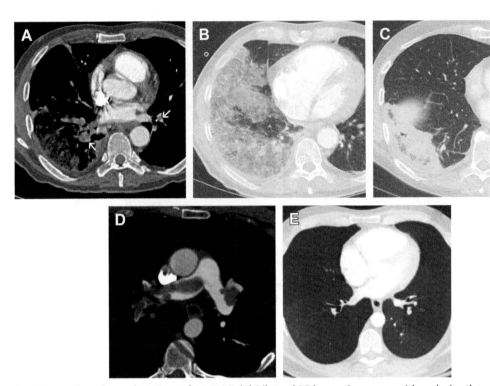

Fig. 2. Parenchymal manifestations of acute PE. (*A*) Bilateral PE (*arrows*) are seen with occlusive thrombus present in the right lower lobar pulmonary artery. (*B*) Lung window image in the same patient demonstrates diffuse ground-glass throughout the right lower lobe with a minimal component of smooth septal line thickening in keeping with pulmonary hemorrhage. (*C*) In a different patient with acute right lower lobe PE, a peripheral area of consolidation centered predominantly in the lateral basal segment of the right lower lobe is seen with central ground-glass opacity characteristic of a pulmonary infarction. (*D*) Another patient with extensive acute central clot burden is noted to have mosaic attenuation on an (*E*) axial minimum intensity projection image with the darker areas reflecting relative vascular hypoperfusion. Mosaic perfusion is a relatively uncommon finding in acute PE seen more frequently in cases with extensive clot burden.

V/Q scan, which typically shows multiple segmental or lobar mismatched perfusion defects, is recommended as the first line of imaging for patients with suspected CTEPH, with a reported sensitivity of 96% and specificity of 90%.[16] Central nonocclusive or recannulized disease may be missed on V/Q.[17] Advanced MDCT is generally reserved for patients with abnormal V/Q scans and may replace catheter pulmonary angiography in centers with significant experience with CTEPH evaluation. MDCT has been shown to have high sensitivity and specificity values at the main and lobar levels in comparison to digital subtraction pulmonary angiography (DSPA) but lower sensitivities at and beyond the segmental level.[17] Obviating the risks of an invasive procedure and the ability to detect alternative diagnoses are key advantages of CTPA, but given the reported lower sensitivity for distal disease, a false-negative diagnosis of CTEPH is possible.[18]

CTPA features of CTEPH can be grouped into vascular, cardiac, and parenchymal findings.[19] Vascular findings include (**Fig. 4**)

- Eccentric or mural thrombus with or without calcification
- Vessel occlusion (pouch deformity) with peripheral attenuation
- Vascular stenoses or beading
- Intraluminal webs or bands
- Bronchial or systemic artery collateralization

Unlike acute emboli in which the thrombus is commonly centrally located in the vessel lumen or, if peripheral, forms acute angles with the vessel wall, chronic organized emboli are eccentric and form obtuse margins with the vessel wall. Calcifications are rare. Bronchial artery enlargement (>2 mm near the aorta) is more characteristic of chronic than acute PE and has been shown to be a marker of more central clot burden.[20]

Cardiac findings (which are seen in pulmonary hypertension not specific for CTEPH) include (**Fig. 5**)

- Dilated main (>29 mm) and central pulmonary arteries

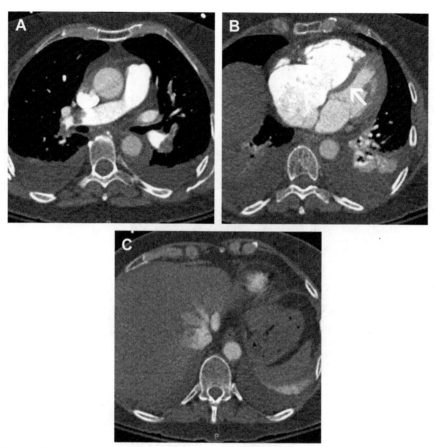

Fig. 3. Cardiac manifestations of acute PE. (*A*) Axial CT images demonstrate acute bilateral PE in the proximal pulmonary arteries. (*B*) There is dilatation of the right atrium and ventricle with leftward bowing of the interventricular septum (*arrow*) indicative of elevated pulmonary artery pressures. (*C*) Reflux of contrast into a mildly dilated intrahepatic inferior vena cava is also noted suggesting tricuspid regurgitation.

- Right ventricular and atrial dilatation
- Right ventricular hypertrophy
- Flattening or leftward bowing of the interventricular septum
- Dilated inferior vena cava and hepatic veins with or without contrast reflux (suggesting tricuspid regurgitation)
- Patent foramen ovale

A main pulmonary artery diameter increase greater than 29 mm and a ratio of main pulmonary artery diameter to ascending aortic diameter greater than 1 strongly suggest elevated pulmonary pressures.[21] An RV:LV diameter ratio greater than or equal to 1 is indicative of right ventricular enlargement, and flattening of the interventricular septum indicates elevated right ventricular pressures.

Pulmonary parenchymal findings include (**Fig. 6**)

- Mosaic attenuation
- Peripheral parenchymal scarring/opacities
- Bronchiectasis

Mosaic attenuation refers to geographic areas of higher and lower attenuation seen within the lung parenchyma when viewed at lung window settings and has been reported in a majority of CTEPH patients. When due to CTEPH, the vessels are often noticeably diminutive in the areas of hyperlucency. The more common cause of mosaic attenuation is small airways disease and, if there is diagnostic uncertainty, exhalation imaging can be performed that would show persistent lucency in the setting of air trapping. Mosaic attenuation has been noted to be more frequent in patients with persistent pulmonary hypertension after pulmonary endarterectomy (PEA), suggesting that it may indicate a more distal distribution of disease, especially when out of proportion to central findings.[22] Parenchymal opacities and pleural thickening are thought to represent sequelae of scarring from prior infarction.

PEA is the only curative treatment of CTEPH. An invasive surgical procedure that involves surgical removal of the organized thrombus and inner arterial wall from the main, lobar, and segmental

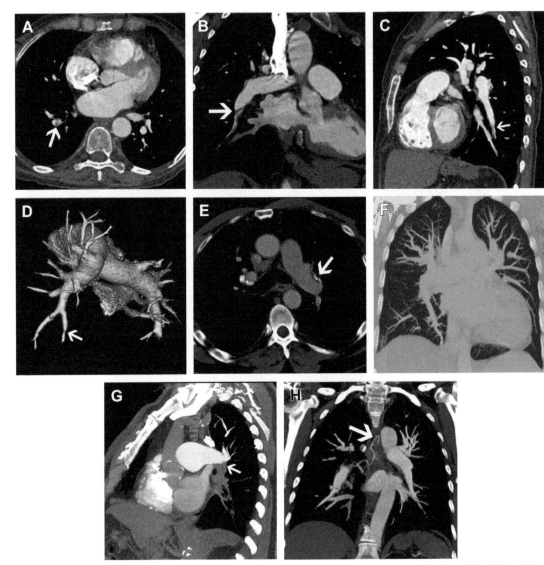

Fig. 4. Vascular manifestations of CTEPH. (*A, B*) Intravascular web (*arrows*), thin central ribbon-like filling defect is seen in the right lower lobar pulmonary artery extending into a segmental branch of a patient with CTEPH. (*C*) Intimal irregularity and eccentric thrombus can be seen in a different patient (*arrow*). (*D*) Focal vascular stenosis (*arrow*) can also occur due to central vascular recanalization. (*E*) Calcification may occasionally occur in eccentric, organized thrombus (*arrow*). (*F*) Increased vascular tortuosity and areas of diminutive vascularity are typical in CTEPH as seen on a coronal MIP image. (*G*) Chronic vascular occlusion as seen on this oblique sagittal CT (*arrow*) can be differentiated from that seen in acute disease by virtue of the concave appearance of the contrast column and the decrease in size of peripheral pulmonary branch vessels. (*H*) Lastly, bronchial artery enlargement may be encountered (*arrow*) and has been shown to correlate with a greater central clot burden.

pulmonary arteries, PEA has a relatively low operative mortality at experienced centers of 4% to 10%.[23] A key factor in operability is the presence of a proximal distribution of clot burden and exclusion of comorbidities, such as chronic obstructive pulmonary disease or interstitial lung disease, left ventricular dysfunction, and malignancy. Up to 40% of patients evaluated are considered nonoperable.[24]

PULMONARY ARTERIOVENOUS MALFORMATIONS

PAVMs are direct vascular communications between pulmonary arterioles and venules without intervening capillary networks. Although rare in the general population, more than 70% of patients who are diagnosed with PAVMs are found to have the autosomal dominant genetic disorder,

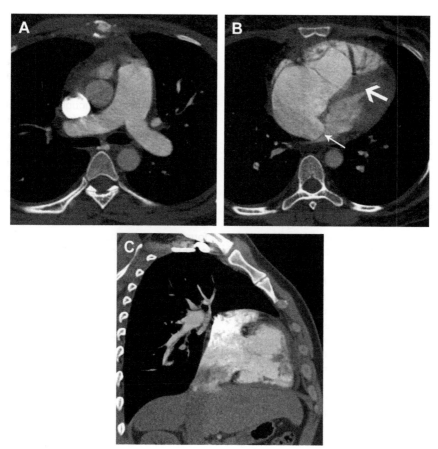

Fig. 5. Cardiac manifestations of CTEPH. (*A*) Enlargement of the main and central pulmonary arteries is noted on axial image with the main pulmonary artery larger than the adjacent aorta. (*B*) The right atrium and right ventricle are enlarged with minimal right ventricular thickening. Flattening of the interventricular septum and leftward bulge of the interatrial septum (*arrows*) are indicative of elevated pulmonary pressures. (*C*) Dilatation and reflux of contrast into the inferior vena cava suggest tricupsid regurgitation as seen on an oblique sagittal image. Note that these findings are not specific for CTEPH but can be seen in any cause of pulmonary hypertension.

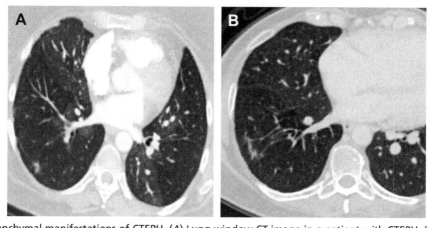

Fig. 6. Parenchymal manifestations of CTEPH. (*A*) Lung window CT image in a patient with CTEPH demonstrates mosaic attenuation (geographic areas of alternating lower and higher attenuation) due to areas of relative hypoperfusion. Note that the vessels in the lower attenuation areas are diminutive in comparison to the higher attenuation regions, indicating a small vessel etiology. (*B*) Peripheral areas of parenchymal consolidation (*right lower lobe*) and pleural thickening with associated architectural distortion are indicative of scarring likely from prior infarction.

hereditary hemorrhagic telangiectasia (HHT).[25] HHT is a consensus diagnosis, using the Curaçao diagnostic criteria[26]:

- Recurrent and spontaneous epistaxis
- Multiple mucocutaneous telangiectasias
- Visceral arteriovenous malformations (AVMs) (pulmonary, hepatic, cerebral, and so forth)
- First-degree relative with HHT (or genetic mutation)

Patients are graded as definite (3 or more), suspected (2), or unlikely (1 or fewer) for HHT. Although AVMs can be seen in virtually any organ, lesions are especially common in the gastrointestinal tract, lung, liver, and brain. More than 40% of patients screened for PAVMs in the setting of HHT are positive.[27]

Acquired PAVMs account for a minority of lesions and can be seen in penetrating chest trauma, hepatic cirrhosis (hepatopulmonary syndrome), and infections, such as schistosomiasis. In patients with univentricular congenital heart disease repaired with a unidirectional or bidirectional Glenn shunt (superior vena cava to pulmonary artery- anastomosis), 25% have been reported to develop PAVMs.[28] Although the mechanism is unclear, it is postulated that hepatic factors responsible for the inhibition of AVM development play a role given the prevalence of lesions in the right lung, which is sometimes excluded from admixture with hepatic venous blood (unilateral Glenn shunt).

Although many remain asymptomatic, PAVMs in HHT can lead to complications, such as transient ischemic attack, stroke, and brain abscess, presumably due to paradoxic embolization.[29] Migraine headaches are another common finding. Less commonly, due to right-to-left shunting in the setting of numerous PAVMs, hypoxia can develop. Lesions along the pleura and tracheobronchial tree can rupture causing hemothorax or hemoptysis, respectively. Hemorrhagic complications are known to be increased during pregnancy, particularly latter stages, due to a combination of factors, such as decreased vascular wall stability and increased cardiac output.[30]

Agitated saline contrast transthoracic echocardiography is the study of choice for screening patients with suspected HHT for PAVM, with a sensitivity of more than 98%.[31] The appearance of the air bubbles in the left atrium after 3 to 8 cardiac cycles is indicative of a shunt at the pulmonary level. MDCT has replaced DSPA for evaluation of patients with suspected abnormality on chest radiography or abnormal echocardiography because it has been shown to have a higher sensitivity (83% vs 70%) for PAVMs.[32] In addition, it obviates repeated invasive examinations in an often younger population, who need repeated screening (generally every 5–10 years for those with an initial negative screen and more frequent in those with treated or untreated PAVM).[26] Although a noncontrast examination with 1-mm reconstructions is adequate for detecting PAVMs, at the authors' center intravenous contrast (similar to PE protocol discussed previously) is used to allow for better vascular assessment, screening for extrapulmonary AVMs such as liver lesions, and 3-D reconstruction of larger lesions in preparation for treatment. A low-dose precontrast examination is still performed at the time of initial screening to avoid confusing calcified granulomas, which frequently have feeding arteries, with PAVMs. IV microfilters are not used because they do not allow for automated high-rate injections; however, a wet-to-wet hookup technique is rigorously applied to avoid the risk of paradoxic air embolization. Data are viewed on a dedicated 3-D workstation with multiplanar thin maximum intensity projection (MIP) images on lung window settings at 4- to 5-mm thickness to optimize detection.

Diagnosing PAVM requires the detection of both a feeding artery and a draining vein coursing to and from the nidus (Fig. 7). Granulomas, certain nonthrombotic emboli, and infections can have feeding arteries and mimic PAVMs (Fig. 8). Rarely, pulmonary vein varices (usually in the setting of fibrosing mediastinitis) can mimic PAVMs.

A majority of PAVMs are classified as simple, meaning that there is a single feeding artery and a single draining vein, whereas 20% are classified as complex with more than 1 feeding artery.[33] A vast majority of PAVMs are fed by the pulmonary arteries but rarely systemic vessels, such as intercostal, phrenic, and internal mammary arteries, can be the feeding source. Atypical lesions are not infrequently encountered, such as ground-glass opacities (telangiectatic PAVM) and pulmonary fissural vessels (Fig. 9). Numerous or diffuse PAVMs are much more common in the setting of HHT.

Characterization of the morphology, anatomic location, number, and size of feeding arteries is required. The size of the feeding artery, measured beyond the segmental portion of the vessel proximal to the nidus, is the most important information provided from MDCT because lesions with feeding arteries measuring 3 mm or greater in size are targeted for embolization with coils or endovascular plugs given the high rate of complications with lesions of this size.[34] Patients with PAVM and feeding arteries in the 2- to 3-mm size range

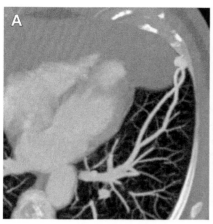
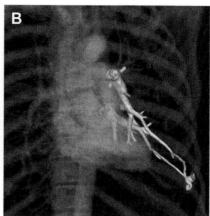

Fig. 7. Simple PAVM. (*A*) In this patient with HHT, a nidus of an arteriovenous malformation is seen in the lingula with a single feeding artery and single draining vein on an axial MIP image. (*B*) Contrast-enhanced examinations permit 3-D image generation that can be useful in preparation for transcatheter treatment.

usually go on to catheter angiography because many are treatable. After transcatheter treatment, a follow-up examination is recommended in 6 to 12 months and every 3 years thereafter due to the known incidence of reperfusion (due to incomplete occlusion, recanalization, or additional feeding artery recruitment) of up to 15% and the interval growth of smaller PAVMs estimated to occur in approximately 18% of patients.[26,35] After embolization, the artery beyond the point of occlusion as well as the nidus should shrink in size and lack enhancement (**Fig. 10**). Enhancement of the draining vein may persist due to retrograde venous flow and should not be mistaken for reperfusion.

Attention to the upper abdominal organs, especially on contrast-enhanced examinations, is important because many patients with PAVM are eventually diagnosed with HHT. At the authors'

institution, the abdomen is routinely imaged in the arterial phase at the time of initial screening. Hepatic AVMs on MDCT have been reported in more than 50% of patients with HHT and can be seen either as vascular blushes, early hepatic or portal vein enhancement, or dilatation of the celiac axis and hepatic artery.[36] Gastrointestinal, pancreatic, and renal AVMs also may be seen and lend support for the diagnosis of HHT.

PULMONARY VASCULITIS

Inflammation and destruction of vascular walls is characteristic of vasculitis and encompasses a wide range of etiologies, including infection, hypersensitivity, and malignancy, although many are idiopathic. The primary vasculitides are categorized according to size of the predominantly

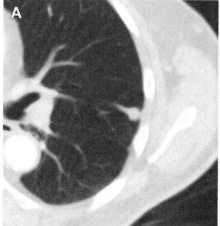
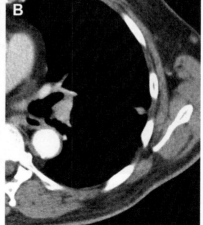

Fig. 8. PAVM mimick. (*A*) A feeding vessel coursing to a nodule in the left upper lobe may be confused for an artery coursing to the nidus of a PAVM. (*B*) On soft tissue window, however, there is no enhancement of the nidus, as this represented a noncalcified granuloma.

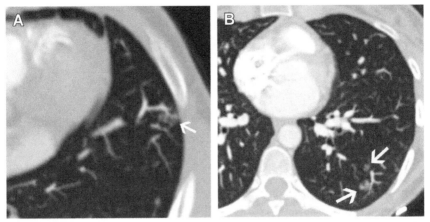

Fig. 9. Telangiectatic PAVMs. (*A, B*) A commonly encountered "atypical" type of PAVM is the cloud-like or purely ground-glass nidus (*arrows*) where numerous tiny vascular connections between the arteriole and venule form that cannot be resolved at the spatial resolution of MDCT.

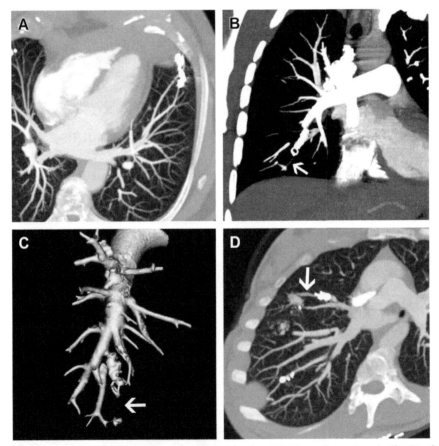

Fig. 10. Treated PAVMs. (*A*) After coil embolization of the simple PAVM from the patient in **Fig. 7**A, the nidus has nearly resolved and no longer is opacified on an axial thin MIP image. In the post-treatment evaluation to assess for reperfusion of a nidus, be aware of the possibility of venous backfilling of the nidus mimicking recanalization. (*B, C*) Note, in a different patient with a treated PAVM, that the feeding artery proximal to the nidus but beyond the coils (*arrows*) is no longer opacified, although there is still some opacification of the nidus itself. (*D*) This is in contrast to a patient with recanalization of a previously treated feeding artery where there is persistent opacification of the feeding artery distal to the coils (*arrow*) and enhancement of the nidus.

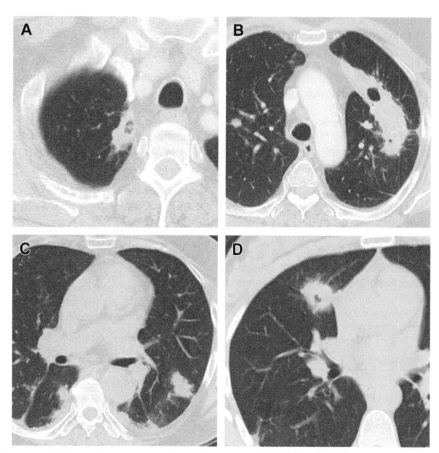

Fig. 11. GPA. In a c-ANCA–positive patient with the diagnosis of GPA (*A–C*), multiple nodules and areas of consolidation are seen, many of which demonstrate central areas of cavitation, a common feature for nodules larger than 2 cm in size. (*D*) Faint perilesional ground-glass is seen around a nodule in the right middle lobe in a different patient indicative of hemorrhage related to the underlying vasculitis.

affected vessels and the nomenclature was recently updated in 2012 to more accurately reflect the underlying diseases.[37] Large-vessel vasculitis involves the aorta and its major branches as well as the accompanying veins, medium vessel vasculitis involves the main visceral branches, and small vessel vasculitis involves the parenchymal arteries, veins, and microvasculature. These are not exclusive categories, and many disease entities have manifestations in various-sized vessels. Although a thorough review of all the pulmonary vasculitides is beyond the scope of this article, the entities more commonly encountered involving the pulmonary circulation are discussed briefly with emphasis on thoracic radiographic manifestations.

Granulomatosis with Polyangitis

The most common of the antineutrophil cytoplasmic antibody (ANCA)-associated vasculitides, granulomatosis with polyangiitis (GPA), formerly referred to as Wegener granulomatosis, is a necrotizing small vessel vasculitis associated with vascular

and extravascular granuloma formation. Although not exclusive, a vast majority of patients with active disease are cytoplasmic (c)-ANCA (proteinase 3–ANCA) positive. Characteristically, there is

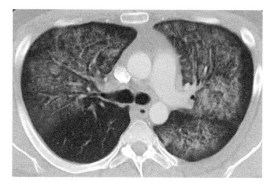

Fig. 12. MPA. Lung window image from a patient who presented with renal failure and dyspnea demonstrating diffuse ground-glass opacity sparing the peripheral portions of the lungs indicative of diffuse alveolar hemorrhage, the most common pulmonary manifestation of MPA.

involvement of the upper and lower respiratory tract and kidneys although many organ systems can be involved at various time points and limited forms involving only the lungs occur in up to 25%.[38]

Upper tract involvement is ubiquitous and characterized by recurrent sinus infections, ulcerations, nasal wall deformities and, within the trachea and mainstem bronchi, wall thickening, masses, and commonly subglottic stenoses.[39] Lower tract disease afflicts small arteries, capillaries, and veins, leading to the development of predominantly peribronchovascular nodules and consolidation and occasionally diffuse ground-glass indicative of diffuse alveolar hemorrhage. Multiple pulmonary nodules are the most common form of pulmonary involvement and when larger than 2 cm have a high propensity to cavitate (**Fig. 11**).[40] Approximately 15% of lesions have associated ground-glass halos indicative of perilesional hemorrhage. As is typical of most vasculitides, pulmonary manifestations often have a waxing, waning, or migratory appearance with or without treatment.

Microscopic Polyangitis

Microscopic polyangitis (MPA) is a necrotizing vasculitis without significant immune deposition features that does not have extravascular inflammation or granuloma formation. It is more closely associated with perinuclear-ANCA (myeloperoxidase-ANCA) and has high rates of rapidly progressive glomerulonephritis. Pulmonary vascular involvement again centers on arteries, capillaries, and veins, with diffuse pulmonary hemorrhage one of the most common pulmonary manifestations, occurring in up to 30%.[41] It is a frequent cause of pulmonary-renal syndrome. Radiographically, diffuse areas of ground-glass and/or high-density consolidation can be seen, often sparing the periphery indicative of hemorrhage due to capillaritis (**Fig. 12**). Repeated episodes of pulmonary hemorrhage can lead to pulmonary fibrosis, similar to idiopathic pulmonary hemosiderosis, and iron deficiency anemia.[42]

Eosinophilic Granulomatosis with Polyangitis (Churg-Strauss)

The least common of the ANCA vasculitides is eosinophilic GPA (EGPA), which is a necrotizing, granulomatous small vessel vasculitis associated with asthma and eosinophilia. American College of Rheumatology criteria require 4 of the following 6 criteria to establish the diagnosis[43]:

- Asthma (often adult onset and severe)
- Greater than 10% eosinophils on a differential leukocyte count
- Mononeuropathy or polyneuropathy
- Radiographic migratory or transient pulmonary opacities
- Paranasal sinus abnormalities (especially nasal polyps)
- Extravascular eosinophil accumulation on biopsy

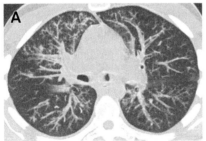
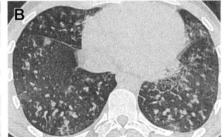
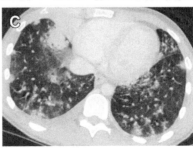

Fig. 13. EGPA. (*A*) Thin MIP lung window image from an asthmatic patient who presented with eosinophilia and dyspnea demonstrates centrilobular nodules and bronchovascular thickening. (*B*) Mosaic attenuation and bronchial wall thickening are noted in the lung bases indicative of small airways involvement. (*C*) Two days later the patient developed a right pleural effusion and areas of peripheral consolidation in the lung bases with surrounding faint ground-glass in keeping with active vasculitis. Biopsy revealed changes consistent with EGPA.

The disease progresses in phases, initially with a prodromal phase predominated by asthma and allergic manifestations, such as allergic rhinitis.[44] The eosinophilic phase is typically when the first radiographic manifestations are seen due to peripheral blood eosinophilia and organ infiltration by eosinophils. The lung and skin are the most commonly affected organ systems. Areas of peripheral, often lobular, consolidation and ground-glass opacity are manifestations of lung involvement and may be transient or migratory, mimicking simple pulmonary eosinophilia and organizing pneumonia or, over time, chronic eosinophilic pneumonia (**Fig. 13**).[45] Centrilobular nodules and bronchial dilatation may also be encountered either due to coexisting asthma or direct eosinophilic infiltration. Nodules and cavitation are rare and more typical of GPA. The vasculitic phase occurs later and can affect a variety of organ systems. Cardiac involvement accounts for approximately 50% of mortality and can manifest as cardiomyopathy, pericarditis, or endomyocarditis. Cardiac magnetic resonance can be used to assess for areas of wall motion abnormality, delayed contrast enhancement, or chamber thrombi.

SUMMARY

It is important to be familiar with the imaging manifestations of pulmonary vascular diseases, especially in an era where there is widespread and routine use of high-quality CTPA. Recognition of imaging features of various diseases is often crucial in assisting clinicians with establishing a diagnosis. Although thromboembolic disease is the most commonly encountered pulmonary vascular disease, other rarer diseases, such as PAVMs and vasculitis, must be kept in mind because they can have a variety of clinical and radiographic presentations. In the end, a comprehensive and multidisciplinary approach is required when dealing with pulmonary vascular disease.

REFERENCES

1. Naess IA, Christiansen SC, Romundstadt P, et al. Incidence and mortality of venous thrombosis: a population-based study. J Thromb Haemost 2007; 5(4):692–9.
2. Komissarova M, Chong S, Frey K, et al. Imaging of acute pulmonary embolism. Emerg Radiol 2013; 20(2):89–101.
3. Moser KM, Fedullo PF, LitteJohn JK, et al. Frequent asymptomatic pulmonary embolism in patients with deep venous thrombosis. JAMA 1994;271(3):223–5.
4. van Belle A, Buller HR, Huisman MV, et al. Effectiveness of managing suspected pulmonary embolism using an algorithm combining clinical probability, D-dimer testing, and computed tomography. JAMA 2006;295(2):172–9.
5. Stein PD, Fowler SE, Goodman LR, et al. Multidetector computed tomography for acute pulmonary embolism. N Engl J Med 2006;354(22):2317–27.
6. Hall WB, Truitt SG, Scheunemann LP, et al. The prevalence of clinically relevant incidental findings on chest computed tomographic angiograms ordered to diagnose pulmonary embolism. Arch Intern Med 2009;169(21):1961–5.
7. Wittram C, Maher MM, Yoo AJ, et al. CT angiography of pulmonary embolism: diagnostic criteria and causes of misdiagnosis. Radiographics 2004;24:1219–38.
8. Patel S, Kazerooni EA. Helical CT for the evaluation of acute pulmonary embolism. AJR Am J Roentgenol 2005;185(1):135–49.
9. Lim KE, Chan CY, Chu PH, et al. Right ventricular dysfunction secondary to acute massive pulmonary embolism detected by helical computed tomography pulmonary angiography. Clin Imaging 2005;29: 16–21.
10. Gosselin MV, Rubin GD, Leung AN, et al. Unsuspected pulmonary embolism: prostective detection on routine helical CT scans. Radiology 1998;208:209–15.
11. Pengo V, Lensing AW, Prins MH, et al. Incidence of chronic thromboembolic pulmonary hypertension after pulmonary embolism. N Engl J Med 2004; 350(22):2257–64.
12. Auger WR, Kim NH, Kerr KM, et al. Chronic thromboembolic pulmonary hypertension. Clin Chest Med 2007;28(1):255–69.
13. Fedullo PF, Rubin LJ, Kerr KM, et al. The natural history of acute and chronic thromboembolic disease: the search for the missing link. Eur Respir J 2000; 15(3):435–7.
14. Moser KM, Bloor CM. Pulmonary vascular lesions occurring in patients with chronic major vessel thromboembolic pulmonary hypertension. Chest 1994;105(5):1619–20.
15. Galie N, Hoeper MM, Humbert M, et al. Guidelines for the diagnosis and treatment of pulmonary hypertension: the task force for the diagnosis and treatment of pulmonary hypertension of the European Society of Cardiology (ESC) and the European Respiratory Society (ERS), endorsed by the International Society of Heart and Lung Transplanatation (ISHLT). Eur Heart J 2009;30:2493–537.
16. Ryan KL, Fedullo PF, Davis GB, et al. Perfusion scan findings understate the severity of angiographic and hemodynamic compromise in chronic thromboembolic pulmonary hypertension. Chest 1988;93(6): 1180–5.
17. Sugiura T, Tanabe N, Matsuura Y, et al. Role of 320-slice CT imaging in the diagnostic workup of patients with chronic thromboembolic pulmonary hypertension. Chest 2013;143:1070–7.

18. Wilkens H, Lang I, Behr J, et al. Chronic thromboembolic pulmonary hypertension (CTEPH): updated recommendations of the Cologne Consensus Conference 2011. Int J Cardiol 2011;154(Suppl 1):S54–60.

19. Willemink MJ, van Es HW, Koobs L, et al. CT evaluation of chronic thromboembolic pulmonary hypertension. Clin Radiol 2012;67(3):277–85.

20. Schimizu H, Tanabe N, Terada J, et al. Dilatation of bronchial arteries correlates with extent of central disease in patients with chronic thromboembolic pulmonary hypertension. Circ J 2008;72(7):1136–41.

21. Frazier AA, Galvin JR, Franks TJ, et al. From the archives of AFIP: pulmonary vasculature: hypertension and infarction. Radiographics 2000;20(2):491–524.

22. Sherrick AD, Swensen SJ, Hartman TE. Mosaic pattern of lung attenuation on CT scans: frequency among patients with pulmonary artery hypertension of different causes. AJR Am J Roentgenol 1997; 169:79–82.

23. Mayer E, Jenkins D, Lindner J, et al. Surgical management and outcome of patients with chronic thromboembolic pulmonary hypertension: results from an international prospective registry. J Thorac Cardiovasc Surg 2011;141:702–10.

24. Jenkins D, Mayer E, Screaton N, et al. State-of-the-art chronic thromboembolic pulmonary hypertension diagnosis and management. Eur Respir Rev 2012; 21(123):32–9.

25. Cottin V, Dupuis-Girod S, Lesca G, et al. Pulmonary vascular manifestations of hereditary hemorrhagic telangiectasia (Rendu-Osler disease). Respiration 2007;74(4):361–78.

26. Faughnan ME, Palda VA, Garcia-Tsao G, et al. International guidelines for the diagnosis and management of hereditary haemorrhagic telangiectasia. J Med Genet 2011;48(2):73–87.

27. Fraughnan ME, Granton JT, Young LH. The pulmonary vascular complications of hereditary haemorrhagic telangiectasia. Eur Respir J 2009;33:1186–94.

28. Duncan BW, Desai S. Pulmonary arteriovenous malformations after cavopulmonary anastomosis. Ann Thorac Surg 2003;76:1759–66.

29. White RI, Lynch-Nyhan A, Terry P, et al. Pulmonary arteriovenous malformations: techniques and long-term outcome of embolotherapy. Radiology 1988; 169(3):663–9.

30. Gossage JR, Kanj G. Pulmonary arteriovenous malformations. A state of the art review. Am J Respir Crit Care Med 1998;158(2):643–61.

31. Gossage JR. Role of contrast echocardiography in screening for pulmonary arteriovenous malformation in patients with hereditary hemorrhagic telangiectasia. Chest 2010;138:769–71.

32. Nawaz A, Litt HI, Stavropoulos W, et al. Digital subtraction pulmonary arteriography versus multidetector CT in the detection of pulmonary arteriovenous malformations. J Vasc Interv Radiol 2008;19:1582–8.

33. White RI, Mitchell SE, Barth KH, et al. Angioarchitecture of pulmonary arteriovenous malformations: an important consideration before embolotherapy. AJR Am J Roentgenol 1983;140(4):681–6.

34. White RI, Pollak JS, Wirth JA. Pulmonary arteriovenous malformations: diagnosis and transcatheter embolotherapy. J Vasc Interv Radiol 1996;7: 787–804.

35. Remy-Jardin M, Dumont P, Brillet PY, et al. Pulmonary arteriovenous malformations treated with embolotherapy: helical CT evaluation of long-term effectiveness after 2-21 year follow-up. Radiology 2006;239(2):576–85.

36. Buscarini E, Plauchu H, Garcia Tsao G, et al. Liver involvement in hereditary hemorrhagic telangiectasia: consensus recommendations. Liver Int 2006; 26:1040–6.

37. Jennette JC, Falk RJ, Bacon PA, et al. 2012 revised International Chapel Hill Consensus Conference Nomenclature of Vasculitides. Arthritis Rheum 2013;65(1):1–11.

38. Stone JH, Wegner's Granulomatosis Etanercept Trial Research Group. Limited versus severe Wegener's granulomatosis: baseline data on patients in the Wegener's granulomatosis etanercept trail. Arthritis Rheum 2003;48(8):2299–309.

39. Martinez F, Chung JH, Digumarthy SR, et al. Common and uncommon manifestations of Wegener granulomatosis at chest CT: radiologic-pathologic correlation. Radiographics 2012;32(1):51–69.

40. Marten K, Schnyder P, Schirg E, et al. Pattern-based differential diagnosis in pulmonary vasculitis using volumetric CT. Am J Roentgenol 2005;184: 720–33.

41. Engelke C, Schaefer-Prokop C, Schirg E, et al. High-resolution CT and CT angiography of peripheral pulmonary vascular disorders. Radiographics 2002; 22(4):739–64.

42. Masi AT, Hunder GG, Lie JT, et al. The American College of Rheumatology 1990 criteria for the classification of Churg-Strauss syndrome (allergic granulomatosis and angiitis). Arthritis Rheum 1990;33(8): 1094–100.

43. Pagnoux C, Guillevin L. Churg-Strauss syndrome: evidence for disease subtypes? Curr Opin Rheumatol 2010;22(1):21–8.

44. Jeong YJ, Kim KI, Seo IJ, et al. Eosinophilic lung diseases: a clinical, radiologic, and pathologic overview. Radiographics 2007;27(3):617–37.

45. Choi YH, Im JG, Han BK, et al. Thoracic manifestation of Churg-Strauss syndrome: radiologic and clinical findings. Chest 2000;117:117–24.

Occupational and Environmental Lung Disease

Danielle M. Seaman, MD[a],*, Cristopher A. Meyer, MD[b],
Jeffrey P. Kanne, MD[b]

KEYWORDS

- Silica • Coal • Asbestos • Hard metal • Beryllium • Occupational asthma
- Hypersensitivity pneumonitis • Biomass

KEY POINTS

- Occupational and environmental lung disease is a major cause of respiratory impairment worldwide.
- Despite regulations, exposures to the "classic" dusts, such as silica, coal, and asbestos, continue to be a worldwide cause of disease.
- New etiologies for occupational lung disease continue to emerge, and known causes are emerging in new industries.
- Nonoccupational environmental lung disease contributes to major respiratory disease, asthma, and chronic obstructive pulmonary disease.
- Knowledge of the imaging patterns of occupational and environmental lung disease is critical in managing patients with suspected or occult exposures.

INTRODUCTION

The association of occupational lung disease (OLD) with mining has been recognized since the 1500s when silica exposure and tuberculosis were described by Agricola.[1] Occupational and environmental lung diseases still remain major causes of pulmonary impairment worldwide. Globally, Driscoll and colleagues[2] report an estimated 386,000 respiratory deaths and almost 6.6 million disability adjusted life years (DALYS) attributable to occupational airborne particulates.

The "classic" mineral dust pneumoconioses, asbestos, silica, and coal, remain a worldwide problem. The Comparative Risk Assessment Study by the World Health Organization estimates that these pneumoconioses resulted in 30,000 deaths and 1,288,000 DALYS; it has been suggested that the methodology in this study grossly underestimated the number of deaths due to strict data collection requirements.[3]

In the United States, industrial regulations have decreased the prevalence of pneumoconioses. Since the introduction of the Coal Miners Health and Safety Act in 1969, the percentage of underground miners with a 20-year to 24-year tenure with radiographic findings of coal worker's pneumoconiosis (CWP) declined from 32.8% in 1970 to 1.9% in 2009. Despite these strict regulations, higher rates of CWP and progressive massive

Disclosures: Dr. DM Seaman is NIOSH Certified B reader. She has received consultant fees in conjunction with medicolegal expert testimony in the field of occupational lung disease. Research grant funding from Bracco Diagnostics Inc. Dr. CA Meyer is NIOSH Certified B reader. He has received grant funding, honoraria for film interpretation and lectures on occupational lung disease as well as consultant fees in conjunction with medicolegal expert testimony. Dr JP Kanne is NIOSH Certified B reader and consultant for Parexel Informatics.
a Duke University Medical Center, 1612 Bivins Street, Durham, NC 27707, USA; b University of Wisconsin School of Medicine and Public Health, 600 Highland Avenue, MC 3252, Madison, WI 53792, USA
* Corresponding author.
E-mail address: seaman.danielle@gmail.com

fibrosis (PMF) are reported in mines with fewer than 50 employees compared with larger mines.[4]

Immunologic factors contribute to OLD. Hypersensitivity pneumonitis (HP) occurs across professions. Hard metal and beryllium result in immune-mediated toxicity. Recent literature proposes the concept of mixed-dust exposure resulting in an immune-mediated chronic interstitial pneumonia pattern, although the impact of smoking and environmental risk factors remain unclear.[5]

Airway-related respiratory disease is the largest category of OLD, with estimates that occupational exposure accounts for 11% of asthma morbidity and mortality, translating globally to 38,000 deaths and 1.6 million DALYS.[6] Occupational diacetyl exposure and nylon flock are recognized causes of airways disease.

Finally, nonoccupational environmental exposures significantly contribute to major respiratory disease, asthma, and chronic obstructive pulmonary disease (COPD). Four major drivers of global lung disease are tobacco, indoor air pollution (biomass fuel burning), external air pollution, and occupational exposure.[6] A thorough evaluation of these factors is beyond the scope of this article. The contribution of tobacco and age in the development of lung fibrosis is briefly discussed.[7,8]

Identifying occupational exposures as a cause of lung injury requires a thorough knowledge of the patient's history, physical examination, laboratory testing, and medical imaging. The low cost and limited radiation exposure of chest radiography make it the most widely used medical imaging examination for workforce screening. High-resolution computed tomography (HRCT) has become the test of choice for characterizing diffuse lung disease, even supplanting the need for surgical lung biopsy in many patients with idiopathic pulmonary fibrosis.[9] The sensitivity and specificity of HRCT exceed those of chest radiography in the setting of pneumoconiosis.[10] This article reviews the findings of the classic mineral dust pneumoconioses, immune-mediated, and airway centric OLDs, and describes several more common environmental lung diseases. Given the often long latency of these diseases and occasionally occult nature of exposures, physicians must anticipate these diseases in their practice and recognize characteristic imaging features.

IMAGING FEATURES OF OCCUPATIONAL LUNG DISEASE
Dusts

Pathophysiology of particulate clearance
Pneumoconiosis, meaning "dusty lungs," is most often due to coal dust, silica dust, and asbestos fiber inhalation and is among the most common causes of OLD. When dust is inhaled, the larger particulates deposit on the mucosa of the nose and large airways and are cleared by mucociliary transport in approximately 8 hours. Smaller particles reach the alveoli and are phagocytized by alveolar macrophages. Macrophages migrate to the lymphatics where they are eliminated. Lymphatic drainage is driven by pulmonary artery pressure (lower in the apices and on the right) and chest wall excursion (lowest in the upper posterior chest wall). The slowest lymphatic clearance and thus greatest retention of particles is in the upper posterior lung, right worse than left. A high particulate burden rapidly overwhelms these mechanisms. Macrophage aggregates may be engulfed by type I pneumocytes and incorporated into the interstitium. Dust particles can cause direct epithelial damage, resulting in bronchitis and impaired ciliary clearance. Alveolar macrophages release inflammatory mediators that produce extracellular matrix components, such as collagen, and stimulate fibroblasts leading to fibrosis. Recruitment of peripheral blood monocytes and neutrophils causes alveolar inflammation and damage to the alveolar epithelial cells. Damage to the airspaces can result in emphysema. Mineral dust exposure is a complex interaction of reactive oxygen species, antioxidants, cytokines, growth factors, eicosanoids, proteases, and antiproteases, leading to lung dysfunction and pathology.[11]

Deposition of fibers depends on the ratio of fiber length and width (aspect ratio), which determines aerodynamic properties. Deposition in larger airways occurs as the ends of inhaled fibers impact the mucosa, particularly at sites of directional change, such as bifurcations. Most fibers deposited in the mucosa are removed via mucociliary clearance, migrating fibers to the larynx to be swallowed and removed by the gastrointestinal tract. In the periphery, airflow is slower, and fibers settle by gravity. Thin fibers tend to penetrate deep into the lung, aligning with laminar flow. Fibers deposited in the nonciliated airways beyond the terminal bronchioles may migrate through the epithelium into the interstitium, ultimately leading to pulmonary fibrosis.[12] Fibers cleared via lymphatic drainage to the pleura accumulate at lymphatic stoma inciting inflammation, ultimately leading to pleural plaque formation and mesothelioma.[13] Longer fibers that cannot be broken down or engulfed by alveolar macrophages remain in the lung as asbestos bodies.

Silica
Silica or silicon dioxide is most commonly encountered in its crystalline form (quartz or cristobalite).

Exposures most commonly occur in industries that cut, grind, or drill silica-containing concrete, masonry, tile, and rock and include brick, concrete, and pottery manufacturing, foundries, and sandblasting operations.[14] A new potential industrial exposure is hydraulic fracking where fine sand is driven into fracture sites in the process of natural gas extraction.[4] The Occupational Safety and Health Administration (OSHA) reported that of 116 full-shift air samples collected at 11 fracturing sites in 5 states, 47% were greater than the calculated OSHA permissible exposure limit (PEL) with 9% greater than 10 times the PEL.[15] A recent outbreak of silicosis occurred in workers in Turkey in the process of sandblasting denim to "distress" jeans.[14] The silicotic or hyalinized nodule is the unit lesion of silicosis resulting when the alveolar macrophage phagocytizes silica, resulting in macrophage death and subsequent release of cytokines that incite fibrosis.[16]

Four main types of lung disease occur as a result of silica exposure: simple silicosis, complicated silicosis, accelerated silicosis, and acute silicoproteinosis. Small airways disease may be the first manifestation of silica exposure, manifesting as air trapping on expiratory HRCT.[16] Simple silicosis occurs 10 to 20 years after low to moderate exposure manifesting radiographically as upper-zone

predominant 1-mm to 9-mm nodules with the highest profusion in the posterior lungs, right greater than left (**Fig. 1**). On HRCT, the nodules are centrilobular or perilymphatic in distribution (see **Fig. 1**). Peripheral coalescent nodules may form pseudoplaques or "candle-wax" lesions (see **Fig. 1**).[16] Hilar lymph nodes may enlarge with a classic rimlike pattern of calcification described as "eggshell" (**Fig. 2**). Classically, simple silicosis does not cause symptoms or respiratory impairment.[14] Isolated lymph node enlargement may be the result of lower-level exposure and may precede the development of simple silicosis.[4]

Complicated silicosis or PMF is defined by the presence of coalescent fibrosis termed a large opacity (**Fig. 3**). Large opacities are 1 cm or larger, typically forming in the lung periphery as nodules coalesce; over time, they enlarge and migrate centrally toward the hilum, often resulting in a decreased profusion of small opacities and paracicatricial emphysema (see **Fig. 3**).[16] This is a debilitating disease with progressive dyspnea and functional impairment. The development of complicated disease is more common with silica than coal, as silica is more fibrogenic. Accelerated silicosis is the rapid development of complicated silicosis as a result of very high exposures over a short period of time. This form of silicosis is more

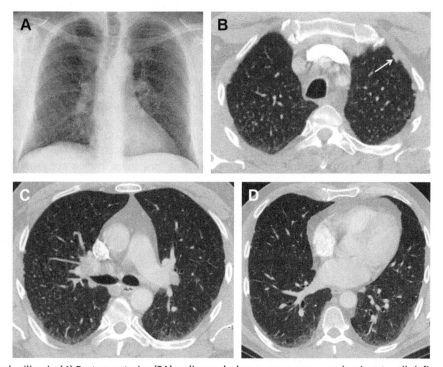

Fig. 1. Simple silicosis. (*A*) Posteroanterior (PA) radiograph shows upper-zone predominant well-defined nodules. (*B–D*) CT images from apex to base confirm solid centrilobular and perilymphatic nodules that are more profuse in the upper lung zones. Note the coalescent subpleural nodules forming pseudoplaques (*arrow*) in (*B*).

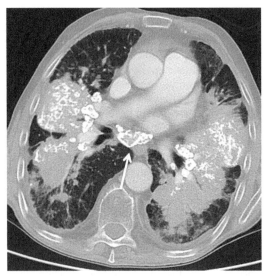

Fig. 2. Silicosis with eggshell calcifications and PMF. CT image showing mediastinal and hilar lymph nodes with peripheral "eggshell" calcifications (*arrow*). Note the calcifications within the large opacities of PMF.

likely to progress, despite removal from the exposure.

Acute silicoproteinosis occurs 1 to 3 years after high levels of silica exposure. Patients typically present with rapidly progressive shortness of breath and constitutional symptoms. Type II pneumocyte proliferation results in excessive surfactant production with lipoproteinaceous material filling the airspaces. On HRCT, a "crazy-paving" pattern is present with extensive ground-glass opacity and interlobular septal thickening (**Fig. 4**). Ill-defined centrilobular nodules and consolidation, which may contain calcification, have been reported. The disease is usually rapidly progressive and fatal.[17]

Silica exposure is associated with an increased risk of mycobacterial infection as a result of damage to alveolar macrophages and impaired

cell-mediated immunity (**Fig. 5**). Although conglomerate masses may spontaneously cavitate, superimposed infection or lung cancer must be suspected (see **Fig. 5**; **Fig. 6**).[4] The International Agency for Research on Cancer classifies silica as a known human carcinogen demonstrating a positive relationship between cumulative silica exposure and mortality from lung cancer.[14] Silica exposure has also been linked to the development of chronic interstitial pneumonia resembling usual interstitial pneumonia (UIP) or nonspecific interstitial pneumonia (NSIP) patterns of fibrosis.[18] Silica has been associated with the development of rheumatoid arthritis, scleroderma, and cytoplasmic antineutrophil cytoplasmic antibody (c-ANCA) associated vasculitis.[4]

Coal dust

Inhalation of coal dust can lead to development of CWP, either simple or complicated. The development of CWP depends on many factors, including coal rank (hardness of the coal), mining method, size of the mine, and the concentration of coal dust exposure.[19] The pathologic lesion of coal dust exposure is the coal macule, a collection of coal dust–laden macrophages (0.5–6 mm) that may be located in the walls of the respiratory bronchioles or adjacent alveoli.[19] Simple CWP is similar radiographically to silicosis with upper-zone, posterior predominant small nodules, greater on the right (**Fig. 7**). With more severe disease, all zones may be involved.[20] Relative to silicosis, the nodules are typically smaller and less well-defined. Similar to silicosis, subpleural pseudoplaques may form as dust accumulates and coalesces in the subpleural lymphatics.[16] Computed tomography (CT) is more sensitive than radiography in detecting low levels of nodule profusion (International Labor Organization classification of profusion 0/1 and 1/0) (**Fig. 8**). The profusion of small nodules on chest radiography in simple CWP

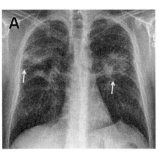
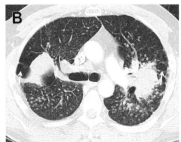
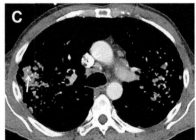

Fig. 3. Complicated silicosis. (*A*) PA radiograph shows upper-zone predominant well-defined nodules and large opacities (≥1 cm) in the mid-lung zones (*arrows*). Note the associated architectural distortion. (*B*) CT image in lung windows confirms the background of small nodules with the large opacities of PMF. Note the paracicatricial emphysema peripheral to the large opacities (*arrows*). (*C*) CT image in soft tissue windows demonstrating that some nodules are calcified (*arrow*).

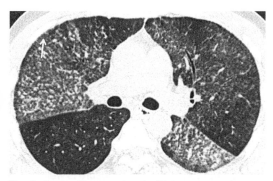

Fig. 4. Acute silicoproteinosis. CT shows extensive centrilobular nodules and ground-glass opacity with scattered areas of interlobular septal thickening (*arrow*). (*Reproduced from* Sirajuddin A, Kanne JP. Occupational lung disease. J Thorac Imaging 2009;24(4):312; with permission.)

does not correlate with the forced expiratory volume in 1 second (FEV1), arterial blood gas values, or subjective dyspnea.[21] This has led to the statement that detection of nodules on HRCT not visible radiographically is a marker of coal dust exposure and not true "disease."[10]

In contrast, complicated CWP can be clinically disabling and potentially fatal. Complicated CWP or PMF is again defined by the presence of an opacity of 1 cm or larger (**Fig. 9**). Large opacities typically begin in the lung periphery with a round or lentiform shape with the lateral border paralleling the pleura. They may enlarge over time and migrate toward the hilum with a decrease in background small nodule profusion (**Fig. 10**). PMF can also cavitate and/or calcify. PMF is less common with coal dust exposure than with silica, as coal is less fibrogenic.[16] MRI is useful in distinguishing

lung cancer, which has high T2 signal as compared with PMF, which is hypointense.[22,23] PET/CT is of limited utility in the diagnosis of lung cancer and mediastinal lymph node staging in the setting of complicated CWP; PMF lesions and malignancy have similar levels of fludeoxyglucose (FDG) avidity (see **Fig. 10**).[24,25] The risk of tuberculosis is also elevated in CWP.

Coal dust exposure can cause chronic bronchitis, emphysema, and COPD, independent of smoking. Rapid declines in FEV1 are reported in miners during their first year of work, even in nonsmokers.[10] Autopsy studies confirm extensive emphysema in coal miners with an emphysema severity index 6 times greater in nonsmoking miners compared with controls.[10] Emphysema score on HRCT correlates better to FEV1, diffusion capacity (DLCO), and symptoms than profusion level of small opacities on chest radiography.[26] Fine linear opacities associated with small nodules at radiography correlate with emphysema (**Fig. 11**).[10]

Rheumatoid pneumoconiosis or Caplan syndrome was first described by Caplan in 1953 and is the presence of large nodules (up to 5 cm) in patients with rheumatoid arthritis. Nodules have a necrotic center and may be cavitary on imaging. Pathologically, the central necrotic core is surrounded by inflammatory cells and dust-filled macrophages, forming a specific ring pattern. Caplan syndrome is also associated with other pneumoconioses caused by asbestos, silica, aluminum, carbon, and dolomite.[16]

Asbestos

Asbestos fibers are a group of fibrous silicates that have high heat resistance, durability, and tensile

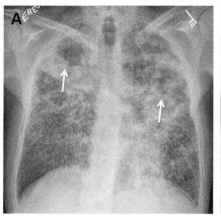

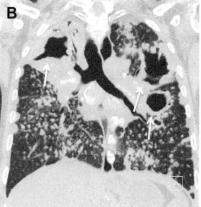

Fig. 5. Complicated silicosis with superimposed nontuberculous mycobacterial infection. (*A*) PA radiograph shows an extensive background of small nodules with large opacities in the right upper zone and left upper and mid zones. There is cavitation within some of the large opacities (*arrows*). Although PMF lesions can cavitate, this should raise the suspicion for the presence of infection or malignancy. (*B*) Coronal reformatted CT image showing the extensive cavitation within the large opacities (*arrows*). Cultures grew *M avium* complex.

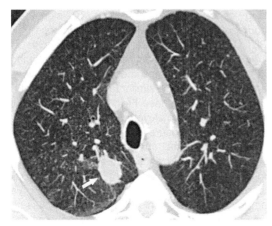

Fig. 6. Silicosis with lung cancer. CT image shows a background of small centrilobular nodules with a mass in the right upper lobe (*arrow*). Although this could represent a large opacity of silicosis, they tend to arise peripherally and have associated architectural distortion. Lung cancer, which was confirmed on biopsy, should be considered in this high-risk population.

strength, and have therefore been used in many industries, including construction and insulation, shipbuilding, and textile manufacturing.[27] The deleterious effects of asbestos exposure have been recognized for decades; nevertheless, the global production of asbestos in 2012 was 2,000,000 tons, with 90% coming from Russia, China, Brazil, and Kazakhstan.[28] There are currently 6 types of regulated asbestos fibers; the serpentine mineral chrysotile and 5 types of amphibole minerals: cummingtonite-grunerite (amosite), riebeckite (crocidolite), actinolite, anthophyllite, and tremolite asbestos.[4] Chrysotile has a serpentine or curly configuration that is more

easily cleared from the lung; amphibole fibers are more rigid and straight and are more fibrogenic and carcinogenic. Some mineral types other than the regulated asbestos fibers can cause the same diseases as asbestos, leading to some controversy regarding how asbestos is defined. Erionite, a mineral used in Turkish home construction, is associated with mesothelioma.[29] Winchite and richterite are a major component of the amphibole fibers contaminating the Libby, MT, vermiculite mine that at one time supplied 80% of the world's supply.[4] Paraoccupational exposure is well recognized, and typically affects occupants in the worker's home as a result of dust accumulation on the worker's hair and clothes.[27] Recently, attention has been given to nonoccupational exposure during home renovations and car maintenance.[27]

The pleura is most frequently affected by asbestos exposure, of which localized pleural thickening or pleural plaque is the most common, occurring in up to 80% of exposed workers (**Fig. 12**). Pleural plaque typically forms 15 to 30 years after exposure and increases with exposure intensity.[16] Plaque almost always localizes to the parietal pleura but can involve the visceral pleura, including the fissures. Plaques are typically bilateral, involving the posterolateral pleura between the 6th through 10th ribs and the diaphragmatic pleura, sparing the apices and costophrenic sulci (see **Fig. 12**).[30] Up to 15% of plaques calcify over time.[16] Chest radiography is less specific and less sensitive than CT for detection of pleural plaque, although calcification makes plaques easier to identify on radiographs. En face pleural plaques have been described as having a holly-leaf configuration (see **Fig. 12**).[30] Extrapleural fat may mimic pleural plaques on chest

A **B**

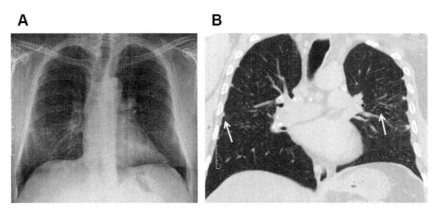

Fig. 7. Simple CWP. (*A*) PA radiograph demonstrates upper-zone predominant nodules. Although nodules of CWP have been described as less well-defined compared with simple silicosis, these entities are radiographically indistinguishable. (*B*) Coronal reformatted CT confirms the upper-zone predominant centrilobular and perilymphatic nodules (*arrows*).

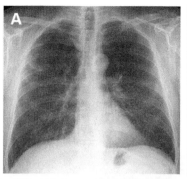
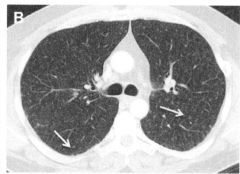

Fig. 8. Simple CWP with low profusion. (*A*) PA radiograph shows upper-zone predominant small nodules with a low level of profusion. (*B*) CT image confirms the presence of small solid centrilobular and perilymphatic nodules (*arrows*).

radiography, although the symmetric, smooth appearance extending into the fissures and over the lung apices are distinguishing features; fat attenuation is easily distinguished on CT (**Fig. 13**).[16] Pleural plaques are composed of acellular collagen in a basket-weave configuration and are not a precursor to mesothelioma.[27] Most studies have shown no association of pleural plaques with lung function abnormalities.[27,31]

Benign pleural effusions are less common (or less recognized), occurring 5 to 10 years after exposure in 3% to 7% of exposed individuals. They are usually exudative and hemorrhagic, resolving spontaneously after 3 to 4 months.[27] Recurrent effusion should raise suspicion for mesothelioma, particularly on a background of pleural plaques, which have a longer latency (15–30 years) than described with benign pleural effusion (**Fig. 14**).

Diffuse pleural thickening (DPT) occurs in up to 22% of asbestos-exposed individuals. It is thought to develop in the setting of pleuritis and benign pleural effusion, ultimately resulting in fibrosis and fusion of the visceral and parietal pleura.[27] There are no CT definitions of DPT, although proposed definitions include uninterrupted pleural thickening greater than or equal to 3 mm, involving up to 25% of the chest wall, with blunting of the costophrenic sulcus (**Fig. 15**).[16] DPT rarely calcifies, and the lung-pleural interface is ill-defined. DPT is associated with restrictive pulmonary physiology that may be relieved with decortication.[27]

Asbestosis is pulmonary fibrosis that occurs as a result of asbestos exposure, with a latency of approximately 15 to 20 years. There is a clear link to intensity and duration of exposure, typically resulting in a UIP pattern of fibrosis with basilar and peripheral predominant septal thickening and traction bronchiectasis (**Fig. 16**). Honeycombing is unusual.[32] Subpleural dotlike and branching opacities of peribronchiolar fibrosis and parenchymal bands are more common in asbestosis

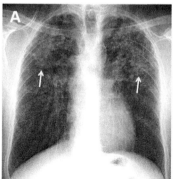
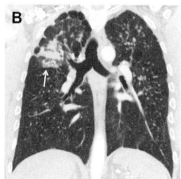
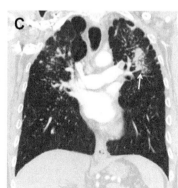

Fig. 9. Complicated CWP. (*A*) PA radiograph shows a background of upper-zone predominant small nodules. There are large opacities (≥1 cm) in the upper lung zones (*arrows*). (*B, C*) Coronal reformatted CT images confirm the background of upper-zone predominant centrilobular nodules. Large opacities are present in the right upper lobe (*arrow, B*) and left upper lobe (*arrow, C*). There is associated architectural distortion and paracicatricial emphysema in the lung apices.

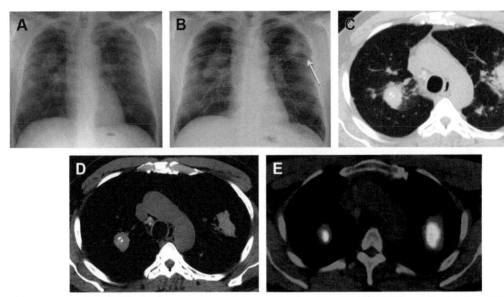

Fig. 10. PMF misdiagnosed as lung cancer in a patient with complicated CWP. (*A*) PA radiograph from 2009 shows a background of small nodules and large opacities in both upper and right mid zones. (*B*) PA radiograph from 2011 shows enlargement of the left upper-zone large opacity (*arrow*). The natural history of large opacities is that they progressively enlarge and migrate toward the hilum. (*C*) CT image in lung windows confirming the presence of large opacities in the upper lobes with a background of small centrilobular nodules. (*D*) CT image in soft tissue windows shows the large opacities to be high attenuation, with the one on the right containing calcification, a feature of large pneumoconiotic opacities. The patient was given a clinical diagnosis of stage 1 lung cancer in the left upper lobe. (*E*) PET/CT showing similar FDG uptake in the large opacities of both upper lobes. PET/CT is not useful in distinguishing lung cancer from large pneumoconiotic opacities, as both are typically FDG-avid. The patient subsequently underwent a left upper lobectomy. Pathology confirmed PMF with no findings of lung cancer.

than idiopathic pulmonary fibrosis (IPF) (see **Fig. 15**). Parenchymal bands are related to visceral pleural fibrosis and should be distinguished from the interstitial fibrosis (see **Fig. 15**).[16] Asbestosis is almost always associated with pleural plaque, as plaque induction occurs with much less exposure (see **Fig. 16**).[33] In the absence of tissue sampling, the diagnosis is made on the basis of occupational and environmental history and pleural plaque as markers of exposure.[30] Prone imaging distinguishes mild asbestosis from dependent atelectasis (**Fig. 17**).[30]

It is important to distinguish lung cancer from rounded atelectasis, the most common mass associated with asbestos exposure (see **Figs. 15 and 16**).[34] Rounded atelectasis presents as a

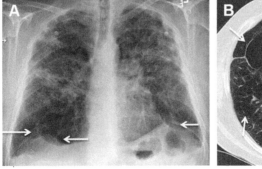
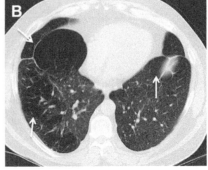

Fig. 11. Complicated CWP with basilar linear opacities. (*A*) PA radiograph shows upper-zone predominant nodules and large opacities in the upper and mid lung zones. Basilar linear opacities have been described in CWP as denoted with arrows. (*B*) CT showing that the linear opacities correspond to areas of paracicatricial emphysema (*arrows*).

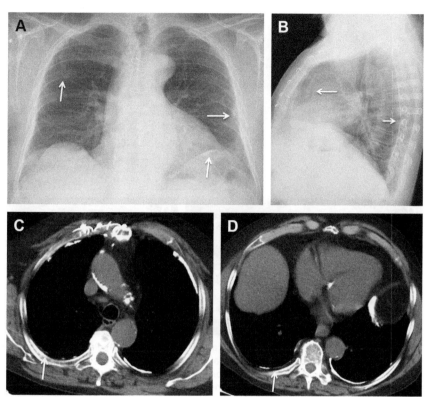

Fig. 12. Asbestos-related pleural plaques. (*A*) PA radiograph shows pleural plaques, including along the left hem-idiaphragm, in profile plaques along the left chest wall, and en face plaques in the right upper zone (*arrows*). En face plaques have been described as having a "holly-leaf" configuration. (*B*) Lateral radiograph shows pleural plaques along the anterior and posterior chest wall (*arrows*). (*C, D*) CT confirms predominantly calcified as well as noncalcified (*arrows*) pleural plaques. Plaques tend to involve the posterolateral parietal pleural between the 6th through 10th ribs and the diaphragm, with sparing of the apices and costophrenic sulci.

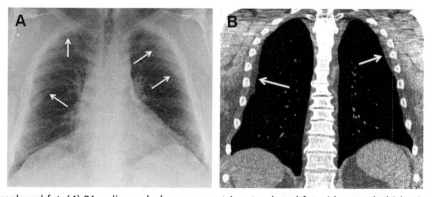

Fig. 13. Extrapleural fat. (*A*) PA radiograph shows symmetric extrapleural fat with smooth thickening extending over the apices and into the fissures (*arrows*); not to be confused with asbestos-related pleural disease. (*B*) Coronal reformatted CT image confirms the presence of extrapleural fat (*arrows*) characterized fat attenuation soft tissue.

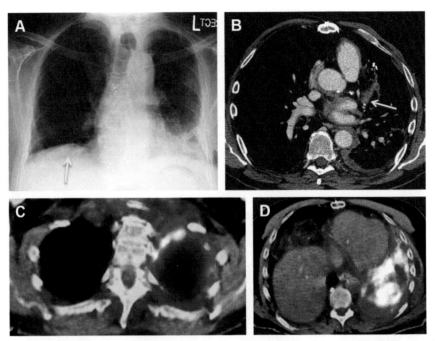

Fig. 14. Epithelioid mesothelioma in a patient with asbestos exposure. (*A*) PA radiograph showing diffuse nodular thickening of the left pleura. Note the pleural plaque along the right hemidiaphragm (*arrow*). New pleural effusion or thickening should raise the suspicion for mesothelioma in the setting of asbestos exposure. (*B*) CT shows nodular left pleural thickening with extension into the mediastinum and involvement of the pericardium (*arrow*). (*C* and *D*) Images from PET/CT showing FDG uptake within the areas of pleural thickening.

rounded subpleural mass adjacent to thickened pleura, particularly DPT, with associated volume loss and swirling of the bronchovascular bundle ("comet tail" sign) (see **Fig. 15**).[30] It is thought that pleural fibrosis causes buckling and infolding of the adjacent lung with associated atelectasis. On PET-CT, rounded atelectasis is usually not FDG-avid.[16]

Inert dust

Inert dust pneumoconiosis results from the inhalation of inorganic dust that does not cause fibrosis and, thus, does not cause symptoms or functional impairment. Siderosis or welder's pneumoconiosis is the result of inhalation of iron oxide particles, which are ingested by alveolar macrophages that accumulate along the perivascular and peribronchial lymphatics.[22] Although typically reported in welders exposed to metal fumes, it is reported in other industries such as steel grinding or silver polishing. The imaging manifestation is 0.5 to 2.0 mm centrilobular perihilar nodules. Interlobular septal thickening and Kerley B lines may be present, as well as patchy areas of ground-glass and emphysema. Accumulation of iron can result in high-attenuation lymph nodes.[35] With cessation of exposure, imaging abnormalities clear as iron dust is eliminated

from the lungs. There are some reports of fibrosis with honeycombing resembling UIP. These patients usually have a prolonged and high-level exposure or other nonwelding occupational inhalation of mixed dust.[36] When iron combines with silica, it is known as silicosiderosis.

Immune-Mediated

Hard metal

Hard metal is an alloy of cobalt and tungsten carbide, occasionally containing other metals, such as nickel, titanium, tantalum, and chromium, primarily used for grinding metal tools, stones, and concrete.[35] Hard metal pneumoconiosis is classically associated with giant cell interstitial pneumonitis (GIP), but also has been associated with occupational asthma, HP, and constrictive bronchiolitis. Cobalt is believed to be the primary toxic exposure. GIP is characterized pathologically by the presence of cannibalistic multinucleated giant cells in the alveolar spaces in addition to intraalveolar macrophages and mononuclear infiltration of the interstitium and alveolar walls.[37] GIP may have fibroblast foci with mature collagen, making it difficult to distinguish from UIP pathologically.[38] In these cases, the presence of cobalt or tungsten at scanning electron microscopy can be

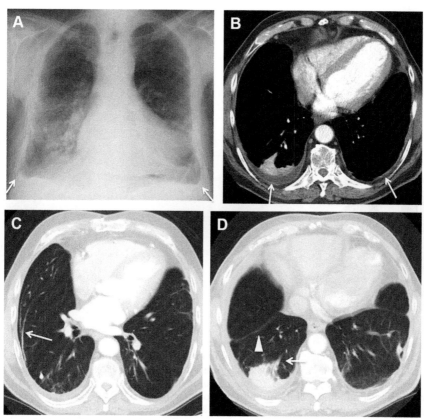

Fig. 15. Asbestos-related DPT, subpleural parenchymal bands, and round atelectasis. (*A*) PA radiograph shows bilateral DPT with blunting of the costophrenic sulci (*arrows*). (*B*) CT shows bilateral smooth uninterrupted pleural thickening and a small right pleural effusion (*arrows*). (*C*) CT image in lung windows shows curvilinear parenchymal band (*arrow*). Parenchymal bands are related to visceral pleural fibrosis and should be distinguished from pulmonary fibrosis secondary to asbestosis. (*D*) CT image more caudad demonstrates masslike consolidation (*arrow*) in the right lower lobe adjacent to thickened pleura. Note the swirling of the bronchovascular structures (comet tail sign). Displacement of the major fissure posteriorly (*arrowhead*) reflects volume loss.

diagnostic. The presence of paucicellular granulomas in the interstitium suggests HP.[38]

Differences in individual susceptibility are suggested by high variation in the levels of disease severity and progression compared with length of exposure. Genetic susceptibility has been described.[38]

The diagnosis of hard metal pneumoconiosis relies on the following[1]: history of exposure to metal dust[2]; symptoms and signs such as dyspnea, cough, and clubbing[3]; radiologic findings of diffuse lung disease; and[4] histologic findings of interstitial lung disease or GIP pattern with at least one hard metal in lung tissue.[30] CT findings typically include bilateral ground-glass or consolidation. Pulmonary fibrosis also has been described with irregular lines and traction bronchiectasis; honeycombing is atypical (**Fig. 18**).[39] Less common imaging manifestations include UIP and desquamative interstitial pneumonia patterns,

centrilobular nodules, and spontaneous pneumothorax.[16,40]

Chronic Beryllium Disease

Chronic beryllium disease (CBD) is a granulomatous lung disease that is most often radiographically indistinguishable from sarcoidosis. A substantial minority (one-third) of cases may resemble HP on imaging.[41–43] Beryllium is a lightweight metal initially used in the manufacture of fluorescent lamps and neon signs but now used in various industries, including aerospace, defense, electronics, dentistry, and recreational equipment. Inhalation of beryllium results in activation of CD4+ T lymphocytes, which migrate to the lungs and incite an inflammatory response with granuloma formation. The epithelioid granuloma, the pathologic hallmark of CBD, is also present in sarcoidosis. The beryllium-specific

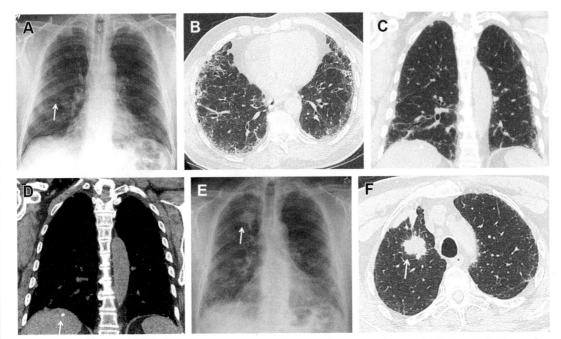

Fig. 16. Asbestosis and lung cancer. (*A*) PA radiograph shows basilar predominant reticulation. Note the en face pleural plaques on the right (*arrow*). (*B*) CT of the lung bases confirms peripheral subpleural reticulation with architectural distortion and traction bronchiectasis, consistent with asbestosis. Note the absence of honeycombing, which is present in a minority of cases. (*C* and *D*) Coronal reformatted CT in lung and soft tissue windows demonstrates the basilar and peripheral distribution of pulmonary fibrosis and calcified plaque along the right hemidiaphragm (*arrow*), respectively. (*E*) PA radiograph 3 years later showing a new right upper lobe mass (*arrow*). (*F*) CT image shows a spiculated right upper lobe mass proven to be non–small cell lung carcinoma (*arrow*).

lymphocyte proliferation test and in vivo patch testing, known as beryllium sensitization (BeS) distinguish CBD from sarcoidosis. BeS progresses to CBD at a rate of 6% to 8% per year, occurring more commonly in genetically susceptible individuals.[44] There is no clear dose-response relationship; CBD may occur with minimal exposure.[44] CBD has been described in a population living near a beryllium manufacturing plant.[45]

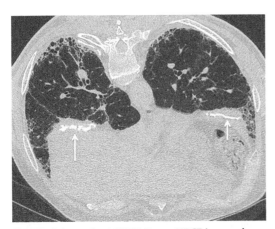

Fig. 17. Asbestosis at HRCT. Prone HRCT image shows peripheral reticulation in the lower lobes. Prone images can be helpful to distinguish early fibrosis from dependent atelectasis, the latter of which resolves on prone imaging. Note the calcified pleural plaques along the diaphragm (*arrows*).

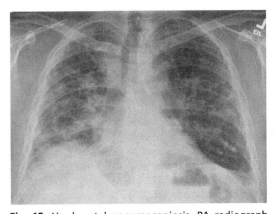

Fig. 18. Hard metal pneumoconiosis. PA radiograph shows diffuse reticulation with architectural distortion reflecting fibrosis. This patient underwent bilateral lung transplantation. Evaluation of the explanted lungs showed GIP.

Before the adoption of OSHA standards in 1949, acute beryllium disease (ABD) was more common.[46] ABD is characterized by a diffuse chemical pneumonitis with widespread airspace opacities developing 1 to 3 weeks after very high exposures.[44] The clinical course of ABD ranges from self-limited to rapidly progressive and fatal.

Although ABD is rare, CBD is now much more common. CBD is characterized clinically by dry cough, dyspnea on exertion, fatigue, and night sweats. Lung function may be normal or may show obstruction, restriction, or abnormal gas exchange.[44] The appearance of CBD on chest radiography and CT is usually similar to sarcoidosis with mid and upper-zone predominant perilymphatic nodules and smooth or nodular septal thickening (**Fig. 19**).[30] The nodules may coalesce along the pleura to form pseudoplaques. Mediastinal and hilar lymphadenopathy is less common than with sarcoidosis, occurring in approximately 32% to 39% of patients.[30] Other imaging manifestations include ground-glass opacities, bronchial wall thickening, and pulmonary fibrosis with associated honeycombing, conglomerate masses, and paracicatricial emphysema (**Fig. 20**). In a recent series, 34 (40%) of 84 patients being reevaluated with a diagnosis of sarcoidosis proved to have CBD[47]; therefore, CBD is an important entity to consider in patients presenting with imaging findings of sarcoidosis.

Airway Centric

Occupational asthma
Occupational asthma is the most common OLD, accounting for approximately 10% to 15% of new-onset asthma in adults with hundreds of recognized inciting agents.[16,48] Work-related asthma is new-onset asthma caused by occupational exposure to airborne dusts, gases, vapors,

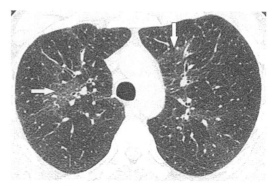

Fig. 20. CBD. CT shows peribronchovascular ground-glass opacity (*arrows*) and bronchial wall thickening.

or fumes; work-exacerbated asthma is preexisting asthma worsened by occupational exposure.[49] The most common occupations include bakers, paint sprayers, health care workers, teachers, miners, chemical workers, animal handlers, welders, agricultural workers, hairdressers, timber workers, and food processing workers.[48–51] Military personnel deployed to Iraq and Afghanistan are at increased risk of developing asthma compared with stateside soldiers.[52] The collapse and burning of the World Trade Center released a complex mixture of dust, smoke, and gas pollutants into the local environment resulting in a high prevalence of lower respiratory symptoms and pulmonary function abnormalities, the most common diagnosis being irritant-induced asthma.[53,54] Surveillance and early detection are key, because early removal from the exposure can reverse the disease. Imaging findings are nonspecific and include bronchial wall thickening, mosaic attenuation, and expiratory air trapping.[33]

Flavor Worker's Lung

Flavor worker's lung is caused by exposure to diacetyl, a diketone flavoring agent, most commonly

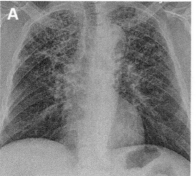

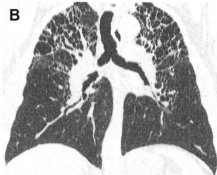

Fig. 19. CBD. (*A*) PA radiograph shows upper-zone predominant fibrosis with reticulation, architectural distortion, and bronchiectasis, similar in appearance to stage 4 sarcoidosis. (*B*) CT demonstrates the upper-zone predominance of the pulmonary fibrosis with extensive traction bronchiectasis, volume loss, and architectural distortion. CBD is important to consider in patients presenting with imaging findings of sarcoidosis.

found in butter-flavored microwave popcorn.[55] It was first described in 2000 when 8 workers in a Missouri popcorn-flavoring plant developed progressive dyspnea and obstructive lung disease.[56] Inhalation of diacetyl causes direct injury to the airway epithelium, leading to bronchiolitis obliterans syndrome (BOS); characterized by inflammation and fibrosis at the bronchiolar level causing luminal obstruction. These patients have irreversible airflow obstruction with a reduction in FEV1 and FEV1/forced vital capacity.[57] On HRCT, as with other causes of BOS, this manifests as mosaic attenuation with expiratory air trapping (**Fig. 21**). Centrilobular nodules, bronchiectasis, and bronchial wall thickening also can be seen.[33]

Flock Worker's Lung

Flock worker's lung disease is caused by inhalation of an ultrafine nylon fiber created when a fiber (primarily nylon) is cut into shorter pieces and applied to a fabric used for clothing and upholstery flocking.[58] This was first described in a plant in Ontario in 1990 when workers developed progressive cough and dyspnea with restrictive pulmonary function tests.[58] HRCT findings include patchy ground-glass and consolidation, diffuse micronodules, or an NSIP or UIP pattern of fibrosis with peripheral honeycombing.[33] Pathologically, a lymphocytic bronchiolitis and peribronchiolitis with lymphoid hyperplasia is observed. Occasionally, diffuse alveolar damage or organizing pneumonia may be present.[58] Although steroid response was variable, all cases showed improvement both clinically and radiographically after cessation of exposure.[58]

Environmental Lung Disease

Hypersensitivity pneumonitis

HP is caused by inhalation of an antigen in a sensitized individual.[59] Since the first description of hypersensitivity pneumonitis in grain workers in 1713 by Bernardino Ramazzini, numerous antigens have been discovered.[60] The most common organic antigens include bacteria, yeasts, fungi, and bird proteins. Examples include thermophilic actinomycetes in farmer's lung and proteins in avian serum, feces, and feathers in bird fancier's lungs. Low molecular weight chemical agents also have been described and include zinc, inks, dyes, and isocyanates.[59]

Classically, HP was divided into acute, subacute, and chronic forms based on symptoms.[61] Lacasse and colleagues[62] evaluated a cohort of patients with HP and performed a cluster analysis revealing significant overlap among the 3 forms. They recommended dividing patients into 2 clusters. Cluster 1 includes acute and subacute presentations and are more likely to have systemic symptoms (fever, chills, myalgia, headache, cough, chest tightness, dyspnea) and reversible disease (**Fig. 22**). Cluster 2 includes subacute and chronic presentations and with higher rates of clubbing, hypoxemia, restrictive physiology, and fibrosis on HRCT (**Fig. 23**).

Acute exacerbations of chronic HP have been recently recognized. Importantly, this occurs without additional antigen exposure and is associated with a poor outcome. It is characterized by worsening dyspnea in the setting of chronic HP with new radiographic opacities that cannot be attributed to another cause (**Fig. 24**). Organizing pneumonia and diffuse alveolar damage have been shown at pathology.[59]

Positive serum-specific antibodies are an important predictor of HP. Bronchoalveolar lavage also can aid in the diagnosis and must show lymphocytosis, although this is a nonspecific finding.[59] Histologically, there is bronchiolocentric interstitial pneumonitis, cellular bronchiolitis, and poorly formed non-necrotizing granulomas. This triad occurs in up to 80% of patients with HP.

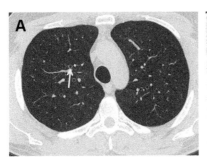
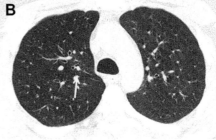

Fig. 21. Flavor worker's lung. (*A*) Inspiratory HRCT image shows mild bronchial dilation (*arrow*) and subtle mosaic attenuation. (*B*) Expiratory HRCT image shows extensive air trapping with areas of spared lung centrally along the bronchovascular structures (*arrow*). Imaging features are consistent with BOS and are indistinguishable from other causes of BOS.

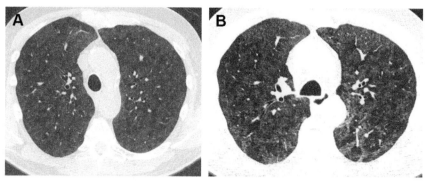

Fig. 22. HP in a patient with multiple pet birds. (*A*) Inspiratory HRCT image shows extensive centrilobular ground-glass nodules and mosaic attenuation ("head-cheese" sign). (*B*) Expiratory HRCT CT image confirms air trapping.

Occasionally, Schaumann bodies, cholesterol clefts, giant cells, and constrictive bronchiolitis may be seen. Chronic HP may be indistinguishable from other causes of pulmonary fibrosis.[63] A recent study demonstrated that 43% of patients referred for evaluation for presumptive IPF were proven to have chronic HP.[64] HRCT features of acute HP include ground-glass opacity, upper-zone predominant centrilobular ground-glass nodules, and air trapping on expiratory imaging (see **Fig. 22**).[59] Lung cysts have occasionally been reported.[65] At HRCT, fibrosis in chronic HP manifests as irregular lines, traction bronchiectasis, and occasional honeycombing (see **Fig. 23**). When fibrosis occurs, the most distinguishing features are a lack of lower zone or peripheral distribution, centrilobular nodules, and air trapping often in 3 or more lobes.[59] The presence and extent of fibrosis, particularly in the presence of auscultatory crackles, confers a poor prognosis.[66]

The most important treatment is identifying and removing the inciting antigen. The inability to identify an antigen has been associated with decreased survival.[67] Systemic corticosteroids may improve symptoms at all stages of disease.

Hot tub lung

Hot tub lung is a hypersensitivitylike reaction in immunocompetent hosts to inhalation of *Mycobacterium* genus, most commonly *Mycobacterium*

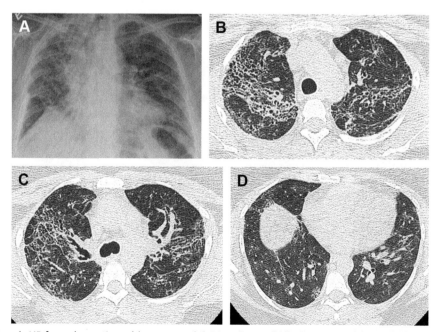

Fig. 23. Chronic HP from domestic mold exposure. (*A*) PA radiograph shows upper-zone predominant pulmonary fibrosis characterized by reticulation and architectural distortion. (*B–D*) Sequential HRCT images demonstrate the upper-zone and peribronchovascular distribution of fibrosis. Air trapping and centrilobular ground-glass nodules (not shown here) can be clues to the diagnosis of chronic HP.

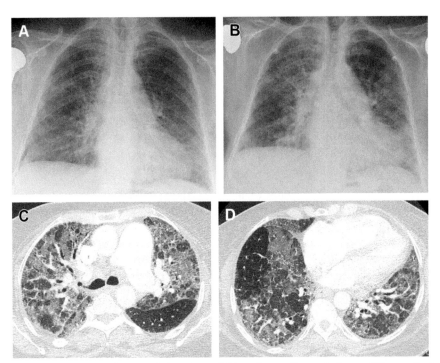

Fig. 24. Woman with acute exacerbation of chronic HP. (*A*) Baseline radiograph shows diffuse reticular opacities. (*B*) PA radiograph obtained during episode of acute dyspnea and hypoxia shows increased diffuse ground-glass opacities superimposed on underlying fibrosis. (*C*, *D*) CT images confirm extensive ground-glass opacity superimposed on peribronchovascular reticulation and traction bronchiectasis.

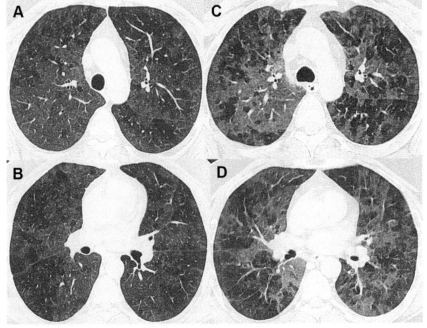

Fig. 25. Hot tub lung from *M avium* complex. (*A*, *B*) Inspiratory HRCT images show mosaic attenuation with ground-glass opacity. (*C*, *D*) Expiratory HRCT images confirm extensive air trapping.

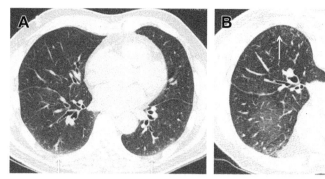

Fig. 26. Incidental mild fibrosis in a 77-year-old man. (*A*) Supine CT image demonstrates mild subpleural reticulation (*arrows*) that persists on prone imaging (*B*). Asymptomatic patients older than 75 have been shown to have an increased incidence of mild fibrosis in the lung bases.

avium complex, found in hot tubs, or less commonly, swimming pools and even household showers.[68] Mycobacteria are aerobic organisms associated with biofilm formation, can aerosolize from water, and are resistant to high temperatures.[69] The clinical presentation is often similar to HP, with fever, dyspnea, and cough. Diagnosis can be made without histopathology on the basis of known hot tub exposure, positive mycobacterial culture, and characteristic radiographic findings.[70] Characteristic CT findings include diffuse centrilobular nodules and ground-glass opacities, as well as expiratory air trapping (**Fig. 25**).[71] Histologically, this is a granulomatous lung disease characterized by small, poorly formed, predominantly non-necrotizing, bronchiolocentric granulomas.[63] There is debate about whether this entity truly represents HP, granulomatous disease, or infection. Factors favoring HP include full clinical, radiologic, and functional recovery after cessation of exposure or steroid therapy and the lack of need for antimycobacterial therapy.[59]

Biomass smoke

Hut lung is a pneumoconiosis resulting from inhalation of smoke from biomass-fueled stoves. Biomass fuels are used widely in the developing world (by up to one-half of the world's population) for cooking and heating, often in poorly ventilated structures.[72] Biomass fuels consist of materials such as wood, grass, corn, and dung.[73] The combustion of biomass releases particulate matter, carbon monoxide, nitrogen oxides, formaldehyde, and polyaromatic hydrocarbons.[74] Inhalation of biomass fumes has been shown to cause a form of mixed-dust pneumoconiosis at histology with macules of dust-laden macrophages and mixed-dust fibrotic lesions consisting of predominantly carbonaceous particles with a smaller amount of silica and silicates.[73] On CT, this correlates with upper-zone predominant centrilobular nodules,

lymphadenopathy, and PMF.[73] Hut lung also has been associated with chronic bronchitis and an airway-predominant COPD phenotype with bronchial wall thickening and air trapping as predominant CT abnormalities.[75]

Other environmental influences

Although review of the effects of environmental exposure to air pollution is beyond the scope of this article, recent studies have linked environmental air pollution to increased mortality, lung cancer, infection, and obstructive lung disease.[76] Global issues related to lung disease as a result of smoking and aging have also received recent attention. Patients older than 75 years have significantly increased incidence of mild basilar fibrosis (**Fig. 26**).[77] There is a strong association of smoking and IPF.[78] Several studies, including a subanalysis from the NLST (National Lung Screening Trial), also have shown ground-glass opacity and reticulation with pulmonary fibrosis in 4% of smokers at baseline.[8]

SUMMARY

Occupational and environmental lung diseases remain major causes of respiratory impairment worldwide. Despite regulations, exposures to "classic" dusts, such as silica, coal, and asbestos, continue to be global causes of pulmonary disease. New sources of OLD are emerging, such as flavor worker's lung. In addition, known dust-related diseases arise in new industries, as seen with silicosis and hydraulic fracking. Nonoccupational environmental lung disease contributes to major respiratory disease, asthma, and COPD, particularly with increasing air pollution and continued use of biomass as a source of fuel. Knowledge of the imaging patterns of occupational and environmental lung diseases is critical in diagnosing patients with occult exposures and managing patients with suspected or known exposures.

REFERENCES

1. Ross MH, Murray J. Occupational respiratory disease in mining. Occup Med 2004;54(5):304–10.
2. Driscoll T, Nelson DI, Steenland K, et al. The global burden of non-malignant respiratory disease due to occupational airborne exposures. Am J Ind Med 2005;48(6):432–45.
3. Fingerhut M, Nelson DI, Driscoll T, et al. The contribution of occupational risks to the global burden of disease: summary and next steps. Med Lav 2006; 97(2):313–21.
4. Laney AS, Weissman DN. The classic pneumoconioses: new epidemiological and laboratory observations. Clin Chest Med 2012;33(4):745–58. Elsevier Inc.
5. Arakawa H. Chronic interstitial pneumonia in silicosis and mix-dust pneumoconiosis: its prevalence and comparison of CT findings with idiopathic pulmonary fibrosis. Chest 2007;131(6):1870–6.
6. Schluger NW, Koppaka R. Lung disease in a global context. A call for public health action. Ann Am Thorac Soc 2014;11(3):407–16.
7. Jin GY, Lynch D, Chawla A, et al. Interstitial lung abnormalities in a CT lung cancer screening population: prevalence and progression rate. Radiology 2013;268(2):563–71.
8. Sverzellati N, Guerci L, Randi G, et al. Interstitial lung diseases in a lung cancer screening trial. Eur Respir J 2011;38(2):392–400.
9. Raghu G, Collard HR, Egan JJ, et al. An official ATS/ERS/JRS/ALAT statement: idiopathic pulmonary fibrosis: evidence-based guidelines for diagnosis and management. Am J Respir Crit Care Med 2011;183:788–824.
10. Gevenois PA, Pichot E, Dargent F, et al. Low grade coal worker's pneumoconiosis. Comparison of CT and chest radiography. Acta Radiol 1994;35(4): 351–6.
11. Schins RP, Borm PJ. Mechanisms and mediators in coal dust induced toxicity: a review. Ann Occup Hyg 1999;43:1–27.
12. Mossman BT, Lippmann M, Hesterberg TW, et al. Pulmonary endpoints (lung carcinomas and asbestosis) following inhalation exposure to asbestos. J Toxicol Environ Health B Crit Rev 2011;14(1–4):76–121.
13. Miserocchi G, Sancini G, Mantegazza F, et al. Translocation pathways for inhaled asbestos fibers. Environ Health 2008;7(1):4.
14. Steenland K, Ward E. Silica: a lung carcinogen. CA Cancer J Clin 2013;64(1):63–9.
15. Hazard A. Worker exposure to silica during hydraulic fracturing. Available at: https://www.osha.gov/dts/hazardalerts/hydraulic_frac_hazard_alert.html. Accessed February 17, 2015.
16. Meyer CA, Lockey JE. Occupational lung disease. Clinically oriented pulmonary imaging. Totowa (NJ): Humana Press; 2012. p. 209–27.
17. Marchiori E, Souza CA, Barbassa TG, et al. Silico-proteinosis: high-resolution CT findings in 13 patients. Am J Roentgenol 2007;189(6):1402–6.
18. Arakawa H, Fujimoto K, Honma K, et al. Progression from near-normal to end-stage lungs in chronic interstitial pneumonia related to silica exposure: long-term CT observations. Am J Roentgenol 2008; 191(4):1040–5.
19. Vallyathan V, Brower PS, Green FH, et al. Radiographic and pathologic correlation of coal workers' pneumoconiosis. Am J Respir Crit Care Med 1996;154:741–8.
20. Laney ES, Petsonk EL. Small pneumoconiotic opacities on US coal worker surveillance chest radiographs are not predominantly in the upper lung zones. Am J Ind Med 2012;55(9):793–8.
21. Bauer TT, Heyer CM, Duchna HW, et al. Radiological findings, pulmonary function and dyspnea in underground coal miners. Respiration 2007;74(1):80–7.
22. Chong S, Lee KS, Chung MJ, et al. Pneumoconiosis: comparison of imaging and pathologic findings. Radiographics 2006;26(1):59–77.
23. Matsumoto S, Miyake H, Oga M, et al. Diagnosis of lung cancer in a patient with pneumoconiosis and progressive massive fibrosis using MRI. Eur Radiol 1998;8(4):615–7.
24. Reichert M, Bensadoun ES. PET imaging in patients with coal workers pneumoconiosis and suspected malignancy. J Thorac Oncol 2009;4(5):649–51.
25. Saydam O, Gokce M, Kilicgun A, et al. Accuracy of positron emission tomography in mediastinal node assessment in coal workers with lung cancer. Med Oncol 2011;29(2):589–94.
26. Santo Tomas LH. Emphysema and chronic obstructive pulmonary disease in coal miners. Curr Opin Pulm Med 2011;17(2):123–5.
27. Prazakova S, Thomas PS, Sandrini A, et al. Asbestos and the lung in the 21st century: an update. Clin Respir J 2013;8(1):1–10.
28. Marsili D, Comba P. Asbestos case and its current implications for global health. Ann Ist Super Sanita 2013;49(3):249–51.
29. Lacourt A, Gramond C, Rolland P, et al. Occupational and non-occupational attributable risk of asbestos exposure for malignant pleural mesothelioma. Thorax 2014;69(6):532–9.
30. Pipavath SN, Godwin JD, Kanne JP. Occupational lung disease: a radiologic review. Semin Roentgenol 2010;45(1):43–52.
31. Rohs AM, Lockey JE, Dunning KK, et al. Low-level fiber-induced radiographic changes caused by Libby vermiculite. Am J Respir Crit Care Med 2008;177(6):630–7.
32. Carrillo MC, Alturkistany S, Roberts H, et al. Low-dose computed tomography (LDCT) in workers previously exposed to asbestos: detection of parenchymal lung disease. J Comput Assist Tomogr 2013; 37(4):626–30.

33. Cox CW, Rose CS, Lynch DA. State of the art: imaging of occupational lung disease. Radiology 2014; 270(3):681–96.

34. Lynch DA, Gamsu G, Ray CS, et al. Asbestos-related focal lung masses: manifestations on conventional and high-resolution CT scans. Radiology 1988;169(3):603–7.

35. Karkhanis VS, Joshi JM. Pneumoconioses. Indian J Chest Dis Allied Sci 2013;55(1):25–34.

36. Antonini JM, Lewis AB, Roberts JR, et al. Pulmonary effects of welding fumes: review of worker and experimental animal studies. Am J Ind Med 2003; 43(4):350–60.

37. Okuno K, Kobayashi K, Kotani Y, et al. A case of hard metal lung disease resembling a hypersensitive pneumonia in radiological images. Intern Med 2010;49(12):1185–9.

38. Naqvi AH, Hunt A, Burnett BR, et al. Pathologic spectrum and lung dust burden in giant cell interstitial pneumonia (hard metal disease/cobalt pneumonitis): review of 100 cases. Arch Environ Occup Health 2008;63(2):51–70.

39. Akira M. Uncommon pneumoconioses: CT and pathologic findings. Radiology 1995;197(2):403–9.

40. Dunlop P, Müller NL, Wilson J, et al. Hard metal lung disease: high resolution CT and histologic correlation of the initial findings and demonstration of interval improvement. J Thorac Imaging 2005;20(4):301–4.

41. Naccache JM, Marchand-Adam S, Kambouchner M, et al. Ground-glass computed tomography pattern in chronic beryllium disease: pathologic substratum and evolution. J Comput Assist Tomogr 2003;27(4):496–500.

42. Daniloff EM, Lynch DA, Bartelson BB, et al. Observer variation and relationship of computed tomography to severity of beryllium disease. Am J Respir Crit Care Med 1997;155(6):2047–56.

43. Newman LS, Buschman DL, Newell JD, et al. Beryllium disease: assessment with CT. Radiology 1994; 190(3):835–40.

44. Mayer A, Hamzeh N, Maier L. Sarcoidosis and chronic beryllium disease: similarities and differences. Semin Respir Crit Care Med 2014;35(3):316–29.

45. Maier LA, Martyny JW, Liang J, et al. Recent chronic beryllium disease in residents surrounding a beryllium facility. Am J Respir Crit Care Med 2008; 177(9):1012–7.

46. Sharma N, Patel J, Mohammed TL. Chronic beryllium disease: computed tomographic findings. J Comput Assist Tomogr 2010;34(6):945–8.

47. Müller-Quernheim J, Gaede KI, Fireman E, et al. Diagnoses of chronic beryllium disease within cohorts of sarcoidosis patients. Eur Respir J 2006;27(6): 1190–5.

48. Stenton SC. Occupational and environmental lung disease: occupational asthma. Chron Respir Dis 2010;7(1):35–46.

49. Mazurek JM, Schleiff PL. Physician recognition of work-related asthma among US farm operators. Fam Med 2010;42(6):408–13.

50. Hashemi N, Boskabady MH, Nazari A. Occupational exposures and obstructive lung disease: a case-control study in hairdressers. Respir Care 2010; 55(7):895–900.

51. McHugh MK, Symanski E, Pompeii LA, et al. Prevalence of asthma by industry and occupation in the US working population. Am J Ind Med 2010;53(5):463–75.

52. Szema AM. Occupational lung diseases among soldiers deployed to Iraq and Afghanistan. Occup Med Health Aff 2013;1.

53. Banauch GI, Dhala A, Prezant DJ. Pulmonary disease in rescue workers at the World Trade Center site. Curr Opin Pulm Med 2005;11(2):160–8.

54. la Hoz de RE. Occupational asthma and lower airway disease among World Trade Center workers and volunteers. Curr Allergy Asthma Rep 2010; 10(4):287–94.

55. Lockey JE, Hilbert TJ, Levin LP, et al. Airway obstruction related to diacetyl exposure at microwave popcorn production facilities. Eur Respir J 2009;34(1):63–71.

56. Sirajuddin A, Kanne JP. Occupational lung disease. J Thorac Imaging 2009;24(4):310–20.

57. Harber P, Saechao K, Boomus C. Diacetyl-induced lung disease. Toxicol Rev 2006;25(4):261–72.

58. Goldyn S, Condos R, Rom W. The burden of exposure-related diffuse lung disease. Semin Respir Crit Care Med 2009;29(6):591–602.

59. Lacasse Y, Girard M, Cormier Y. Recent advances in hypersensitivity pneumonitis. Chest 2012;142(1): 208–17.

60. Hirschmann JV, Pipavath SN, Godwin JD. Hypersensitivity pneumonitis: a historical, clinical, and radiologic review. Radiographics 2009;29(7):1921–38.

61. Richerson HB, Bernstein IL, Fink JN, et al. Guidelines for the clinical evaluation of hypersensitivity pneumonitis. Report of the subcommittee on hypersensitivity pneumonitis. J Allergy Clin Immunol 1989; 84(5 Pt 2):839–44.

62. Lacasse Y, Selman M, Costabel U, et al. Classification of hypersensitivity pneumonitis: a hypothesis. Int Arch Allergy Immunol 2009;149(2):161–6.

63. Barrios RJ. Hypersensitivity pneumonitis: histopathology. Arch Pathol Lab Med 2008;132(2):199–203.

64. Morell F, Villar A, Montero MÁ, et al. Chronic hypersensitivity pneumonitis in patients diagnosed with idiopathic pulmonary fibrosis: a prospective case-cohort study. Lancet Respir Med 2013;1(9):685–94.

65. Franquet T, Hansell DM, Senbanjo T, et al. Lung cysts in subacute hypersensitivity pneumonitis. J Comput Assist Tomogr 2003;27(4):475–8.

66. Mooney JJ, Elicker BM, Urbania TH, et al. Radiographic fibrosis score predicts survival in hypersensitivity pneumonitis. Chest 2013;144(2):586–92.

67. Fernández Pérez ER, Swigris JJ, Forssén AV, et al. Identifying an inciting antigen is associated with improved survival in patients with chronic hypersensitivity pneumonitis. Chest 2013;144(5):1644–51.

68. Marras TK, Wallace RJ, Koth LL, et al. Hypersensitivity pneumonitis reaction to *Mycobacterium avium* in household water. Chest 2005;127(2):664–71.

69. Johnson MM, Odell JA. Nontuberculous mycobacterial pulmonary infections. J Thorac Dis 2014;6(3):210–20.

70. Fjällbrant H, Akerstrom M, Svensson E, et al. Hot tub lung: an occupational hazard. Eur Respir Rev 2013; 22(127):88–90.

71. Hartman TE, Jensen E, Tazelaar HD, et al. CT findings of granulomatous pneumonitis secondary to *Mycobacterium avium*-intracellulare inhalation: "hot tub lung." AJR Am J Roentgenol 2007;188(4):1050–3.

72. Bosson JA, Blomberg A. Update in environmental and occupational medicine 2012. Am J Respir Crit Care Med 2013;188(1):18–22.

73. Mukhopadhyay S, Gujral M, Abraham JL, et al. A case of hut lung: scanning electron microscopy with energy dispersive x-ray spectroscopy analysis of a domestically acquired form of pneumoconiosis. Chest 2013;144(1):323–7.

74. Diaz JV, Koff J, Gotway MB, et al. Case report: a case of wood-smoke-related pulmonary disease. Environ Health Perspect 2006;114(5):759–62.

75. Camp PG, Ramirez-Venegas A, Sansores RH, et al. COPD phenotypes in biomass smoke- versus tobacco smoke-exposed Mexican women. Eur Respir J 2014;43(3):725–34.

76. Carlsten C, Georas SN. Update in environmental and occupational lung diseases 2013. Am J Respir Crit Care Med 2014;189(9):1037–43.

77. Faner R, Rojas M, Macnee W, et al. Abnormal lung aging in chronic obstructive pulmonary disease and idiopathic pulmonary fibrosis. Am J Respir Crit Care Med 2012;186(4):306–13.

78. Cormier Y, Brown M, Worthy S, et al. High-resolution computed tomographic characteristics in acute farmer's lung and in its follow-up. Eur Respir J 2000;16(1):56–60.

Radiologic Evaluation of Idiopathic Interstitial Pneumonias

Tilman L. Koelsch, MD*, Jonathan H. Chung, MD,
David A. Lynch, MB

KEYWORDS

- Idiopathic interstitial pneumonia • Interstitial lung disease • High-resolution CT

KEY POINTS

- Many known secondary causes can produce changes identical those seen in the idiopathic interstitial pneumonias, most commonly collagen vascular diseases, hypersensitivity pneumonitis, and drug reactions.
- Findings required for a confident radiologic diagnosis of usual interstitial pneumonia (UIP) are predominant distribution of fibrosis in the peripheral and posterior-basilar lung with associated honeycombing.
- Lung cancer in the setting of pulmonary fibrosis is often subtle, and careful inspection is mandatory to exclude early malignancy.
- Mild UIP and mild nonspecific interstitial pneumonia (NSIP) may seem similar; given the worse prognosis of UIP versus NSIP, these mild patterns are frequently grouped into the possible UIP category.
- A surgical biopsy may be required.

INTRODUCTION

The idiopathic interstitial pneumonias (IIPs) are a group of fibrosing and inflammatory pulmonary conditions that share many similar clinical features.[1] The classification of IIPs is based on specific histologic changes, each of which is related to a specific idiopathic condition. It is important to remember that many known secondary causes can produce histologic changes identical to those seen in the IIPs, most commonly collagen vascular diseases, hypersensitivity pneumonitis (HP), and drug reactions.[2,3] The IIPs are grouped into the chronic fibrotic conditions (usual interstitial pneumonia [UIP] and nonspecific interstitial pneumonia [NSIP]), the subacute and acute conditions (cryptogenic organizing pneumonia [COP] and acute interstitial pneumonia [AIP]), the smoking-related conditions (respiratory bronchiolitis interstitial lung disease [RB-ILD] and desquamative interstitial pneumonia [DIP]), and, last, the rare conditions (lymphocytic interstitial pneumonia [LIP] and idiopathic pleuroparenchymal fibroelastosis).[2]

Given the many similarities between these conditions in terms of clinical presentation and radiologic/histologic findings, a collaborative multidisciplinary approach between the clinician, radiologist, and pathologist is paramount to achieve an accurate diagnosis. A collaborative diagnostic approach may not only lead to obtaining a more confident diagnosis in a shorter time, but also may often preclude the need for surgical lung biopsy.[4–6] Additionally, a collaborative approach is essential to exclude a known cause of lung disease.[2,7,8] The following is a discussion of the radiologic contribution to the multidisciplinary

Disclosures: None.
Department of Radiology, National Jewish Health, 1400 Jackson Street, Denver, CO 80206, USA
* Corresponding author.
E-mail address: KoelschT@NJHealth.org

Clin Chest Med 36 (2015) 269–282
http://dx.doi.org/10.1016/j.ccm.2015.02.009
0272-5231/15/$ – see front matter © 2015 Elsevier Inc. All rights reserved.

chestmed.theclinics.com

evaluation, with description of the typical radiologic findings seen in each of the IIPs and important associated caveats.

FIBROSING INTERSTITIAL PNEUMONIAS
Usual Interstitial Pneumonia

UIP is the most common of the IIPs and statistically carries the worst long term prognosis.[9,10] It is the histologic and radiologic correlate for idiopathic pulmonary fibrosis (IPF). A UIP-type pattern of pulmonary fibrosis can also be secondary to other conditions, including collagen vascular disease, chronic HP, drug reaction, and asbestosis. The UIP-type pattern induced by other underlying conditions may be indistinguishable from truly idiopathic UIP/IPF. Careful clinical evaluation for potential underlying causes of UIP is essential, because patients with a known secondary cause have a much better prognosis compared with patients with idiopathic UIP, where secondary causes have been excluded.[2,11]

The diagnosis of UIP can frequently be made solely by high-resolution CT (HRCT) evaluation. Multiple studies have shown that expert thoracic radiologists confidently diagnosing UIP have a positive predictive value of 95% to 100%. However, a less confident diagnosis of UIP drops the positive predictive value to as low as 70%.[4,12–14] A typical UIP pattern on HRCT with the appropriate clinical picture can often eliminate a surgical biopsy.[5,15] The guideline-based criteria for radiologic diagnosis of UIP now reflect the level of confidence in the diagnosis and should help to guide further diagnostic steps.[2]

On HRCT, the hallmark features of UIP are a peripheral predominant reticulation in a predominantly posterior and basilar lung distribution, with associated honeycombing (**Fig. 1**). Regions of reticulation represent fine fibrosis on histology.[16] Ground-glass opacity may also be seen, but is less prominent than the associated reticulation and represents microscopic pulmonary fibrosis

beyond the resolution of HRCT.[17] The fibrotic features of UIP may be asymmetric compared with NSIP, which is usually symmetric.[18,19] Traction bronchiectasis and bronchiolectasis may develop in areas of reticulation, indicating that reticulation reflects fibrosis.[20,21] Unfortunately, in a substantial proportion of biopsy-proven cases of UIP/IPF, imaging findings are not specific for UIP.[22]

As UIP progresses, honeycombing develops in the subpleural lungs, representing end-stage fibrosis.[16] Honeycombing in a basal and peripheral distribution of fibrosis is highly supportive of a UIP diagnosis and should be considered definite UIP based on recently released guidelines (**Tables 1** and **2**).[22] Differentiating paraseptal emphysema from honeycombing, although usually straightforward, can be challenging and is a not uncommon dilemma given that smoking is associated with both entities. Honeycombing usually manifests as a regular pattern of thin-walled cysts, often in the lower lungs, whereas paraseptal emphysema most often manifests as several longer cysts often in the upper lungs and may contain subtle internal septations. However, confident differentiation of honeycombing from paraseptal emphysema may not be possible in a few cases.[23–25]

Although typical HRCT features may obviate the need for biopsy, the lack of typical findings does not rule out this diagnosis. It is recognized that in a substantial minority of cases the diagnosis of UIP cannot be made solely on CT. Up to 30% to 50% of UIP cases diagnosed by histology do not carry a confident radiologic diagnosis of UIP.[4,26] Equivocal radiologic features or clinical uncertainty should prompt consideration of surgical biopsy.[20,27–29]

Imaging is helpful in detecting complications of UIP/IPF. Acute respiratory decline in IPF patients are often a result of accelerated deterioration or opportunistic infections. Both of these conditions may have an overlapping appearance, demonstrating new regions of prominent ground-glass opacification, possibly with associated

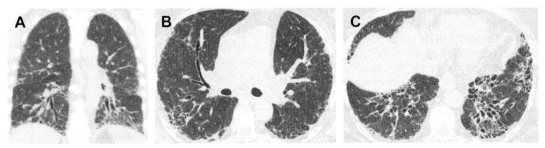

Fig. 1. Usual interstitial pneumonia (UIP) pattern of fibrosis. Coronal (A), axial mid lung (B), and axial lower lung (C) images showing peripheral and basilar predominant reticulation, honeycombing and traction bronchiectasis. Note the asymmetric pattern of fibrosis which is more common in UIP than nonspecific interstitial pneumonia.

Table 1
High-resolution computed tomography features of IIP patterns

	Distribution	Imaging Features
Usual interstitial pneumonia	Basal, peripheral predominant May be asymmetric and patchy	Reticulation, traction bronchiectasis/bronchiolectasis Honeycombing
Nonspecific interstitial pneumonia	Basal predominant Often symmetric and homogeneous Subpleural sparing highly suggestive	Ground-glass opacity and reticulation Honeycombing uncommon, minimal if present
Cryptogenic organizing pneumonia	Peribronchial, peripheral, perilobular Often basilar and peripheral, but can be any anywhere Often bilateral, but can be unilateral	Consolidation with wispy borders and ground-glass opacity Transient bronchial dilation and distortion of lung architecture Look for atoll/reverse halo sign and perilobular thickening, which can be suggestive
Acute interstitial pneumonia	Diffuse	Patchy consolidation and ground-glass opacity Consolidation greater in dependent lung
Respiratory bronchiolitis/respiratory bronchiolitis interstitial lung disease	Upper lung predominant	Centrilobular ground-glass nodules Can have patchy diffuse ground glass opacity if severe
Desquamative interstitial pneumonia	Often basilar and peripheral, but can be anywhere	Ground-glass opacity Look for superimposed tiny cysts
Lymphocytic interstitial pneumonia	Basilar predominant	Cysts, often peribronchovascular and/or subpleural Ground-glass opacity Nodules
Idiopathic pleuroparenchymal fibroelastosis	Upper lung predominant	Dense subpleural pleural and parenchymal scarring Often associated volume loss/architectural distortion

Data from Refs.[26,29]

consolidation superimposed on underlying fibrosis. The new regions of ground glass and consolidation may be located diffusely, patchy, or in peripheral predominant distribution (**Fig. 2**).[30–33]

Patients with IPF are at an increased risk of developing lung cancer, with lung cancer rates ranging from 5% to 50%.[34–38] Lung cancer in UIP typically develops in areas of fibrosis and appears as a slowly enlarging area of consolidation.[38] Because small areas of consolidation are common findings adjacent to dense fibrosis, follow-up imaging to assess for progressive growth or fluorodeoxyglucose positron emission tomography/CT imaging to assess for focal metabolic activity is prudent before considering tissue sampling.[30] Lung cancer in the setting of pulmonary fibrosis is often subtle; therefore, careful inspection is mandatory to exclude early malignancy in pulmonary fibrosis. In particular, the junction of normal lung and pulmonary fibrosis in the lower lung zones should be assessed meticulously given the tendency for lung cancers to arise in these areas (**Fig. 3**).[34]

Many cases of IPF have a strong genetic component, with almost 20% of patients who undergo lung transplant for IPF having a family history of lung fibrosis.[39] Several studies have shown that the genetic inheritance is suggestive of autosomal-dominant transmission with incomplete penetrance,[40–42] which emphasizes the importance of family history in this setting. Several genetic loci have been have been shown to be linked to pulmonary fibrosis.[43–46] Despite the suggestion of an underlying genetic component, these cases are still considered idiopathic.[2] In familial pulmonary fibrosis, the pattern of lung disease may not always conform to a classic lower lung–predominant, UIP-type fibrosis pattern. Frequently, the pattern of fibrosis may be diffuse in a cranial–caudal plane,

Table 2
High-resolution CT features of usual interstitial pneumonia (UIP)

UIP Pattern	Possible UIP Pattern	Inconsistent with UIP
All 4 features	*All 3 features*	*Any of the 7 features*
Subpleural, basal predominance	Subpleural, basal predominance	Upper or mid-lung predominance
Reticular abnormality	Reticular abnormality	Peribronchovascular predominance
Honeycombing with or without traction bronchiectasis	Absence of features listed as inconsistent with UIP pattern (see third column)	Extensive ground-glass abnormality (greater than reticular abnormality)
Absence of features listed as inconsistent with UIP pattern (see third column)		Profuse micronodules (bilateral, predominantly upper lobes)
		Discrete cysts (multiple, bilateral, away from areas of honeycombing)
		Diffuse mosaic attenuation/air trapping (bilateral, in ≥3 lobes)
		Consolidation in bronchopulmonary segment(s)/lobe(s)

Data from Raghu G, Collard HR, Egan JJ, et al. An official ATS/ERS/JRS/ALAT statement: idiopathic pulmonary fibrosis: evidence-based guidelines for diagnosis and management. Am J Respir Crit Care Med 2011;183(6):788–824.

or, in a smaller subset, may even be upper lung predominant (**Fig. 4**).[41]

Nonspecific Interstitial Pneumonia

NSIP is another chronic fibrosing interstitial pneumonia that most commonly has basilar zonal distribution.[47–49] In contrast with UIP, it frequently carries a significantly better prognosis.[2,50] The NSIP-type pattern of pulmonary fibrosis is often secondary to known conditions, most importantly collagen vascular disease. In fact, even when patients do not have a known underlying cause, there are frequently nonspecific laboratory and clinical

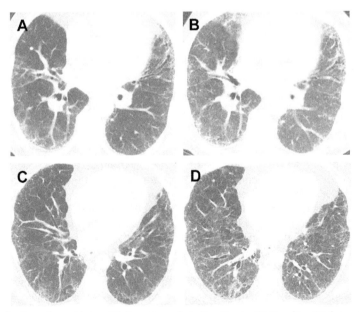

Fig. 2. Acute exacerbation of usual interstitial pneumonia in 2 patients. (*A*) Baseline CT shows peripheral reticular abnormality. (*B*) Follow-up CT shows diffuse increased ground glass, indicating acute exacerbation or infection. Detecting diffuse increases in ground glass can be challenging. Comparison with a baseline CT is useful. Baseline (*C*) and follow-up (*D*) images from a different patient show a similar pattern of bilateral patchy increased ground glass (*D*). Again, comparison with a baseline is useful for this often subtle finding.

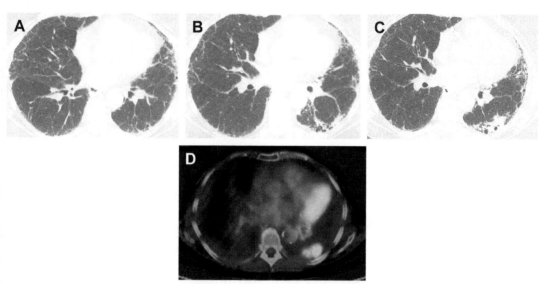

Fig. 3. Usual interstitial pneumonia (UIP) complicated by adenocarcinoma in left lower lobe. (*A*) Baseline CT shows a UIP pattern of fibrosis. (*B*) Follow-up CT 2 years later shows progressive fibrosis and a new, small region of consolidation in the posterior left lower lobe. Differential diagnosis of this finding includes focal dense fibrosis versus adenocarcinoma. A follow-up examination was recommended. (*C*) On follow-up examination 12 months later, this region has enlarged, and positron emission tomography–CT (*D*) demonstrated hypermetabolism in this consolidation. Adenocarcinoma was diagnosed on biopsy. This figure demonstrates the importance of careful evaluation for enlarging consolidations in UIP patients.

features that suggest but do not fulfill criteria of a specific collagen vascular disease.[51,52] Additionally, other important secondary causes of NSIP include HP, drug toxicity, and inhalation exposures.[2,7]

Histologic findings of NSIP tend to be more homogenous than UIP, with similar areas of parenchymal changes throughout a biopsy specimen. This contrasts with UIP, which has a more heterogeneous appearance where areas of end-stage fibrosis are often in proximity to areas of fairly normal lung. Histologically, NSIP has been divided into 2 subtypes: cellular NSIP and fibrotic NSIP. The cellular NSIP subtype demonstrates a greater degree of inflammatory cells without significant fibrosis, and the fibrotic subtype demonstrates greater fibrosis with or without a prominence of inflammatory cells. These subtypes have been used traditionally for prognostic purposes, with the cellular subtype having a relative better treatment response and long-term outcomes.[2,7,53] This differentiation may be less useful from a radiologic perspective, because it has been shown that even areas of prominent ground glass in NSIP most

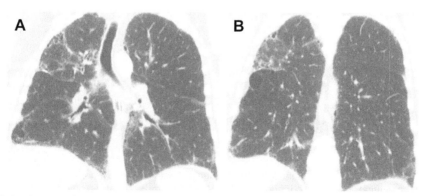

Fig. 4. Familial pulmonary fibrosis (FPF). A mid coronal image (*A*) and a posterior coronal image (*B*) of a patient with FPF. Note that honeycombing and reticulation is more predominant in the right upper lobe and less marked in the lung bases. Most patients with FPF have a classic usual interstitial pneumonia pattern; however, a significant subset have upper lung predominant fibrosis.

frequently represents fine pulmonary fibrosis. Nevertheless, HRCT demonstrating more advanced fibrosis is associated with a poorer prognosis.[33]

Chest radiographs show abnormalities in 90% of NSIP cases, mostly bibasilar findings and volume loss.[54] HRCT evaluation is more specific, and typically shows basilar predominant ground-glass opacity and/or reticulation.[17,47,55] These findings are typically more symmetric and homogeneous compared with the subtle asymmetry often seen in UIP. Additionally, the distribution of disease is often peribronchovascular, which is generally a specific differentiator of NSIP from UIP.[7] In a minority of cases, there is a clear region of symmetric subpleural sparing; when present; this is highly indicative of NSIP.[28,56] A relatively greater degree of traction bronchiectasis relative to the degree of pulmonary parenchymal disease is also an important finding in NSIP. Like the parenchymal disease, prominent traction bronchiectasis should also be symmetric. Honeycombing is a much less common finding in NSIP and, when present, should be relatively mild. Honeycombing may progress over time in NSIP, likely reflecting evolution of NSIP into a UIP pattern, which is not uncommon (**Fig. 5**).[7,17,47,49,57]

NSIP often coexists with organizing pneumonia (OP), with areas of OP seen in up to 50% of histologic samples.[56] Areas of consolidation in NSIP most frequently represent coexisting OP, which

usually have a peribronchovascular or subpleural distribution as seen in isolated cases of OP, as discussed elsewhere in this article.[7,29]

Despite the differences between NSIP and other IIPs, there can be overlapping features that can lead to diagnostic uncertainty. Particularly, mild UIP and mild NSIP may have overlapping features. Given the worse prognosis of UIP compared with NSIP, these mild patterns are frequently grouped into the possible UIP category with definitive diagnosis usually requiring surgical biopsy.[2,22,58]

ACUTE/SUBACUTE INTERSTITIAL PNEUMONIAS
Cryptogenic Organizing Pneumonia

COP, formerly known as bronchiolitis obliterans with OP, typically presents with subacute pulmonary symptoms.[3] On histology, COP is characterized by organizing cellular infiltrate and fibroblastic foci in the distal alveoli, which extend into the distal bronchioles.[59,60] COP refers to idiopathic disease; secondary causes of OP include infections, collagen vascular disease, drug toxicity, and lung or stem cell transplantation.

The inclusion of COP in the American Thoracic Society/European Respiratory Society classification of IIPs is controversial, because cellular pneumonia is prominent in the distal air spaces and is less marked in the interstitium. It remains in the

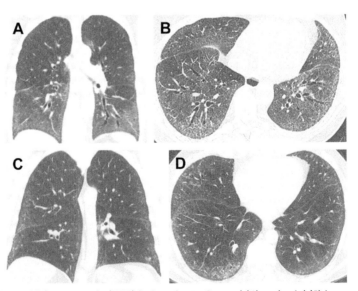

Fig. 5. Nonspecific interstitial pneumonia (NSIP) in 2 patients. Coronal (*A*) and axial (*B*) images with an NSIP-type pattern. Note the symmetric basilar peripheral pattern of reticulation and marked associated traction bronchiectasis. Minimal honeycombing is present in the posterior right lower lobe, which is a feature that should not be a prominent finding in NSIP. Coronal (*C*) and axial (*D*) images from a second patient with NSIP showing symmetric peripheral reticulation with immediate subpleural sparing. Subpleural sparing is present in a minority of patients with NSIP, but when present is highly suggestive of NSIP the diagnosis.

classification scheme because COP has many overlapping clinical and histologic features with the other IIPs, particularly with NSIP.[1,3] It also is often present in the setting of collagen vascular disease, similar to other IIPs.

The imaging features of COP are somewhat diverse; however, there are specific imaging patterns that are highly suggestive of the diagnosis. The most common pattern is of one or more areas of consolidation in a peribronchovascular and/or subpleural distribution, often with irregular or wispy borders; there may be associated components of ground-glass opacity (**Fig. 6**). COP may also be associated with perilobular thickening.[61] There may be transient bronchial dilatation in areas of consolidation. Classically, pulmonary consolidation is migratory, appearing in one area and resolving in another.[62,63]

A relatively specific finding in COP is the atoll or reversed halo sign, which manifests as a central region of ground-glass opacity with a surrounding rim of consolidation.[64] Although uncommon (19% of patients with COP), in the correct clinical setting, this imaging finding is characteristic of COP. However, it is not pathognomonic for COP because the reversed halo sign may also be seen in other conditions, such as mucormycosis, granulomatosis with polyangiitis, sarcoidosis, and pulmonary infarct.[65]

COP typically has a very good prognosis, with a marked response to corticosteroids. However, relapse and recurrence are common. Longer treatment courses and treatment of any underlying condition may help in achieving long-term remission. A significant degree of reticulation portends poor treatment response and a greater tendency to progress to overt pulmonary fibrosis or NSIP.[62,66,67]

Acute Interstitial Pneumonia

AIP is a condition with histology of diffuse alveolar damage, identical to acute respiratory distress syndrome (ARDS). Patients often have a viral-like prodrome followed by rapid respiratory failure, often requiring intubation over days. The diagnosis requires exclusion of secondary causes of ARDS including infection, trauma, reaction to blood transfusion, transplant rejection, or collagen vascular disease.[3,68]

Imaging findings in AIP correlate with the disease stage. On radiography, the early exudative phase is characterized by patchy bilateral consolidation, which often spares the costophrenic sulci. On CT, there is often superimposed patchy ground-glass opacity and consolidation with focal areas of lobular sparing (**Fig. 7**). Dependent consolidation is common. Most often the findings are diffuse, although there may be a slight basilar predominance. In the later organizing stage, there is generally radiographic improvement in the consolidation. On CT, improvement in consolidation and ground-glass opacity is usually present; air-space opacity often demonstrates a

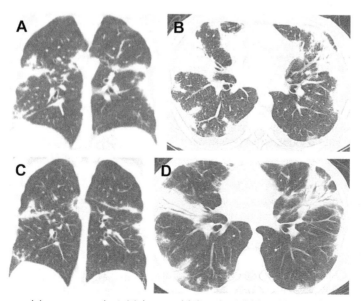

Fig. 6. Cryptogenic organizing pneumonia. Initial coronal (*A*) and axial (*B*) CT images show bilateral peribronchovascular and subpleural consolidation with irregular borders, and small bilateral plural effusions. After 3 weeks of corticosteroid therapy, the multifocal consolidations and pleural effusions have improved markedly (*C, D*).

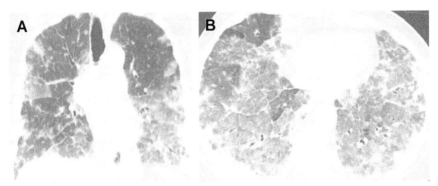

Fig. 7. Acute interstitial pneumonia in the acute phase. Coronal (*A*) and axial (*B*) CT images show widespread ground-glass attenuation, with areas of lobular sparing. There are focal areas of consolidation in the dependent lung.

peribronchovascular distribution. There may be associated bronchial dilatation.[69,70] Patients who survive show progressive clearing of consolidation and ground-glass opacity, although residual fibrosis from the late fibrotic phase may develop. Residual fibrotic findings are often more prominent in the anterior lungs. Fibrosis may range from subtle reticulation to overt architectural distortion and honeycombing.[68,70,71]

Overall, the imaging findings of AIP are similar to ARDS. There is a greater tendency of AIP to be in a basilar predominant distribution. Some studies have shown a slightly greater tendency of AIP to progress to fibrosis. However, these trends are not useful in practice in differentiating AIP from ARDS.[39]

SMOKING-RELATED INTERSTITIAL PNEUMONIAS
Respiratory Bronchiolitis Interstitial Lung Disease

The smoking-related interstitial pneumonias are currently thought to represent a spectrum of lung injury from asymptomatic RB to RB-ILD to DIP. Although these diseases exist on a spectrum, their clinical symptoms, histologic and radiologic findings, and treatment differ enough that they remain categorized separately.[72–74]

RB is a largely asymptomatic condition, which is found at autopsy in most smokers. Patients with longer and more extensive exposure, typically with more than a 30-pack-year smoking history,[75] may develop respiratory symptoms and are diagnosed with RB-ILD. Both of these conditions have similar histologic and radiologic findings, with RB-ILD being distinguished by the presence of clinical symptoms and often more severe imaging findings. Pigmented macrophage accumulation in the first- and second-order respiratory bronchioles is present in both conditions.[74,76,77]

HRCT findings of RB are mild, upper lung–predominant centrilobular ground glass nodularity, which is best seen on thin slice, high-resolution images. These subtle RB findings may be hidden by volume averaging in thicker slice reconstruction.[74,78] Similar upper lung fine centrilobular ground-glass nodularity can also be seen with HP; however, these patients are typically non-smokers and not uncommonly an exposure history supportive of an HP diagnosis is found.[72,79,80]

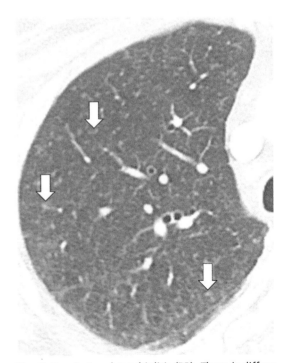

Fig. 8. Respiratory bronchiolitis (RB). There is diffuse centrilobular ground-glass nodularity (few indicated by *arrows*) in the upper lungs on this axial CT image, which is essentially diagnostic of RB in this patient with long smoking history.

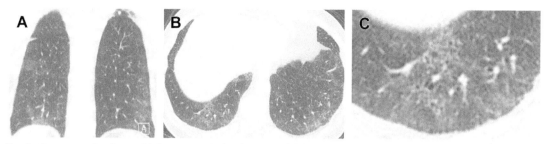

Fig. 9. Desquamative interstitial pneumonia (DIP). Coronal (*A*) and axial (*B*) CT images show patchy lower lung predominant ground glass in this smoker. Note the tiny internal cysts seen in a few of these ground-glass regions (*C*). These small cysts are not present in all DIP cases, but when present are highly indicative of the diagnosis.

Cigarette smoke is known to be a mild immunosuppressant, and perhaps for that reason is relatively protective for some autoimmune lung conditions, including HP and sarcoidosis.

Patients with RB-ILD have more extensive upper lung predominant centrilobular ground-glass nodularity, and may have patchy areas of confluent ground-glass opacity in the upper lungs as compared with those with RB (**Fig. 8**). Although more extensive CT findings may be suggestive of RB-ILD over RB, the diagnosis of RB-ILD should be made clinically. Typically, the diagnosis can be made by history, physical examination, pulmonary function test, and presence of pigmented macrophages on bronchoalveolar lavage without lymphocytes. Surgical lung biopsy is usually not required.[72,73,77,81]

The response to smoking cessation is variable. RB frequently demonstrates resolution of the fine centrilobular ground-glass nodules over years. RB-ILD also frequently improves clinically and by radiologic evaluation; however, a sizable minority of patients do not improve after smoking cessation and some will even continue to progress.

Desquamative Interstitial Pneumonia

DIP is a rare smoking-related disease. A minority of DIP cases are not related to smoking, because up to 40% of those afflicted are nonsmokers.[73,82] Other known causes include autoimmune disease (particularly rheumatoid arthritis), infection including hepatitis C virus, and drug toxicity.[29,83] Like in RB and RB-ILD, patients have pigmented macrophages in their airways; however, in DIP, the distribution of pigmented macrophages is much more extensive. Additionally, aggregated macrophages are often seen. Historically, these aggregated macrophages were thought to represent desquamated respiratory epithelium, and although it is now known what they actually are, the misnomer of DIP persists.[72,84]

Chest radiographs can be normal in up to 20% of patients; findings when present are nonspecific.[85] HRCT findings are also not entirely specific; however, in patients with a long smoking history, DIP should always be a consideration. HRCT typically reveals areas of ground-glass opacity that often are more extensive than in RB-ILD and span several pulmonary lobules typically in a lower and peripheral lung distribution.[74,86,87] A helpful finding, present in up to 70% of cases, is the presence of multiple small clustered cysts within areas of ground-glass opacity (**Fig. 9**).[88] Imaging features of DIP do overlap with other conditions, including chronic aspiration, subacute HP, and NSIP. Owing to diagnostic uncertainty, these patients may require surgical biopsy for diagnosis.[29]

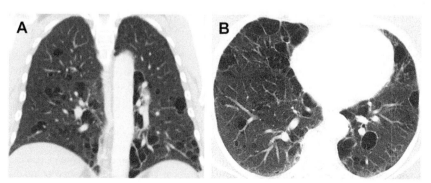

Fig. 10. Lymphocytic interstitial pneumonitis. Coronal (*A*) and axial (*B*) images show lower lung–predominant peribronchovascular and perilymphatic cysts consistent with lymphocytic interstitial pneumonitis.

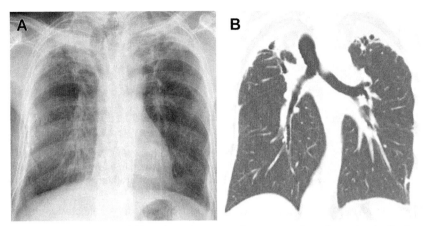

Fig. 11. Idiopathic pleuroparenchymal fibroelastosis. Dense pleuroparenchymal scarring in the lung apices with associated volume loss as indicated by hilar retraction and traction bronchiectasis is shown on this chest radiograph (*A*) and coronal CT (*B*).

RARE ENTITIES
Lymphocytic Interstitial Pneumonia

LIP is a rare condition that is almost always non-idiopathic. Known secondary causes include Sjögren syndrome, human immunodeficiency virus (particularly in children), and prior bone marrow transplantation. Histologically, LIP represents a polymorphic lymphocyte infiltration in the lung interstitium and within the pulmonary lymphatics. Clinically, the presentation of LIP is similar to the subacute or chronic IIPs.[89–91]

The most specific and suggestive finding of LIP on HRCT is the presence of lower lung–predominant perilymphatic cysts, typically adjacent to the peribronchovascular bundles (**Fig. 10**). These cysts are seen in 82% of patients. Other less specific findings are show patchy bilateral ground glass, with subtle subpleural and perilymphatic nodularity.[89,92,93]

Idiopathic Pleuroparenchymal Fibroelastosis

Idiopathic pleuroparenchymal fibroelastosis is a rare interstitial pneumonia that was recently included in the IIP classification.[2] Histologically, upper lobe–predominant subpleural fibrosis is seen, with fibroelastic bundles and intraalveolar fibrosis.[8] On CT, typical findings are dense subpleural upper lung consolidations and exuberant pleural thickenings with associated volume loss and architectural distortion (**Fig. 11**). It is a rare diagnosis, with only a few reported cases in the literature.[94–98] As with other IIPs, patients may present with progressive dyspnea and dry cough. Presentation with chest pain and pneumothorax has been also reported.[96,97,99] There may be a familial association. In addition, bone marrow transplant or chronic recurrent infections have been implicated as a secondary cause.[94,97] Differential considerations include other causes of upper lung fibrosis, including sarcoidosis, chronic HP, and familial pulmonary fibrosis. As a recent addition to the American Thoracic Society/European Respiratory Society classification of IIPs, this entity remains poorly understood in terms of associated causes and long term prognosis. Our anecdotal experience suggests that many patients have a rapid worsening clinical course, which may be triggered by surgical lung biopsy.

REFERENCES

1. Hansell DM. Classification of diffuse lung diseases: why and how. Radiology 2013;268(3):628–40.
2. Travis WD, Costabel U, Hansell DM, et al. An official American Thoracic Society/European Respiratory Society Statement: update of the international multidisciplinary classification of the idiopathic interstitial pneumonias. Am J Respir Crit Care Med 2013; 188(6):733–48.
3. American Thoracic Society, European Respiratory Society. American Thoracic Society/European Respiratory Society international multidisciplinary consensus classification of the idiopathic interstitial pneumonias. This joint statement of the American Thoracic Society (ATS), and the European Respiratory Society (ERS) was adopted by the ATS board of directors, June 2001 and by the ERS Executive Committee, June 2001. Am J Respir Crit Care Med 2002;165:277–304.
4. Hunninghake GW, Zimmerman MB, Schwartz DA, et al. Utility of a lung biopsy for the diagnosis of idiopathic pulmonary fibrosis. Am J Respir Crit Care Med 2001;164(2):193–6.

5. Frankel SK, Schwarz MI. Update in idiopathic pulmonary fibrosis. Curr Opin Pulm Med 2009;15(5): 463–9.

6. Misumi S, Lynch DA. Idiopathic pulmonary fibrosis/ usual interstitial pneumonia: imaging diagnosis, spectrum of abnormalities, and temporal progression. Proc Am Thorac Soc 2006;3(4):307–14.

7. Kligerman SJ, Groshong S, Brown KK, et al. Nonspecific interstitial pneumonia: radiologic, clinical, and pathologic considerations. Radiographics 2009;29(1):73–87.

8. Ryerson CJ, Collard HR. Update on the diagnosis and classification of ILD. Curr Opin Pulm Med 2013;19(5):453–9.

9. Ryerson CJ, Vittinghoff E, Ley B, et al. Predicting survival across chronic interstitial lung disease: the ILD-GAP model. Chest 2014;145(4):723–8.

10. Collard HR, King TE. Demystifying idiopathic interstitial pneumonia. Arch Intern Med 2003;163(1): 17–29.

11. Kim HC, Ji W, Kim MY, et al. Interstitial pneumonia related to undifferentiated connective tissue disease: pathologic pattern and prognosis. Chest 2014;147(1):165–72.

12. Grenier P, Valeyre D, Cluzel P, et al. Chronic diffuse interstitial lung disease: diagnostic value of chest radiography and high-resolution CT. Radiology 1991;179(1):123–32.

13. Lee KS, Primack SL, Staples CA, et al. Chronic infiltrative lung disease: comparison of diagnostic accuracies of radiography and low- and conventional-dose thin-section CT. Radiology 1994; 191(3):669–73.

14. Swensen SJ, Aughenbaugh GL, Myers JL. Diffuse lung disease: diagnostic accuracy of CT in patients undergoing surgical biopsy of the lung. Radiology 1997;205(1):229–34.

15. Peikert T, Daniels CE, Beebe TJ, et al. Interstitial Lung Diseases Network of the American College of Chest Physicians. Assessment of current practice in the diagnosis and therapy of idiopathic pulmonary fibrosis. Respir Med 2008;102(9):1342–8.

16. Arakawa H, Fujimoto K, Honma K, et al. Progression from near-normal to end-stage lungs in chronic interstitial pneumonia related to silica exposure: long-term CT observations. AJR Am J Roentgenol 2008; 191(4):1040–5.

17. Sumikawa H, Johkoh T, Ichikado K, et al. Usual interstitial pneumonia and chronic idiopathic interstitial pneumonia: analysis of CT appearance in 92 patients. Radiology 2006;241(1):258–66.

18. Silva CIS, Müller NL. Idiopathic interstitial pneumonias. J Thorac Imaging 2009;24(4):260–73.

19. Gruden JF, Panse PM, Leslie KO, et al. UIP diagnosed at surgical lung biopsy, 2000–2009: HRCT patterns and proposed classification system. AJR Am J Roentgenol 2013;200(5):W458–67.

20. Lynch DA, Travis WD, Müller NL, et al. Idiopathic interstitial pneumonias: CT features. Radiology 2005;236(1):10–21.

21. Nishimura K, Kitaichi M, Izumi T, et al. Usual interstitial pneumonia: histologic correlation with high-resolution CT. Radiology 1992;182(2):337–42.

22. Raghu G, Collard HR, Egan JJ, et al. An official ATS/ ERS/JRS/ALAT statement: idiopathic pulmonary fibrosis: evidence-based guidelines for diagnosis and management. Am J Respir Crit Care Med 2011;183(6):788–824.

23. Cottin V, Cordier JF. Combined pulmonary fibrosis and emphysema: an experimental and clinically relevant phenotype. Am J Respir Crit Care Med 2005;172(12):1605 [author reply: 1605–6].

24. Sverzellati N, De Filippo M, Bartalena T, et al. High-resolution computed tomography in the diagnosis and follow-up of idiopathic pulmonary fibrosis. Radiol Med 2010;115(4):526–38.

25. Mura M, Zompatori M, Pacilli AM, et al. The presence of emphysema further impairs physiologic function in patients with idiopathic pulmonary fibrosis. Respir Care 2006;51(3):257–65.

26. Lynch DA, Godwin JD, Safrin S, et al. High-resolution computed tomography in idiopathic pulmonary fibrosis: diagnosis and prognosis. Am J Respir Crit Care Med 2005;172(4):488–93.

27. Hodnett PA, Naidich DP. Fibrosing interstitial lung disease. A practical high-resolution computed tomography–based approach to diagnosis and management and a review of the literature. Am J Respir Crit Care Med 2013;188(2):141–9.

28. Sumikawa H, Johkoh T, Colby TV, et al. Computed tomography findings in pathological usual interstitial pneumonia: relationship to survival. Am J Respir Crit Care Med 2008;177(4):433–9.

29. Hobbs S, Lynch D. The idiopathic interstitial pneumonias: an update and review. Radiol Clin North Am 2014;52(1):105–20.

30. Lloyd CR, Walsh SL, Hansell DM. High-resolution CT of complications of idiopathic fibrotic lung disease. Br J Radiol 2011;84(1003):581–92.

31. Churg A, Müller NL, Silva CI, et al. Acute exacerbation (acute lung injury of unknown cause) in UIP and other forms of fibrotic interstitial pneumonias. Am J Surg Pathol 2007;31(2):277–84.

32. Hyzy R, Huang S, Myers J, et al. Acute exacerbation of idiopathic pulmonary fibrosis. Chest 2007;132(5): 1652–8.

33. Akira M, Kozuka T, Yamamoto S, et al. Computed tomography findings in acute exacerbation of idiopathic pulmonary fibrosis. Am J Respir Crit Care Med 2008;178(4):372–8.

34. Yoshida R, Arakawa H, Kaji Y. Lung cancer in chronic interstitial pneumonia: early manifestation from serial CT observations. AJR Am J Roentgenol 2012;199(1):85–90.

35. Archontogeorgis K, Steiropoulos P, Tzouvelekis A, et al. Lung cancer and interstitial lung diseases: a systematic review. Pulm Med 2012;2012(1):315918.

36. Ma Y, Seneviratne CK, Koss M. Idiopathic pulmonary fibrosis and malignancy. Curr Opin Pulm Med 2001;7(5):278–82.

37. Ozawa Y, Suda T, Naito T, et al. Cumulative incidence of and predictive factors for lung cancer in IPF. Respirology 2009;14(5):723–8.

38. Bouros D, Hatzakis K, Labrakis H, et al. Association of malignancy with diseases causing interstitial pulmonary changes. Chest 2002;121(4):1278–89.

39. Tomiyama N, Müller NL, Johkoh T, et al. Acute respiratory distress syndrome and acute interstitial pneumonia: comparison of thin-section CT findings. J Comput Assist Tomogr 2001;25(1):28–33.

40. Lee HL, Ryu JH, Wittmer MH, et al. Familial idiopathic pulmonary fibrosis: clinical features and outcome. Chest 2005;127(6):2034–41.

41. Lee HY, Seo JB, Steele MP, et al. High-resolution CT scan findings in familial interstitial pneumonia do not conform to those of idiopathic interstitial pneumonia. Chest 2012;142(6):1577–83.

42. Chung JH, Chawla A, Peljto AL, et al. CT findings of probable UIP have a high predictive value for histologic UIP. Chest 2014;147(2):450–9.

43. Fingerlin TE, Murphy E, Zhang W, et al. Genome-wide association study identifies multiple susceptibility loci for pulmonary fibrosis. Nat Genet 2013;45(6):613–20.

44. Alder JK, Chen JJ, Lancaster L, et al. Short telomeres are a risk factor for idiopathic pulmonary fibrosis. Proc Natl Acad Sci U S A 2008;105(35):13051–6.

45. Barlo NP, van Moorsel CH, Ruven HJ, et al. Surfactant protein-D predicts survival in patients with idiopathic pulmonary fibrosis. Sarcoidosis Vasc Diffuse Lung Dis 2009;26(2):155–61.

46. Hunninghake GM, Hatabu H, Okajima Y, et al. MUC5B promoter polymorphism and interstitial lung abnormalities. N Engl J Med 2013;368(23):2192–200.

47. Elliot TL, Lynch DA, Newell JD, et al. High-resolution computed tomography features of nonspecific interstitial pneumonia and usual interstitial pneumonia. J Comput Assist Tomogr 2005;29(3):339–45.

48. Jeong YJ, Lee KS, Müller NL, et al. Usual interstitial pneumonia and non-specific interstitial pneumonia: serial thin-section CT findings correlated with pulmonary function. Korean J Radiol 2005;6(3):143–52.

49. Sumikawa H, Johkoh T, Fujimoto K, et al. Pathologically proved nonspecific interstitial pneumonia: CT pattern analysis as compared with usual interstitial pneumonia CT pattern. Radiology 2014;272(2):549–56.

50. Jegal Y, Kim DS, Shim TS, et al. Physiology is a stronger predictor of survival than pathology in fibrotic interstitial pneumonia. Am J Respir Crit Care Med 2005;171(6):639–44.

51. Suda T, Kono M, Nakamura Y, et al. Distinct prognosis of idiopathic nonspecific interstitial pneumonia (NSIP) fulfilling criteria for undifferentiated connective tissue disease (UCTD). Respir Med 2010;104(10):1527–34.

52. Corte TJ, Copley SJ, Desai SR, et al. Significance of connective tissue disease features in idiopathic interstitial pneumonia. Eur Respir J 2012;39(3):661–8.

53. Travis WD, Matsui K, Moss J, et al. Idiopathic nonspecific interstitial pneumonia: prognostic significance of cellular and fibrosing patterns: survival comparison with usual interstitial pneumonia and desquamative interstitial pneumonia. Am J Surg Pathol 2000;24(1):19–33.

54. Park JS, Lee KS, Kim JS, et al. Nonspecific interstitial pneumonia with fibrosis: radiographic and CT findings in seven patients. Radiology 1995;195(3):645–8.

55. Flaherty KR, Thwaite EL, Kazerooni EA, et al. Radiological versus histological diagnosis in UIP and NSIP: survival implications. Thorax 2003;58(2):143–8.

56. Travis WD, Hunninghake G, King TE Jr, et al. Idiopathic nonspecific interstitial pneumonia. Am J Respir Crit Care Med 2008;177(12):1338–47.

57. Akira M, Inoue Y, Arai T, et al. Long-term follow-up high-resolution CT findings in non-specific interstitial pneumonia. Thorax 2011;66(1):61–5.

58. Lynch DA, Huckleberry JM. Usual interstitial pneumonia: typical and atypical high-resolution computed tomography features. Semin Ultrasound CT MR 2014;35(1):12–23.

59. Epler GR, Colby TV, McLoud TC, et al. Bronchiolitis obliterans organizing pneumonia. N Engl J Med 1985;312(3):152–8.

60. Davison AG, Heard BE, McAllister WA, et al. Cryptogenic organizing pneumonitis. Q J Med 1983;52(207):382–94.

61. Ujita M, Renzoni EA, Veeraraghavan S, et al. Organizing pneumonia: perilobular pattern at thin-section CT. Radiology 2004;232(3):757–61.

62. Lee JS, Lynch DA, Sharma S, et al. Organizing pneumonia: prognostic implication of high-resolution computed tomography features. J Comput Assist Tomogr 2003;27(2):260–5.

63. Lee KS, Kullnig P, Hartman TE, et al. Cryptogenic organizing pneumonia: CT findings in 43 patients. AJR Am J Roentgenol 1994;162(3):543–6.

64. Kim SJ, Lee KS, Ryu YH, et al. Reversed halo sign on high-resolution CT of cryptogenic organizing pneumonia: diagnostic implications. AJR Am J Roentgenol 2003;180(5):1251–4.

65. Walker CM, Mohammed TL, Chung JH. Reversed halo sign. J Thorac Imaging 2011;26(3):W80.

66. Cottin V, Cordier JF. Cryptogenic organizing pneumonia. Semin Respir Crit Care Med 2012;33(5): 462–75.

67. Roberton BJ, Hansell DM. Organizing pneumonia: a kaleidoscope of concepts and morphologies. Eur Radiol 2011;21(11):2244–54.

68. Vourlekis JS. Acute interstitial pneumonia. Clin Chest Med 2004;25(4):739–47.

69. Johkoh T, Müller NL, Cartier Y, et al. Idiopathic interstitial pneumonias: diagnostic accuracy of thin-section CT in 129 patients. Radiology 1999;211(2): 555–60.

70. Ichikado K, Suga M, Müller NL, et al. Acute interstitial pneumonia: comparison of high-resolution computed tomography findings between survivors and nonsurvivors. Am J Respir Crit Care Med 2002;165(11):1551–6.

71. Desai SR, Wells AU, Rubens MB, et al. Acute respiratory distress syndrome: CT abnormalities at long-term follow-up. Radiology 1999;210(1):29–35.

72. Hidalgo A, Franquet T, Giménez A, et al. Smoking-related interstitial lung diseases: radiologic-pathologic correlation. Eur Radiol 2006;16(11): 2463–70.

73. Ryu JH, Myers JL, Capizzi SA, et al. Desquamative interstitial pneumonia and respiratory bronchiolitis-associated interstitial lung disease. Chest 2005; 127(1):178–84.

74. Heyneman LE, Ward S, Lynch DA, et al. Respiratory bronchiolitis, respiratory bronchiolitis-associated interstitial lung disease, and desquamative interstitial pneumonia: different entities or part of the spectrum of the same disease process? AJR Am J Roentgenol 1999;173(6):1617–22.

75. Fraig M, Shreesha U, Savici D, et al. Respiratory bronchiolitis: a clinicopathologic study in current smokers, ex-smokers, and never-smokers. Am J Surg Pathol 2002;26(5):647–53.

76. Remy-Jardin M, Remy J, Gosselin B, et al. Lung parenchymal changes secondary to cigarette smoking: pathologic-CT correlations. Radiology 1993; 186(3):643–51.

77. Nair A, Hansell DM. High-resolution computed tomography features of smoking-related interstitial lung disease. Semin Ultrasound CT MR 2014; 35(1):59–71.

78. Reddy TL, Mayo J, Churg A. Respiratory bronchiolitis with fibrosis. High-resolution computed tomography findings and correlation with pathology. Ann Am Thorac Soc 2013;10(6):590–601.

79. McSharry C, Banham SW, Boyd G. Effect of cigarette smoking on the antibody response to inhaled antigens and the prevalence of extrinsic allergic alveolitis among pigeon breeders. Clin Allergy 1985; 15(5):487–94.

80. Warren CP. Extrinsic allergic alveolitis: a disease commoner in non-smokers. Thorax 1977;32(5): 567–9.

81. Ryu JH, Colby TV, Hartman TE, et al. Smoking-related interstitial lung diseases: a concise review. Eur Respir J 2001;17(1):122–32.

82. Godbert B, Wissler MP, Vignaud JM. Desquamative interstitial pneumonia: an analytic review with an emphasis on aetiology. Eur Respir Rev 2013; 22(128):117–23.

83. Kroll RR, Flood DA, Srigley J. Desquamative interstitial pneumonitis in a non-smoker: a rare diagnosis. Can Respir J 2014;21(2):86–8.

84. Palmucci S, Roccasalva F, Puglisi S, et al. Clinical and radiological features of idiopathic interstitial pneumonias (IIPs): a pictorial review. Insights Imaging 2014;5(3):347–64.

85. Carrington CB, Gaensler EA, Coutu RE, et al. Natural history and treated course of usual and desquamative interstitial pneumonia. N Engl J Med 1978; 298(15):801–9.

86. Hartman TE, Primack SL, Kang EY, et al. Disease progression in usual interstitial pneumonia compared with desquamative interstitial pneumonia. Assessment with serial CT. Chest 1996;110(2):378–82.

87. Hartman TE, Primack SL, Swensen SJ, et al. Desquamative interstitial pneumonia: thin-section CT findings in 22 patients. Radiology 1993;187(3): 787–90.

88. Koyama M, Johkoh T, Honda O, et al. Chronic cystic lung disease: diagnostic accuracy of high-resolution CT in 92 patients. AJR Am J Roentgenol 2003; 180(3):827–35.

89. Swigris JJ, Berry GJ, Raffin TA, et al. Lymphoid interstitial pneumonia: a narrative review. Chest 2002; 122(6):2150–64.

90. Cha SI, Fessler MB, Cool CD, et al. Lymphoid interstitial pneumonia: clinical features, associations and prognosis. Eur Respir J 2006;28(2):364–9.

91. Hare SS, Souza CA, Bain G, et al. The radiological spectrum of pulmonary lymphoproliferative disease. Br J Radiol 2012;85(1015):848–64.

92. Silva CI, Flint JD, Levy RD, et al. Diffuse lung cysts in lymphoid interstitial pneumonia: high-resolution CT and pathologic findings. J Thorac Imaging 2006; 21(3):241–4.

93. Tian X, Yi ES, Ryu JH. Lymphocytic interstitial pneumonia and other benign lymphoid disorders. Semin Respir Crit Care Med 2012;33(5):450–61.

94. Reddy TL, Tominaga M, Hansell DM, et al. Pleuroparenchymal fibroelastosis: a spectrum of histopathological and imaging phenotypes. Eur Respir J 2012;40(2):377–85.

95. Becker CD, Gil J, Padilla ML. Idiopathic pleuroparenchymal fibroelastosis: an unrecognized or misdiagnosed entity? Mod Pathol 2008;21(6):784–7.

96. Frankel SK, Cool CD, Lynch DA, et al. Idiopathic pleuroparenchymal fibroelastosis: description of a novel clinicopathologic entity. Chest 2004;126(6):2007–13.

97. Thüsen von der JH, Hansell DM, Tominaga M, et al. Pleuroparenchymal fibroelastosis in patients with pulmonary disease secondary to bone marrow transplantation. Mod Pathol 2011;24(12):1633–9.

98. Enomoto N, Kusagaya H, Oyama Y, et al. Quantitative analysis of lung elastic fibers in idiopathic pleuroparenchymal fibroelastosis (IPPFE): comparison of clinical, radiological, and pathological findings with those of idiopathic pulmonary fibrosis (IPF). BMC Pulm Med 2014;14(1):91.

99. Piciucchi S, Tomassetti S, Casoni G, et al. High resolution CT and histological findings in idiopathic pleuroparenchymal fibroelastosis: features and differential diagnosis. Respir Res 2011; 12(1):111.

Connective Tissue Disease–related Thoracic Disease

Yutaka Tsuchiya, MD[a,b,*], Aryeh Fischer, MD[c],
Joshua J. Solomon, MD[d], David A. Lynch, MB[a]

KEYWORDS

- Airways disease • Connective tissue disease • Interstitial lung disease
- Nonspecific interstitial pneumonia • Usual interstitial pneumonia

KEY POINTS

- Understanding the prevalence of each entity and the characteristic imaging patterns of each connective tissue disease (CTD) manifestation helps to make the correct diagnosis for CTD-related thoracic disease.
- Drug-induced toxicity, pulmonary infection, and malignancy are frequently seen in patients with CTD. These complications should be excluded when thoracic involvement newly occurs.
- Innovative approaches for evaluating severity and therapeutic effect for patients with CTD-associated thoracic disease have been under development.

INTRODUCTION

Connective tissue disease (CTD) is a group of systemic disorders characterized by autoimmunity and autoimmune-mediated organ damage. It frequently targets the lungs and other thoracic manifestations. CTD-related thoracic disease comprises features directly related to the CTD (including interstitial lung diseases [ILDs], airway diseases, vascular diseases, lymphoproliferative disease, and pleural diseases) and indirect complications (including infections, drug toxicity, and malignancy).

Thoracic disease in CTD has several unique features (**Box 1**):

- It is often asymptomatic, discovered as a consequence of routine radiologic evaluation of a patient with collagen vascular disease.

- In contrast, thoracic disease may be the first manifestation of a CTD, which may develop up to 5 years after initial presentation with CTD.[1–4]
- Although CTD may involve a single lung compartment (pulmonary interstitium, airways, vessels, or pleura), it is common to have involvement of several compartments (eg, interstitial abnormality with pulmonary hypertension [PH] or pleural effusion).
- Although overlap occurs, each CTD has a characteristic pattern of pulmonary involvement, and the prevalence of each thoracic complication entity varies according to the specific CTD (**Table 1**).
- Clues to the diagnosis may be apparent on chest radiograph or computed tomography (CT). For example, a dilated esophagus

[a] Department of Radiology, National Jewish Health, 1400 Jackson Street, Denver, CO 80206, USA;
[b] Department of Respiratory Medicine, Showa University Fujigaoka Hospital, 1-30 Fujigaoka, Yokohama 227-8501, Japan; [c] Department of Rheumatology, National Jewish Health, 1400 Jackson Street, Denver, CO 80206, USA; [d] Department of Respiratory and Critical Care Medicine, National Jewish Health, 1400 Jackson Street, Denver, CO 80206, USA
* Corresponding author. Department of Radiology, National Jewish Health, 1400 Jackson Street, Denver, CO 80206.
E-mail address: caeser-salad.2corn-soups@nifty.com

Clin Chest Med 36 (2015) 283–297
http://dx.doi.org/10.1016/j.ccm.2015.02.010

Table 1
Relative frequency of CTD-related manifestations in different diseases

	SSc	RA	pSS	MCTD	PM/DM	SLE
Airways	−	++	++	+	−	+
ILD	+++	++	++	++	+++	+
Pleural	−	++	+	+	−	+++
Vascular	+++	−	+	++	+	+
DAH	−	−	−	−	−	++

Abbreviations: DAH, diffuse alveolar hemorrhage; MCTD, mixed CTD; PM/DM, polymyositis/dermatomyositis; pSS, primary Sjögren syndrome; RA, rheumatoid arthritis; SLE, systemic lupus erythematosus; SSc, scleroderma.

Data from Fischer A, du Bois R. Interstitial lung disease in connective tissue disorders. Lancet 2012;380(9842): 689–98.

should suggest scleroderma, and joint erosions suggest rheumatoid arthritis (RA).

Understanding the prevalence of each entity and the characteristic patterns of each CTD manifestation contributes to the correct diagnosis for CTD-related thoracic disease. This article discusses the characteristic radiologic findings of each CTD-related thoracic disease.

IMAGING TECHNIQUES

Chest CT is helpful not only for diagnosis but also for evaluation for progression and treatment in patients with CTD-related thoracic disease.

The use of thin sections (0.5–1.5 mm) is essential if spatial resolution and lung detail are to be optimized. Also, using a high-resolution CT (HRCT) algorithm is a critical element in performing HRCT. Prone imaging is helpful for identifying early lung fibrosis in the posterior lungs.[5] Multiplanar CT reconstructions may be helpful in identifying distribution of disease. Postexpiratory HRCT scans are helpful for showing significant air trapping in patients with suspected airways or obstructive lung diseases, such as bronchiolitis obliterans (BO) (**Fig. 1**).

IMAGING PATTERNS

Most of the parenchymal manifestations of CTD are similar to those found in idiopathic interstitial pneumonias (IIPs),[6] and can be classified using the same system.[7] The most common pattern of interstitial fibrosis seen in CTD is nonspecific interstitial pneumonia (NSIP) (**Fig. 2**).[8] However, usual interstitial pneumonia (UIP) (**Fig. 3**), organizing pneumonia (OP) (**Fig. 4**), and lymphocytic interstitial pneumonia (LIP) (**Fig. 5**) may also be seen. In addition to interstitial pneumonia, there may be evidence of airways disease, including bronchiectasis, obliterative bronchiolitis, or follicular bronchiolitis (FB). Bronchiectasis, usually found in RA, is usually cylindrical and must be distinguished from the traction bronchiectasis found in lung fibrosis. Obliterative bronchiolitis is characterized by mosaic attenuation and air trapping (see **Fig. 1**). FB may be associated with tree-in-bud pattern. In addition, clinicians should seek evidence of pleural disease and PH. Enlargement of the central pulmonary arteries is common in

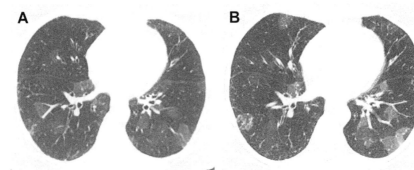

Fig. 1. BO in RA. (*A*) CT at full inspiration shows mosaic perfusion pattern as a result of BO. (*B*) End-expiratory CT shows marked lung inhomogeneity as a result of air trapping.

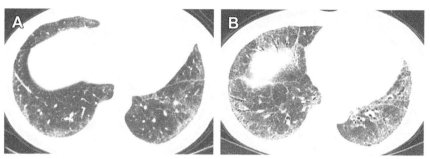

Fig. 2. Progressive lung fibrosis (NSIP pattern) in systemic scleroderma. (*A*) Initial CT shows moderate basal ground-glass opacities and reticular abnormality in lower lungs. (*B*) CT 6 years later shows marked progression of reticular abnormality with increased traction bronchiectasis.

patients with PH, but normal-sized pulmonary arteries do not exclude this diagnosis.

SPECIFIC CONNECTIVE TISSUE DISEASES
Rheumatoid Arthritis

RA is associated with a wide variety of pleuropulmonary, airway, and vascular manifestations (**Box 2**). The prevalence of radiologically detectable ILD with RA is 10% to 12%.[9–11] The most common pattern of lung fibrosis in RA is UIP (50%–60%) (see **Fig. 3**); less common are NSIP (40%–50%) and OP (10%).[12–16] A few cases of diffuse alveolar damage (DAD)[17] and desquamative interstitial pneumonia (DIP)[15] have also been described. CT findings in interstitial pneumonia associated with RA are similar to those of the idiopathic variety.[18–20] However, associated nodules, mosaic attenuation, pulmonary arterial enlargement, and pleural abnormality may provide a clue to the underlying diagnosis. There is growing evidence that the radiologic UIP pattern in RA-ILD is associated with significantly shortened survival compared with that in patients without the UIP pattern.[21,22] Assayag and colleagues[23] suggested in a recent study of RA-ILD that, when the radiologic UIP pattern is present on CT, histopathologic UIP can be determined with a high degree of confidence.

RA is considered the most frequent CTD associated with large and small airway disease, with prevalence ranging from 8% to 65%.[24–28] The major complications are BO, FB, and bronchiectasis. The characteristic CT finding of BO is mosaic perfusion with expiratory air trapping, often associated with evidence of mild bronchial dilatation (see **Fig. 1**).[29–31] The CT finding of FB is centrilobular nodules and tree-in-bud pattern, often associated with peribronchial nodules, and with areas of ground-glass abnormality.[24,27] PH commonly occurs in patients with RA, but is usually mild.[32] Pleural disease is common in patients who have RA, being seen in up to 40% at autopsy; however, symptomatic pleural disease is less common.[10,33] Necrobiotic nodules, similar to subcutaneous rheumatoid nodules, uncommonly occur in the lung. They are usually round, well defined, and may cavitate (**Fig. 6**). Drug-induced lung disease and pulmonary infection are discussed later.

Systemic Sclerosis (Scleroderma)

Systemic sclerosis (SSc) has a higher prevalence of pulmonary involvement than the other CTDs (**Box 3**).

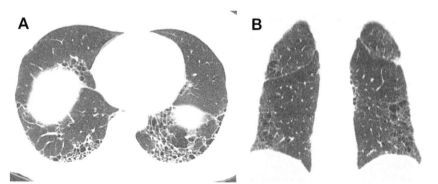

Fig. 3. UIP in RA. (*A*, *B*) Axial and coronal CT images through the lower lungs show typical pattern of basal, peripheral predominant reticular abnormality, and honeycombing.

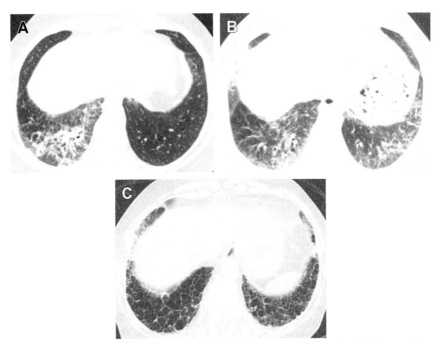

Fig. 4. Characteristic CT patterns in dermatomyositis. (*A*) CT shows consolidation in right lower lobe, compatible with OP. (*B*) Consolidation evolved to bilateral reticular and ground-glass opacities, which is more suggestive of NSIP. (*C*) The abnormalities found in (*B*) evolved into honeycombing.

NSIP is more frequently seen in SSc (see **Fig. 2**) than UIP,[34,35] and other histologic patterns (eg, OP and DAD) are very rare. CT findings of SSc-ILD reflect the dominant NSIP histology, and are characterized by confluent ground-glass opacification and fine reticular pattern, often posterior and subpleural, usually associated with traction bronchiectasis and bronchiolectasis.[36–38] Honeycombing, when present, is usually mild.[39] However, patients with honeycombing are more likely to progress on serial evaluation.[37] The lung fibrosis associated with SSc is associated with a much better prognosis than that found in idiopathic lung fibrosis,[40–42] most likely, in part, because of the predominant NSIP histology. However, patients with scleroderma who have more than 20% involvement by fibrosis on initial CT have a much higher mortality than those with lesser degrees of fibrosis.

The prevalence of PH in patients with SSc, when the diagnosis is based on rigorous right-sided heart catheter for assessment of filling pressures, is about 8% to 14%,[43,44] either as an isolated finding or in association with lung fibrosis. PH is

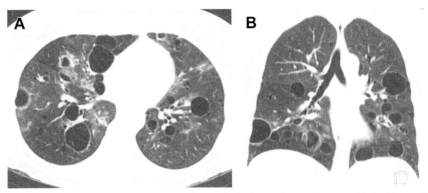

Fig. 5. LIP in Sjögren syndrome. (*A*) Axial CT image through the lower lungs shows multiple thin-walled peribronchovascular cysts, with some associated ground-glass abnormality. (*B*) Coronal images show that the cystic abnormality is predominantly in the lower lobes.

Box 2
RA-related thoracic disease
• Interstitial pneumonia (eg, UIP [most common], NSIP, OP, DAD, and DIP)
• Airways disease (eg, FB, BO, and bronchiectasis)
• PH
• Pleuritis
• Necrobiotic nodules
• Drug-induced lung disease (eg, methotrexate and the tumor necrosis factor alpha inhibitors)
• Infection (eg, tuberculosis, nontuberculosis mycobacteriosis, *Pneumocystis jiroveci* pneumonia)
Abbreviations: DAD, diffuse alveolar damage; DIP, desquamative interstitial pneumonia.

Box 3
SSc-related thoracic disease
• Lung fibrosis (40%–100%)
• NSIP pattern (80%–90%)
• UIP (10%–20%)
• Patients with honeycombing and those with more than 20% involvement are more likely to progress
• PH (particularly in CREST)
• PH out of proportion to extent of lung fibrosis
• Esophageal dysmotility

particularly common in patients with limited scleroderma (CREST syndrome).[45] PH usually causes enlargement of the main and proximal pulmonary arteries on chest radiographs or CT (**Fig. 7**); however, normal-sized pulmonary arteries do not exclude the diagnosis. Esophageal dilation is found in up to 80% of cases with SSc on CT.[46] Patients with SSc with severe esophageal dysfunction have an increased frequency of apparent ILD on CT.[47,48]

Polymyositis/Dermatomyositis

Polymyositis/dermatomyositis (PM/DM) are idiopathic inflammatory myopathies characterized by weakness in the proximal limb muscles.[49] Pulmonary involvement is one of the most frequent complications and is associated with high morbidity and mortality in PM/DM (**Box 4**).[50] The

antisynthetase antibody syndrome, which is a variant of PM/DM, is characterized by a positive serologic test for antiaminoacyl transfer RNA synthetase antibodies and less severe disease.[51,52] The characteristic CT pattern with PM/DM or with the antisynthetase syndrome is most commonly the NSIP and OP pattern, often occurring in combination (see **Fig. 4**).[52] Therefore, the most common abnormalities are confluent ground-glass opacities and consolidation in the lower lobes, superimposed on a background of reticular abnormality with traction bronchiectasis.[53–55] On serial evaluation, the changes of ground-glass opacities, consolidation, reticular abnormality, and traction bronchiectasis may all be partially reversible with treatment.[53,54,56] In contrast, some patients have clinically amyopathic dermatomyositis (CADM) characterized by little or no evidence of muscular manifestations with anti–CADM-140 antibody positivity. This variant commonly has a rapidly progressive form with acute respiratory failure from DAD or fulminant OP.[51,57] When the CT features of DM patients with anti–CADM-140 antibody are compared with those without this antibody, the prevalence of lower lung consolidation or ground-glass opacities is higher, and the prevalence of reticular opacity is lower.[58]

Systemic Lupus Erythematosus

Systemic lupus erythematosus (SLE) is commonly associated with pleural and pulmonary abnormalities. Pleural effusion is the most common thoracic finding. However, pulmonary fibrosis is uncommon. The most common cause of a pulmonary opacity in SLE is infection. Pulmonary hemorrhage and pulmonary thromboembolism may also occur (**Box 5**).[59,60]

Pleuritis is the most specific thoracic manifestation, occurring in 40% to 85% of patients with SLE,[61–63] and is one of the diagnostic criteria for

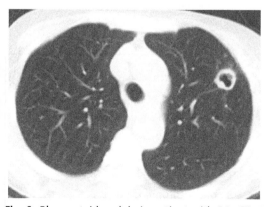

Fig. 6. Rheumatoid nodule in patient with RA. CT at the level of the upper lobes shows round, well-defined, cavitary nodule in left upper lobe.

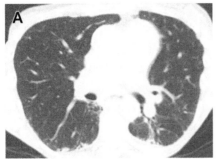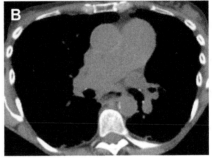

Fig. 7. PH in SSc. (*A*) CT through the midlungs shows minimal fibrosis. (*B*) Mediastinal window settings at the same level show dilated pulmonary trunk. Note the dilated, food-filled esophagus.

SLE (**Fig. 8**).[64] Acute lupus pneumonitis is a poorly defined entity, characterized by a variable degree of respiratory impairment accompanied by focal or diffuse pulmonary consolidation.[63] It is now thought that most cases previously identified as lupus pneumonitis probably represented acute interstitial pneumonia with or without pulmonary hemorrhage.[65] Diffuse alveolar hemorrhage is associated with diffuse or patchy consolidation and ground-glass abnormality.[66] Because many cases of alveolar hemorrhage are not associated with hemoptysis, it is important to consider this as a potential cause of ground-glass abnormality on CT in patients with lupus.

The frequency of SLE-related PH is from 0.5% to 17.5%. Mechanisms of development of PH may include acute or chronic thromboembolic disease associated with antiphospholipid antibody syndrome, increased pulmonary vascular resistance, inflammation, immune dysregulation, and vascular remodeling.[67] Shrinking lung syndrome is characterized by unexplained dyspnea, small lung volumes, and restrictive lung physiology, with or without diaphragmatic elevation, in the absence of other pulmonary diseases (**Fig. 9**).[68,69]

Sjögren Syndrome

Sjögren syndrome (SS) is characteristically associated with LIP (**Box 6**, see **Fig. 5**). Peribronchovascular, centrilobular, and subpleural nodules may be seen. The cystic changes of LIP are often not associated with significant symptoms or physiologic impairment, which may explain why NSIP is the most frequently seen histologic pattern (61%) in patients who undergo biopsy.[70,71] FB is the most frequent airway disease in SS (**Fig. 10**).[72] It is characterized by lymphoid aggregates, with or without germinal centers, situated in the walls of bronchioles and possibly compressing their lumens.[27] FB typically shows small nodular opacities in centrilobular and peribronchovascular distribution or lung cysts.[27] Patients with SS are at increased risk of developing non-Hodgkin lymphomas, which include mucosa-associated lymphoid tissue (MALT) lymphoma[73,74] and other subtypes of lymphoma such as nodal marginal zone lymphomas and diffuse large B-cell lymphoma.[75,76] The radiographic presentation of MALT lymphomas is lung nodules; airspace consolidation with or without air bronchograms that is bilateral in more than half of the patients. Lymphadenopathy is characteristically absent.

Box 4
PM/DM-related thoracic disease

- Basal predominant, NSIP, or confluent OP pattern is the most common
- May evolve to NSIP pattern
- DAD or UIP may also occur
- Similar features seen with antisynthetase syndrome
- DAD or fulminant OP is seen in CADM

Abbreviation: CADM, clinically amyopathic dermatomyositis.

Box 5
SLE-related thoracic disease

- Opportunistic infection (the most common)
- Pleural effusion or thickening (40%–85%)
- Diffuse alveolar hemorrhage
- ILD (uncommon)
- PH
- Pulmonary thromboembolism
- Rare manifestations (eg, shrinking lung syndrome)

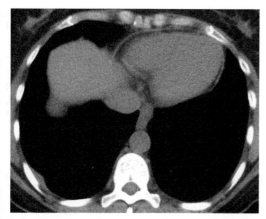

Fig. 8. Pleuritis with SLE. CT at the level of the lung bases shows right pleural thickening and mild pericardial thickening.

Other types of lymphoma should be suspected if consolidation, solitary or multifocal large nodules (>1 cm), lymphadenopathy, or effusions are present.[77] Pulmonary amyloidosis is a rare complication of SS. Large, irregular, smooth-bordered, and often calcified nodules are randomly distributed in commonly bilateral, peripheral, and lower-lobe locations (**Fig. 11**). Amyloid may also be associated with multiple cysts and septal thickening, similar to those seen with lymphoid interstitial pneumonia.[78,79] Pleural effusion, pleural thickening[80,81] and PH are rare manifestations of SS.

Mixed Connective Tissue Disease

Mixed CTD (MCTD) is an overlap syndrome that is a distinct clinicopathologic entity.[82] The principal characteristics are the presence of (1) features of SLE, scleroderma, and PM/DM, occurring together or evolving sequentially during observation; and (2) antibodies to an extractable nuclear antigen (ribonucleoprotein).[82] The imaging findings of MCTD are driven by the dominant connective disease manifestation (**Box 7**).[83] Thus,

patients with MCTD who have a lupuslike presentation tend to present with pleural effusions, whereas patients with a pattern similar to scleroderma are associated with NSIP.[7,84]

Ground-glass attenuation is the most common parenchymal abnormality in patients with MCTD-ILD,[85,86] which corresponds most closely with NSIP. Less common findings include honeycombing, consolidation, and poorly defined centrilobular nodules. Pleural thickening and pleural and pericardial effusions are also seen in patients with MCTD.[87] Other important complications include PH,[88–90] which occurs in 10% to 45% of patients with MCTD,[87] and esophageal dysmotility.[89]

PEARLS AND PITFALLS
Drug-induced Pneumonitis

Because most patients with CTD are treated with antiinflammatory or immunosuppressive drugs, drug-induced pneumonitis must always be considered as a cause of pulmonary abnormality. Various drugs, in particular methotrexate (**Fig. 12**) and the tumor necrosis factor alpha inhibitors, have been associated with drug-induced pneumonitis with CTD, although it is often difficult to distinguish association from causality. Drugs can result in a variety of histopathologic reaction patterns in the lung parenchyma. The most common CT patterns of drug toxicity in CTD are NSIP and OP. However, some patients have more than 1 histopathologic pattern and overlap,[91,92] which may result in the various patterns on CT. Drug-induced pneumonitis should always be considered in a patient with CTD presenting with new parenchymal abnormalities.

Respiratory Infections

Patients with CTD are at increased risk of respiratory infections. Predisposition to infection in patients with CTD is both inherent, in the form of

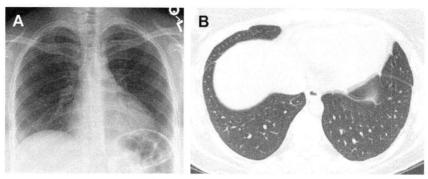

Fig. 9. Shrinking lung syndrome in SLE. (A) Chest radiograph shows bilateral reduced lung volumes. The heart is moderately enlarged. (B) CT image through the lower lungs shows the absence of other pulmonary diseases that might account for decreased lung volume.

Box 6
SS–related thoracic disease

- ILD, most commonly LIP
- Airway disease (eg, FB and BO)
- Malignant lymphoma
- Amyloidosis
- Rare complications (eg, pleuritis or PH)

---

had UIP. Because early lung cancer is hard to detect on chest radiographs in the context of CTD-ILD, routine use of CT is recommended for early detection of lung cancer as well as for evaluating serial changes in CTD-ILD. Lung cancer related to ILD can be difficult to detect even on CT, because it tends to begin in areas of fibrosis, so small malignant lung nodules may be difficult to distinguish from focal fibrosis.

disease-related immune dysregulation, and acquired, caused by immunosuppressive treatment regimens. In particular, newer biologic agents, such as antitumor necrosis factor antibodies (etanercept, infliximab, and adalimumab), predispose to tuberculosis, nontuberculous mycobacteria, or fungal infection, including pneumocystis, and these should be strongly suspected when new parenchymal abnormalities are identified in these patients (**Fig. 13**).[93–95] Screening for occult infection and careful follow-up with chest radiographs or CT are needed for patients with CTD throughout their treatment periods.

Thoracic Malignancy

The rate of lung cancer is greater in patients with CTDs than in the general population.[96–101] RA, SSc, and SS are also associated with a higher risk of non-Hodgkin lymphoma.[96,99–101] Malignancy can be associated with DM as paraneoplastic syndrome. In review of 153 reported cases of lung cancer associated with CTDs[102] there was a correlation between smoking and development of lung cancer in patients with RA and PM/DM. Most patients with SSc who developed lung cancer had underlying interstitial fibrosis (**Fig. 14**).[103] Takayanagi and colleagues[104] reported that 19.4% of patients with RA/UIP had lung cancer and 50% of patients with RA with lung cancer

CONTROVERSIES
Do Suggestive Forms of Connective Tissue Disease–associated Interstitial Lung Disease Exist?

It is common to encounter patients with ILD who have some features that suggest the possibility of an underlying CTD, such as autoantibody positivity or symptoms such as Raynaud phenomenon or arthritis. However, many of these patients do not fulfil existing criteria for the classifiable CTDs and are thus considered as idiopathic by default. Several recent studies have proposed different names and criteria to characterize these individuals with an autoimmune character of ILD,[2,105–107] but as yet there are no consensus-derived or validated criteria.

Undifferentiated CTD (UCTD) is a category with a long history in the rheumatologic literature and is considered to encompass patients with symptoms and signs that suggest a CTD with antinuclear antibody positivity, but not fulfilling existing classification criteria for a specific CTD, in the absence of major organ involvement or damage.[105] In 2007, a broader set of UCTD classification criteria were proposed by Kinder and colleagues[106] and retrospectively applied to a cohort of patients with IIPs. Patients who met the broader criteria of UCTD were more likely to have a pattern of NSIP (**Fig. 15**). Fischer and colleagues[2] proposed the term lung-dominant CTD, and a set of novel classification criteria, for cases in which ILD has a rheumatologic character as supported by specific autoantibodies or histopathologic features but does not meet existing criteria for a defined CTD. Such a classification was intended to provide a framework by which natural history, pathobiology, treatment, and prognostic studies can be implemented.[2] In addition, Vij and colleagues[107] described a cohort of patients with ILD retrospectively identified as having what they termed autoimmune-featured ILD, and offered a further set of proposed classification criteria that included the presence of a sign or symptom that suggested a CTD and a serologic test that reflected an autoimmune process.[107]

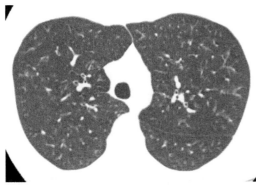

Fig. 10. FB in SS. CT through the upper lungs shows ill-defined centrilobular nodules.

A
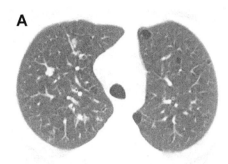

B
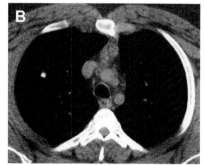

Fig. 11. Nodular amyloidosis in SS. (*A*) Axial CT through the upper lungs shows small nodules and well-defined, thin-walled cysts. (*B*) Mediastinal window setting at the level of *A* shows calcification within a nodule.

Each of these categories has a unique set of proposed criteria and has yet to be prospectively validated. In response, the American Thoracic Society/European Respiratory Society Task Force, An International Working Group on Undifferentiated Forms of CTD-ILD, has recently been formed to develop a consensus regarding the nomenclature and criteria for the classification of suggestive forms of CTD-ILD.[108] The intention of the task force is to achieve multidisciplinary consensus on how to classify this amorphous ILD subgroup and enable the much-needed prospective, multicenter, and multidisciplinary studies to further the understanding of these individuals with ILD and features that suggest an underlying CTD.

Is Rheumatoid Arthritis Initiated in Airways?

Airways disease is common in RA. Studies show that the prevalence of airway disease on HRCT in patients with RA is 60% to 80%.[109–111] With the recent attention to the lungs as a possible site of the pathogenesis of RA, the airways may play a central role.

The preclinical phase of RA is defined as a period of seropositivity (eg, the presence of rheumatoid factor or antibodies to citrullinated protein antigens [ACPAs] without evidence of clinical synovitis).[112,113] Patients with preclinical RA have a higher incidence of airways disease. Demoruelle

and colleagues[111] showed a significantly higher prevalence of airways disease in this subset on HRCT compared with autoantibody-negative controls (76% vs 33% respectively). Moreover, Fischer and colleagues[114] reported on a cohort of patients with ACPA positivity and no evidence of RA, and airways disease was the most common HRCT finding, seen in 81% of patients.

There is biological plausibility to support the airways as a possible site of initial immune dysregulation. At mucosal surfaces, exposure to environmental factors such as tobacco or bacteria can result in induction of a local as well as systemic immunoglobulin A response,[115] and such a process provides an opportunity for a potential dysregulated immune response that could result in the development of autoimmunity. In patients

Box 7
MCTD-related thoracic disease

- Features of SS, polymyositis, scleroderma, SLE
- Lung fibrosis (NSIP pattern is common)
- PH
- Pleural effusion

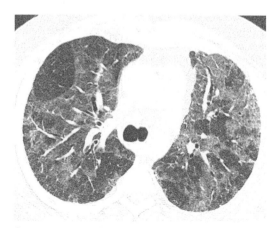

Fig. 12. Pneumonitis caused by methotrexate in a patient with RA. Axial CT image through the midlungs shows extensive ground-glass abnormality, which is new compared with prior studies. There are multiple spared lobules, suggesting a mosaic attenuation pattern, but these did not show air trapping on expiratory images.

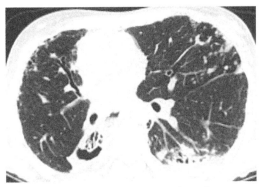

Fig. 13. *Mycobacterium avium* complex infection in a patient receiving anti–tumor necrosis factor alpha therapy for RA. Axial images at the level of the mid-lobe and lingula show multiple nodular opacities, and a cavity in the right lower lung. There is mild subpleural reticular abnormality with honeycombing.

with RA, submucosal collections of B and T cells called bronchus-associated lymphoid tissue have been described and hypothesized as a site of generation of autoantibodies in these patients.[116] Patients with preclinical RA have been found to have RA-related autoantibodies in sputum and these antibodies can predate autoantibodies in serum.[117] These data suggest that the airways may play a central role in the initiation of RA, with a mechanism hypothesized to be gene-environmental interactions at the mucosal surface in the airways.

FUTURE DIRECTIONS
Quantitative Lung Imaging

Quantitative lung imaging is increasingly used by researchers for evaluating the severity of ILD, and assessing change over time and therapeutic effects. In a longitudinal study of lung CT densitometry in 48 patients with SSc, quantitative lung imaging analysis was significantly reproducible and more correlated with pulmonary function testing, 6-minute walking testing, and quality-of-life questionnaire parameters than visual assessment of lung changes in thin-section CT.[118] The Scleroderma Lung Study[119] reported that significant correlations were noted between changes in quantitative lung fibrosis scores and changes in both forced vital capacity and dyspnea. Yabuuchi and colleagues[120] reported in a study of 17 patients with SSc-ILD after autoperipheral blood stem cell transplant that the change in extent of ground-glass opacities measured quantitatively showed strong correlation with the therapeutic response. Although quantitative lung imaging has been used only for patients with SSc among the CTD-ILDs, development of the technique could offer the potential for reviewing the severity and evaluating the effect of treatments of other CTDs.

MRI

Pulmonary MRI, in contrast with the morphologic approach using thin-section CT, has been used to noninvasively quantitate various pulmonary diseases. Recently, pulmonary functional MRI was suggested as a new approach for assessment in various pulmonary diseases.[121–128] For example, with oxygen-enhanced MRI, the percentage of oxygen-enhanced pixels was strongly correlated with measurements of gas transfer in patients with CTD with ILD.[129] Ohno and colleagues[130] recently showed that the oxygen enhancement ratio on MRI was correlated with pulmonary functional parameters and serum Krebs von den Lungen-6 (KL-6) in CTD-ILD. These techniques can be considered a potential biomarker for management of patients with CTD, and may play a complementary role to thin-section CT.

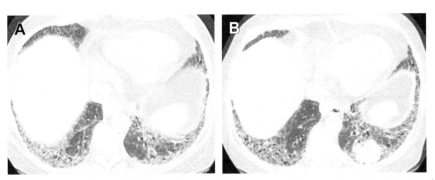

Fig. 14. Lung cancer in a patient with SSc associated with pulmonary fibrosis. (*A*) Initial CT image through the lower lungs shows moderate basal reticular abnormality with ground-glass opacities. (*B*) CT 3 years later shows a 3-cm mass in the fibrotic left lower lobe.

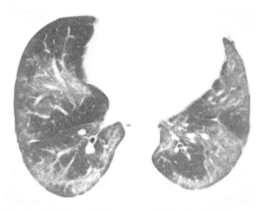

Fig. 15. NSIP in undifferentiated CTD. Axial CT images through the lower lungs show extensive bilateral ground-glass opacities and mild superimposed reticulation. Subpleural sparing is present, which is characteristic of NSIP.

SUMMARY

Pulmonary involvement is a frequent manifestation of CTD-related thoracic disease. It is important to characterize the underlying pattern when pulmonary involvement occurs in a patient with CTD, and to exclude other causes, such as infections, drug toxicity, and malignancy. A systematic approach, evaluating each compartment of the lung (airway, interstitium, pleura, pulmonary vasculature) may be helpful. In complex cases, a multidisciplinary approach should be considered, potentially including the pulmonologist, rheumatologist, radiologist, pathologist, and sometimes the infectious disease specialist or oncologist. New techniques, such as quantitative CT and MRI, are expected to be helpful for evaluation and management of CTD-associated thoracic disease.

REFERENCES

1. Fischer A. Interstitial lung disease: a rheumatologist's perspective. J Clin Rheumatol 2009;15:95–9.
2. Fischer A, West SG, Swigris JJ, et al. Connective tissue disease-associated interstitial lung disease: a call for clarification. Chest 2010;138:251–6.
3. Antoniou KM, Margaritopoulos G, Economidou F, et al. Pivotal clinical dilemmas in collagen vascular diseases associated with interstitial lung involvement. Eur Respir J 2009;33:882–96.
4. Tzelepis GE, Toya SP, Moutsopoulos HM. Occult connective tissue diseases mimicking idiopathic interstitial pneumonias. Eur Respir J 2008;31:11–20.
5. Volpe J, Storto ML, Lee K, et al. High-resolution CT of the lung: determination of the usefulness of CT scans obtained with the patient prone based on plain radiographic findings. AJR Am J Roentgenol 1997;169:369–74.
6. American Thoracic Society, European Respiratory Society. American Thoracic Society/European Respiratory Society International multidisciplinary consensus classification of the idiopathic interstitial pneumonias. This joint statement of the American Thoracic Society (ATS), and the European Respiratory Society (ERS) was adopted by the ATS Board of Directors, June 2001 and by the ERS Executive Committee, June 2001. Am J Respir Crit Care Med 2002;165:277–304.
7. Kim EA, Lee KS, Johkoh T, et al. Interstitial lung diseases associated with collagen vascular diseases: radiologic and histopathologic findings. Radiographics 2002;22(Spec No):S151–65.
8. Travis WD, Costabel U, Hansell DM, et al, ATS/ERS Committee on Idiopathic Interstitial Pneumonias. An official American Thoracic Society/European Respiratory Society statement: update of the international multidisciplinary classification of the idiopathic interstitial pneumonias. Am J Respir Crit Care Med 2013;188:733–48.
9. Mori S, Cho I, Koga Y, et al. Comparison of pulmonary abnormalities on high-resolution computed tomography in patients with early versus longstanding rheumatoid arthritis. J Rheumatol 2008;35:1513–21.
10. Shannon TM, Gale ME. Noncardiac manifestations of rheumatoid arthritis in the thorax. J Thorac Imaging 1992;7:19–29.
11. Frank ST, Weg JG, Harkleroad LE, et al. Pulmonary dysfunction in rheumatoid disease. Chest 1973;63:27–34.
12. Yousem SA, Colby TV, Carrington CB. Lung biopsy in rheumatoid arthritis. Am Rev Respir Dis 1985;131:770–7.
13. Tanaka N, Kim JS, Newell JD, et al. Rheumatoid arthritis-related lung diseases: CT findings. Radiology 2004;232:81–91.
14. Yoshinouchi T, Ohtsuki Y, Fujita J, et al. Nonspecific interstitial pneumonia pattern as pulmonary involvement of rheumatoid arthritis. Rheumatol Int 2005;26:121–5.
15. Hakala M, Paakko P, Huhti E, et al. Open lung biopsy of patients with rheumatoid arthritis. Clin Rheumatol 1990;9:452–60.
16. Mroz BJ, Sexauer WP, Meade A, et al. Hemoptysis as the presenting symptom in bronchiolitis obliterans organizing pneumonia. Chest 1997;111:1775–8.
17. Parambil JG, Myers JL, Ryu JH. Diffuse alveolar damage: uncommon manifestation of pulmonary involvement in patients with connective tissue diseases. Chest 2006;130:553–8.
18. Steinberg DL, Webb WR. CT appearances of rheumatoid lung disease. J Comput Assist Tomogr 1984;8:881–4.

19. Bergin CJ, Muller NL. CT of interstitial lung disease: a diagnostic approach. AJR Am J Roentgenol 1987;148:9–15.

20. Fewins HE, McGowan I, Whitehouse GH, et al. High definition computed tomography in rheumatoid arthritis associated pulmonary disease. Br J Rheumatol 1991;30:214–6.

21. Kim EJ, Elicker BM, Maldonado F, et al. Usual interstitial pneumonia in rheumatoid arthritis-associated interstitial lung disease. Eur Respir J 2010;35:1322–8.

22. Tsuchiya Y, Takayanagi N, Sugiura H, et al. Lung diseases directly associated with rheumatoid arthritis and their relationship to outcome. Eur Respir J 2011;37:1411–7.

23. Assayag D, Elicker BM, Urbania TH, et al. Rheumatoid arthritis-associated interstitial lung disease: radiologic identification of usual interstitial pneumonia pattern. Radiology 2014;270:583–8.

24. Hayakawa H, Sato A, Imokawa S, et al. Bronchiolar disease in rheumatoid arthritis. Am J Respir Crit Care Med 1996;154:1531–6.

25. Cortet B, Perez T, Roux N, et al. Pulmonary function tests and high resolution computed tomography of the lungs in patients with rheumatoid arthritis. Ann Rheum Dis 1997;56:596–600.

26. Perez T, Remy-Jardin M, Cortet B. Airways involvement in rheumatoid arthritis: clinical, functional, and HRCT findings. Am J Respir Crit Care Med 1998;157:1658–65.

27. Howling SJ, Hansell DM, Wells AU, et al. Follicular bronchiolitis: thin-section CT and histologic findings. Radiology 1999;212:637–42.

28. Leslie KO, Trahan S, Gruden J. Pulmonary pathology of the rheumatic diseases. Semin Respir Crit Care Med 2007;28:369–78.

29. Sweatman MC, Millar AB, Strickland B, et al. Computed tomography in adult obliterative bronchiolitis. Clin Radiol 1990;41:116–9.

30. Aquino SL, Webb WR, Golden J. Bronchiolitis obliterans associated with rheumatoid arthritis: findings on HRCT and dynamic expiratory CT. J Comput Assist Tomogr 1994;18:555–8.

31. Schwarz MI, Lynch DA, Tuder R. Bronchiolitis obliterans: the lone manifestation of rheumatoid arthritis? Eur Respir J 1994;7:817–20.

32. Dawson JK, Goodson NG, Graham DR, et al. Raised pulmonary artery pressures measured with Doppler echocardiography in rheumatoid arthritis patients. Rheumatology (Oxford) 2000;39:1320–5.

33. Gamsu G. Radiographic manifestations of thoracic involvement by collagen vascular diseases. J Thorac Imaging 1992;7:1–12.

34. Bouros D, Wells AU, Nicholson AG, et al. Histopathologic subsets of fibrosing alveolitis in patients with systemic sclerosis and their relationship to outcome. Am J Respir Crit Care Med 2002;165:1581–6.

35. Kim DS, Yoo B, Lee JS, et al. The major histopathologic pattern of pulmonary fibrosis in scleroderma is nonspecific interstitial pneumonia. Sarcoidosis Vasc Diffuse Lung Dis 2002;19:121–7.

36. Schurawitzki H, Stiglbauer R, Graninger W, et al. Interstitial lung disease in progressive systemic sclerosis: high-resolution CT versus radiography. Radiology 1990;176:755–9.

37. Remy-Jardin M, Remy J, Wallaert B, et al. Pulmonary involvement in progressive systemic sclerosis: sequential evaluation with CT, pulmonary function tests, and bronchoalveolar lavage. Radiology 1993;188:499–506.

38. Desai SR, Veeraraghavan S, Hansell DM, et al. CT features of lung disease in patients with systemic sclerosis: comparison with idiopathic pulmonary fibrosis and nonspecific interstitial pneumonia. Radiology 2004;232:560–7.

39. Goldin JG, Lynch DA, Strollo DC, et al, Scleroderma Lung Study Research Group. High-resolution CT scan findings in patients with symptomatic scleroderma-related interstitial lung disease. Chest 2008;134:358–67.

40. Wells AU, Cullinan P, Hansell DM, et al. Fibrosing alveolitis associated with systemic sclerosis has a better prognosis than lone cryptogenic fibrosing alveolitis. Am J Respir Crit Care Med 1994;149:1583–90.

41. Renzoni E, Rottoli P, Coviello G, et al. Clinical, laboratory and radiological findings in pulmonary fibrosis with and without connective tissue disease. Clin Rheumatol 1997;16:570–7.

42. Muir TE, Tazelaar HD, Colby TV, et al. Organizing diffuse alveolar damage associated with progressive systemic sclerosis. Mayo Clin Proc 1997;72:639–42.

43. Hachulla E, Gressin V, Guillevin L, et al. Early detection of pulmonary arterial hypertension in systemic sclerosis: a French nationwide prospective multicenter study. Arthritis Rheum 2005;52:3792–800.

44. Mukerjee D, St George D, Coleiro B, et al. Prevalence and outcome in systemic sclerosis associated pulmonary arterial hypertension: application of a registry approach. Ann Rheum Dis 2003;62:1088–93.

45. Hunzelmann N, Genth E, Krieg T, et al, Registry of the German Network for Systemic Scleroderma. The registry of the German Network for Systemic Scleroderma: frequency of disease subsets and patterns of organ involvement. Rheumatology (Oxford) 2008;47:1185–92.

46. Bhalla M, Silver RM, Shepard JA, et al. Chest CT in patients with scleroderma: prevalence of asymptomatic esophageal dilatation and mediastinal

lymphadenopathy. AJR Am J Roentgenol 1993; 161:269–72.

47. Lock G, Pfeifer M, Straub RH, et al. Association of esophageal dysfunction and pulmonary function impairment in systemic sclerosis. Am J Gastroenterol 1998;93:341–5.

48. Marie I, Dominique S, Levesque H, et al. Esophageal involvement and pulmonary manifestations in systemic sclerosis. Arthritis Rheum 2001;45: 346–54.

49. Dalakas MC, Hohlfeld R. Polymyositis and dermatomyositis. Lancet 2003;362:971–82.

50. Fathi M, Lundberg IE. Interstitial lung disease in polymyositis and dermatomyositis. Curr Opin Rheumatol 2005;17:701–6.

51. Connors GR, Christopher-Stine L, Oddis CV, et al. Interstitial lung disease associated with the idiopathic inflammatory myopathies: what progress has been made in the past 35 years? Chest 2010;138:1464–74.

52. Koreeda Y, Higashimoto I, Yamamoto M, et al. Clinical and pathological findings of interstitial lung disease patients with anti-aminoacyl-tRNA synthetase autoantibodies. Intern Med 2010;49:361–9.

53. Akira M, Hara H, Sakatani M. Interstitial lung disease in association with polymyositis-dermatomyositis: long-term follow-up CT evaluation in seven patients. Radiology 1999;210:333–8.

54. Mino M, Noma S, Taguchi Y, et al. Pulmonary involvement in polymyositis and dermatomyositis: sequential evaluation with CT. AJR Am J Roentgenol 1997;169:83–7.

55. Ikezoe J, Johkoh T, Kohno N, et al. High-resolution CT findings of lung disease in patients with polymyositis and dermatomyositis. J Thorac Imaging 1996;11:250–9.

56. Arakawa H, Yamada H, Kurihara Y, et al. Nonspecific interstitial pneumonia associated with polymyositis and dermatomyositis: serial high-resolution CT findings and functional correlation. Chest 2003;123:1096–103.

57. Mukae H, Ishimoto H, Sakamoto N, et al. Clinical differences between interstitial lung disease associated with clinically amyopathic dermatomyositis and classic dermatomyositis. Chest 2009;136: 1341–7.

58. Tanizawa K, Handa T, Nakashima R, et al. HRCT features of interstitial lung disease in dermatomyositis with anti-CADM-140 antibody. Respir Med 2011;105:1380–7.

59. Primack SL, Muller NL. Radiologic manifestations of the systemic autoimmune diseases. Clin Chest Med 1998;19:573–86, vii.

60. Kim JS, Lee KS, Koh EM, et al. Thoracic involvement of systemic lupus erythematosus: clinical, pathologic, and radiologic findings. J Comput Assist Tomogr 2000;24:9–18.

61. Harvey AM, Shulman LE, Tumulty PA, et al. Systemic lupus erythematosus: review of the literature and clinical analysis of 138 cases. Medicine (Baltimore) 1954;33:291–437.

62. Murin S, Wiedemann HP, Matthay RA. Pulmonary manifestations of systemic lupus erythematosus. Clin Chest Med 1998;19:641–65, viii.

63. Wiedemann HP, Matthay RA. Pulmonary manifestations of systemic lupus erythematosus. J Thorac Imaging 1992;7:1–18.

64. Tan EM, Cohen AS, Fries JF, et al. The 1982 revised criteria for the classification of systemic lupus erythematosus. Arthritis Rheum 1982;25:1271–7.

65. Swigris JJ, Fischer A, Gillis J, et al. Pulmonary and thrombotic manifestations of systemic lupus erythematosus. Chest 2008;133:271–80.

66. Fishbein GA, Fishbein MC. Lung vasculitis and alveolar hemorrhage: pathology. Semin Respir Crit Care Med 2011;32:254–63.

67. Kishida Y, Kanai Y, Kuramochi S, et al. Pulmonary venoocclusive disease in a patient with systemic lupus erythematosus. J Rheumatol 1993; 20:2161–2.

68. Rolla G, Brussino L, Bertero MT, et al. Respiratory function in systemic lupus erythematosus: relation with activity and severity. Lupus 1996;5:38–43.

69. Rolla G, Brussino L, Bertero MT, et al. Increased nitric oxide in exhaled air of patients with systemic lupus erythematosus. J Rheumatol 1997; 24:1066–71.

70. Ito I, Nagai S, Kitaichi M, et al. Pulmonary manifestations of primary Sjogren's syndrome: a clinical, radiologic, and pathologic study. Am J Respir Crit Care Med 2005;171:632–8.

71. Parambil JG, Myers JL, Lindell RM, et al. Interstitial lung disease in primary Sjogren syndrome. Chest 2006;130:1489–95.

72. Newball HH, Brahim SA. Chronic obstructive airway disease in patients with Sjogren's syndrome. Am Rev Respir Dis 1977;115:295–304.

73. Voulgarelis M, Dafni UG, Isenberg DA, et al. Malignant lymphoma in primary Sjogren's syndrome: a multicenter, retrospective, clinical study by the European Concerted Action on Sjogren's Syndrome. Arthritis Rheum 1999;42:1765–72.

74. Papiris SA, Kalomenidis I, Malagari K, et al. Extranodal marginal zone B-cell lymphoma of the lung in Sjogren's syndrome patients: reappraisal of clinical, radiological, and pathology findings. Respir Med 2007;101:84–92.

75. Theander E, Henriksson G, Ljungberg O, et al. Lymphoma and other malignancies in primary Sjogren's syndrome: a cohort study on cancer incidence and lymphoma predictors. Ann Rheum Dis 2006;65:796–803.

76. Tonami H, Matoba M, Kuginuki Y, et al. Clinical and imaging findings of lymphoma in patients with

Sjogren syndrome. J Comput Assist Tomogr 2003; 27:517–24.

77. Honda O, Johkoh T, Ichikado K, et al. Differential diagnosis of lymphocytic interstitial pneumonia and malignant lymphoma on high-resolution CT. AJR Am J Roentgenol 1999;173:71–4.

78. Jeong YJ, Lee KS, Chung MP, et al. Amyloidosis and lymphoproliferative disease in Sjogren syndrome: thin-section computed tomography findings and histopathologic comparisons. J Comput Assist Tomogr 2004;28:776–81.

79. Chen KT. Amyloidosis presenting in the respiratory tract. Pathol Annu 1989;24(Pt 1):253–73.

80. Uffmann M, Kiener HP, Bankier AA, et al. Lung manifestation in asymptomatic patients with primary Sjogren syndrome: assessment with high resolution CT and pulmonary function tests. J Thorac Imaging 2001;16:282–9.

81. Teshigawara K, Kakizaki S, Horiya M, et al. Primary Sjogren's syndrome complicated by bilateral pleural effusion. Respirology 2008;13:155–8.

82. Sharp GC, Irvin WS, Tan EM, et al. Mixed connective tissue disease–an apparently distinct rheumatic disease syndrome associated with a specific antibody to an extractable nuclear antigen (ENA). Am J Med 1972;52:148–59.

83. Hunninghake GW, Fauci AS. Pulmonary involvement in the collagen vascular diseases. Am Rev Respir Dis 1979;119:471–503.

84. Franquet T. High-resolution CT of lung disease related to collagen vascular disease. Radiol Clin North Am 2001;39:1171–87.

85. Bodolay E, Szekanecz Z, Devenyi K, et al. Evaluation of interstitial lung disease in mixed connective tissue disease (MCTD). Rheumatology (Oxford) 2005;44:656–61.

86. Kozuka T, Johkoh T, Honda O, et al. Pulmonary involvement in mixed connective tissue disease: high-resolution CT findings in 41 patients. J Thorac Imaging 2001;16:94–8.

87. Prakash UB. Respiratory complications in mixed connective tissue disease. Clin Chest Med 1998; 19:733–46.

88. Fagan KA, Badesch DB. Pulmonary hypertension associated with connective tissue disease. Prog Cardiovasc Dis 2002;45:225–34.

89. Sullivan WD, Hurst DJ, Harmon CE, et al. A prospective evaluation emphasizing pulmonary involvement in patients with mixed connective tissue disease. Medicine (Baltimore) 1984;63:92–107.

90. Wiener-Kronish JP, Solinger AM, Warnock ML, et al. Severe pulmonary involvement in mixed connective tissue disease. Am Rev Respir Dis 1981;124: 499–503.

91. Camus P, Bonniaud P, Fanton A, et al. Drug-induced and iatrogenic infiltrative lung disease. Clin Chest Med 2004;25:479–519, vi.

92. Flieder DB, Travis WD. Pathologic characteristics of drug-induced lung disease. Clin Chest Med 2004;25:37–45.

93. Mutlu GM, Mutlu EA, Bellmeyer A, et al. Pulmonary adverse events of anti-tumor necrosis factor-alpha antibody therapy. Am J Med 2006;119:639–46.

94. Tsiodras S, Samonis G, Boumpas DT, et al. Fungal infections complicating tumor necrosis factor alpha blockade therapy. Mayo Clin Proc 2008;83:181–94.

95. Komano Y, Harigai M, Koike R, et al. Pneumocystis jiroveci pneumonia in patients with rheumatoid arthritis treated with infliximab: a retrospective review and case-control study of 21 patients. Arthritis Rheum 2009;61:305–12.

96. Bouros D, Hatzakis K, Labrakis H, et al. Association of malignancy with diseases causing interstitial pulmonary changes. Chest 2002;121:1278–89.

97. Bin J, Bernatsky S, Gordon C, et al. Lung cancer in systemic lupus erythematosus. Lung Cancer 2007; 56:303–6.

98. Huang YL, Chen YJ, Lin MW, et al. Malignancies associated with dermatomyositis and polymyositis in Taiwan: a nationwide population-based study. Br J Dermatol 2009;161:854–60.

99. Onishi A, Sugiyama D, Kumagai S, et al. Cancer incidence in systemic sclerosis: meta-analysis of population-based cohort studies. Arthritis Rheum 2013;65:1913–21.

100. Lazarus MN, Robinson D, Mak V, et al. Incidence of cancer in a cohort of patients with primary Sjogren's syndrome. Rheumatology 2006;45:1012–5.

101. Zinzani PL, Magagnoli M, Galieni P, et al. Nongastrointestinal low-grade mucosa-associated lymphoid tissue lymphoma: analysis of 75 patients. J Clin Oncol 1999;17:1254.

102. Yang Y, Fujita J, Tokuda M, et al. Lung cancer associated with several connective tissue diseases: with a review of literature. Rheumatol Int 2001;21:106–11.

103. Le Jeune I, Gribbin J, West J, et al. The incidence of cancer in patients with idiopathic pulmonary fibrosis and sarcoidosis in the UK. Respir Med 2007;101:2534–40.

104. Takayanagi N, Tokunaga D, Tsuchiya Y, et al. Lung cancer associated with rheumatoid arthritis and usual interstitial pneumonia. Nihon Kokyuki Gakkai Zasshi 2008;46:438–42 [in Japanese].

105. Mosca M, Neri R, Bombardieri S. Undifferentiated connective tissue diseases (UCTD): a review of the literature and a proposal for preliminary classification criteria. Clin Exp Rheumatol 1999;17:615–20.

106. Kinder BW, Collard HR, Koth L, et al. Idiopathic nonspecific interstitial pneumonia: lung manifestation of undifferentiated connective tissue disease? Am J Respir Crit Care Med 2007;176:691–7.

107. Vij R, Noth I, Strek ME. Autoimmune-featured interstitial lung disease: a distinct entity. Chest 2011; 140:1292–9.

108. Fischer A, Brown KK. Interstitial lung disease in undifferentiated forms of connective tissue disease. Arthritis Care Res 2014;67:4–11.

109. Wilsher M, Voight L, Milne D, et al. Prevalence of airway and parenchymal abnormalities in newly diagnosed rheumatoid arthritis. Respir Med 2012; 106:1441–6.

110. Metafratzi ZM, Georgiadis AN, Ioannidou CV, et al. Pulmonary involvement in patients with early rheumatoid arthritis. Scand J Rheumatol 2007;36:338–44.

111. Demoruelle MK, Weisman MH, Simonian PL, et al. Brief report: airways abnormalities and rheumatoid arthritis-related autoantibodies in subjects without arthritis: early injury or initiating site of autoimmunity? Arthritis Rheum 2012;64:1756–61.

112. Deane KD, Norris JM, Holers VM. Preclinical rheumatoid arthritis: identification, evaluation, and future directions for investigation. Rheum Dis Clin North Am 2010;36:213–41.

113. Majka DS, Deane KD, Parrish LA, et al. Duration of preclinical rheumatoid arthritis-related autoantibody positivity increases in subjects with older age at time of disease diagnosis. Ann Rheum Dis 2008;67:801–7.

114. Fischer A, Solomon JJ, du Bois RM, et al. Lung disease with anti-CCP antibodies but not rheumatoid arthritis or connective tissue disease. Respir Med 2012;106:1040–7.

115. Moldoveanu Z, Clements ML, Prince SJ, et al. Human immune responses to influenza virus vaccines administered by systemic or mucosal routes. Vaccine 1995;13:1006–12.

116. Rangel-Moreno J, Hartson L, Navarro C, et al. Inducible bronchus-associated lymphoid tissue (iBALT) in patients with pulmonary complications of rheumatoid arthritis. J Clin Invest 2006;116: 3183–94.

117. Willis VC, Demoruelle MK, Derber LA, et al. Sputum autoantibodies in patients with established rheumatoid arthritis and subjects at risk of future clinically apparent disease. Arthritis Rheum 2013;65: 2545–54.

118. Camiciottoli G, Orlandi I, Bartolucci M, et al. Lung CT densitometry in systemic sclerosis: correlation with lung function, exercise testing, and quality of life. Chest 2007;131:672–81.

119. Kim HJ, Brown MS, Elashoff R, et al. Quantitative texture-based assessment of one-year changes in fibrotic reticular patterns on HRCT in scleroderma lung disease treated with oral cyclophosphamide. Eur Radiol 2011;21:2455–65.

120. Yabuuchi H, Matsuo Y, Tsukamoto H, et al. Evaluation of the extent of ground-glass opacity on high-resolution CT in patients with interstitial pneumonia associated with systemic sclerosis: comparison between quantitative and qualitative analysis. Clin Radiol 2014;69:758–64.

121. Muller CJ, Schwaiblmair M, Scheidler J, et al. Pulmonary diffusing capacity: assessment with oxygen-enhanced lung MR imaging preliminary findings. Radiology 2002;222:499–506.

122. Ohno Y, Iwasawa T, Seo JB, et al. Oxygen-enhanced magnetic resonance imaging versus computed tomography: multicenter study for clinical stage classification of smoking-related chronic obstructive pulmonary disease. Am J Respir Crit Care Med 2008;177:1095–102.

123. Ohno Y, Hatabu H, Takenaka D, et al. Dynamic oxygen-enhanced MRI reflects diffusing capacity of the lung. Magn Reson Med 2002;47: 1139–44.

124. Salerno M, Altes TA, Brookeman JR, et al. Dynamic spiral MRI of pulmonary gas flow using hyperpolarized (3)He: preliminary studies in healthy and diseased lungs. Magn Reson Med 2001;46:667–77.

125. Driehuys B, Cofer GP, Pollaro J, et al. Imaging alveolar-capillary gas transfer using hyperpolarized 129Xe MRI. Proc Natl Acad Sci U S A 2006; 103:18278–83.

126. Stephen MJ, Emami K, Woodburn JM, et al. Quantitative assessment of lung ventilation and microstructure in an animal model of idiopathic pulmonary fibrosis using hyperpolarized gas MRI. Acad Radiol 2010;17:1433–43.

127. Ohno Y, Koyama H, Nogami M, et al. Dynamic perfusion MRI: capability for evaluation of disease severity and progression of pulmonary arterial hypertension in patients with connective tissue disease. J Magn Reson Imaging 2008;28: 887–99.

128. Ohno Y, Hatabu H, Murase K, et al. Quantitative assessment of regional pulmonary perfusion in the entire lung using three-dimensional ultrafast dynamic contrast-enhanced magnetic resonance imaging: preliminary experience in 40 subjects. J Magn Reson Imaging 2004;20:353–65.

129. Molinari F, Eichinger M, Risse F, et al. Navigator-triggered oxygen-enhanced MRI with simultaneous cardiac and respiratory synchronization for the assessment of interstitial lung disease. J Magn Reson Imaging 2007;26:1523–9.

130. Ohno Y, Nishio M, Koyama H, et al. Pulmonary MR imaging with ultra-short TEs: utility for disease severity assessment of connective tissue disease patients. Eur J Radiol 2013;82:1359–65.

Cystic and Nodular Lung Disease

J. Caleb Richards, MD*, David A. Lynch, MB, Jonathan H. Chung, MD

KEYWORDS

- Cystic lung disease • Nodular lung disease • High-resolution computed tomography

KEY POINTS

- A lung cyst is a lucent structure with a thin perceptible wall. When multiple lung cysts are present, the spectrum of cystic lung disease should be considered.
- Recognizing zonal predominance and cyst morphology is helpful in reaching an accurate diagnosis of cystic lung disease. Abnormalities within the intervening lung parenchyma and outside the thorax may also be helpful.
- Entities such as emphysema, honeycombing, cavities, and bronchiectasis can mimic true cystic lung disease.
- Nodular lung disease is best characterized by the relationship to the secondary pulmonary lobule (SPL), with the 3 main patterns being centrilobular, perilymphatic, and random.
- A multimodality approach including clinical history, physical examination, and imaging is often essential to narrow down the differential diagnosis of nodular lung disease.

INTRODUCTION

Diffuse cystic and nodular lung diseases often have characteristic imaging findings, which may allow the radiologist to be the first to suggest the diagnosis. Diffuse cystic lung diseases are rare entities. The most common causes of cystic lung disease are lymphangioleiomyomatosis (LAM) and Langerhans cell histiocytosis (LCH); differentiation of LAM from LCH on computed tomography (CT) of the chest is readily made in most clinical cases. Other less common cystic lung diseases include Birt-Hogg-Dube syndrome, lymphocytic interstitial pneumonitis, and light chain deposition disease. Although emphysema, honeycombing, cavities, and bronchiectasis mimic cystic lung disease, careful inspection of CT images usually allows one to differentiate true cystic lung disease from these entities. Diffuse nodular lung disease are categorized into 3 main categories based on nodule relationship to the SPL: centrilobular,

perilymphatic, and random. Each of these categories carries a unique differential diagnosis. In diffuse nodular lung disease, a specific diagnosis can be achieved through a combination of history, physical examination, and imaging findings.

CYSTIC LUNG DISEASE

The Fleischner Society defines a cyst as a round parenchymal lucency or low-attenuating area with a well-defined interface with normal lung.[1] The presence of multiple cysts throughout the lung signals the presence of cystic lung disease, which carries a short differential diagnosis. A specific diagnosis can be made based on the imaging appearance of lung cysts and their axial and zonal distribution.

Lymphangioleiomyomatosis

LAM is a rare multiorgan disorder, which occurs almost exclusively in women of childbearing

---

Department of Radiology, National Jewish Health, 1400 Jackson Street, Denver, CO 80206, USA
* Corresponding author.
E-mail address: RichardsJ@NJHealth.org

Clin Chest Med 36 (2015) 299–312
http://dx.doi.org/10.1016/j.ccm.2015.02.011
0272-5231/15/$ – see front matter © 2015 Elsevier Inc. All rights reserved.

age.[2,3] Pathologically, LAM is characterized by smooth muscle proliferation along the pulmonary interstitium affecting the lymphatics, vessels, airways, alveolar septa, and pleura.[4] LAM can occur sporadically or in association with tuberous sclerosis complex (TSC-LAM), although TSC-LAM is 5 to 10 times more common than sporadic LAM. LAM occurs in 30% of women with TSC.[2] Clinically, patients present with progressing dyspnea on exertion, recurrent pleural effusions (chylothorax), and spontaneous pneumothoraces.[5] In a series of 32 patients with LAM, exertional dyspnea (47%) and spontaneous pneumothorax (53%) were the most common findings at presentation, whereas 81% of patients within this cohort exhibited spontaneous pneumothorax at some point during the course of the disease.[6]

Appearance on chest radiography varies with disease severity. The radiograph may show normal results or increased reticular markings related to superimposition of cyst walls. As the disease progresses-, the cysts become more apparent and may have a lower lung zone predominance. Lung volumes are normal to increased. Pleural effusion or spontaneous pneumothorax can occur and is usually readily apparent on imaging.[3,6–8]

Results on CT are almost always abnormal, and CT can demonstrate parenchymal abnormality even when the radiograph shows normal results.[9] High-resolution computed tomography (HRCT) is superior to traditional CT in defining the parenchymal abnormality in LAM, with the characteristic features being diffuse, thin-walled cysts with normal intervening parenchyma (**Fig. 1**). The cysts tend to be round and uniform in shape measuring 3 to 5 mm, although cysts measuring up to 25 to 30 mm have been reported.[3,4,9] Occasionally, the cysts may appear polygonal in shape or fused.[10,11] Cysts enlarge and become more numerous as the disease progresses.[9–11]

The prevalence of LAM in patients with TSC varies, although age seems to be a critical risk factor for the development of cystic lung disease, as Cudzilo and colleagues[12] reported a cystic lung disease prevalence of 81% in subjects with TSC older than 40 years. Multifocal micronodular pneumocyte hyperplasia (MMPH) is an additional feature seen in patients with TSC. MMPH is a hamartomatous process of the lungs, which manifests at imaging with diffusely scattered, randomly distributed nodules measuring 1 to 8 mm in diameter.[13,14]

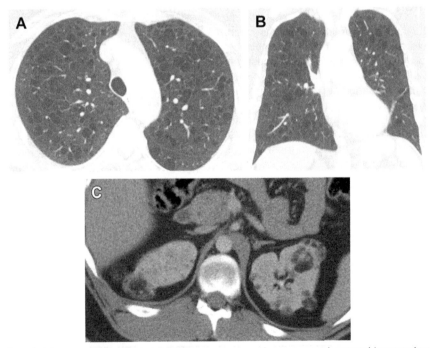

Fig. 1. Lymphangioleiomyomatosis. (*A*) Axial CT shows round, uniform cysts with normal intervening lung parenchyma. (*B*) Coronal reformation showing diffuse distribution of cysts without zonal predominance. (*C*) Axial CT of the abdomen showing multiple fat-attenuation lesions in both kidneys, consistent with angiomyolipomas in a patient with tuberous sclerosis. Grossly, one can infer that the lesions are fatty by comparing the internal density with that of adjacent abdominal fat.

Renal angiomyolipomas (AMLs) are the most common extrathoracic manifestation of LAM and are seen more commonly in TSC-LAM.[15] AMLs characteristically appear as partially fat-attenuating lesions on CT (see **Fig. 1**).[16] AMLs larger than 4 cm are at greater risk for spontaneous or traumatic rupture, which is the most common cause of death.[17,18] Thus, embolization has been advocated in AMLs larger than 4 cm.[19] Other extrathoracic manifestations include abdominal lymphadenopathy, lymphangioleiomyomas, ascites, and extrarenal AMLs.[15,20,21]

Langerhans Cell Histiocytosis

Pulmonary LCH is a smoking-related lung disease, most frequently seen in young adults, with 80% to 100% of cases reporting a current or prior smoking history.[4,22] The Langerhans cell is a dendritic cell occurring in epithelial surfaces, first described by Paul Langerhans in 1868.[23] These cells have since been linked to several disorders, with isolated pulmonary involvement first described in 1951.[24] Isolated pulmonary LCH was later categorized as an LCH variant, different from the pulmonary involvement seen in multisystem disease, and now is recognized as the more common form.[22,25] Histopathologically, pulmonary LCH is characterized by infiltration of bronchiolar walls and epithelium by LCH cells, which develop into discrete bronchiolocentric, stellate interstitial nodules.[22] Kambouchner and colleagues[26] demonstrated that cavitation of nodules represents bronchiolar luminal enlargement from inflammation, fibrosis and destruction of the bronchiolar wall, coalescence of adjacent affected airways, and traction emphysema or paracicatricial airspace enlargement in peribronchiolar alveolar spaces.[27]

The exact incidence and prevalence of pulmonary LCH is unknown, as some patients may be asymptomatic or the disorder may spontaneously resolve.[22,28] Clinically, patients most commonly present with nonproductive cough and dyspnea and less commonly weight loss, fatigue, chest pain, and fever.[24,29] Spontaneous pneumothorax is a recognized feature, which can have a high recurrence rate when managed without pleurodesis.[30] About 25% of patients are asymptomatic and diagnosed incidentally at imaging.[22,24]

Most patients demonstrate abnormalities on chest radiography.[31,32] Radiographic findings include symmetric, upper lung predominant abnormality including nodules, reticulonodular opacity, and cysts.[22,33] Nodules are considered an early manifestation and tend to become less apparent as cystic change becomes more prominent.[34] Pneumothorax can be the initial manifestation of pulmonary LCH, even in the absence of other recognizable radiographic abnormality.[34]

HRCT is superior to radiography in demonstrating lung abnormalities in LCH, often allowing for a confident diagnosis.[35] The most useful feature distinguishing LCH from other cystic lung diseases is its upper lung zone predominance with relative or complete sparing of the costophrenic sulci (**Fig. 2**).[36] Nodules, when present, are a helpful feature distinguishing LCH from LAM, which does not typically present with nodules except in TSC-related MMPH. Early LCH may appear similar to respiratory bronchiolitis (RB) with small, ill-defined bronchiolocentric nodules.[26,37] Cyst formation develops as the disease progresses.[38] Cysts can coalesce to form irregular, bizarre shapes, which is characteristic of LCH.[22,26,36] Brauner and colleagues[39] postulated the sequential progression of abnormality seen on CT as follows: nodules, cavitary nodules, thick-walled cysts, thin-walled cysts, and confluent cysts.

Clinical and radiographic course of LCH is variable, with stabilization occurring in 50% of patients and spontaneous regression in 25%.[22] On follow-up imaging, nodules, even when

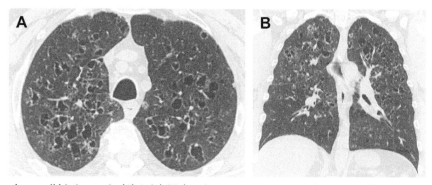

Fig. 2. Langerhans cell histiocytosis. (*A*) Axial CT showing numerous cysts with irregular, bizarre shapes and small nodules in the intervening lung parenchyma. (*B*) Coronal reformation demonstrating upper lung predominance with relative sparing of the lung bases.

cavitary, were found to be potentially reversible. Cysts do not typically show improvement on follow-up.[40] In general, more extensive cystic disease on initial presentation corresponds to worse outcome.[37]

Lymphocytic Interstitial Pneumonia

Lymphocytic interstitial pneumonia (LIP) is a benign lymphoproliferative disorder characterized histologically by a diffuse cellular interstitial infiltrate composed of mature small lymphocytes and plasma cells, which have a propensity for the perilymphatic interstitium.[41–43] This disease process is associated with numerous conditions, most commonly autoimmune syndromes or immune deficiency such as Sjögren syndrome, autoimmune thyroid syndrome, human immunodeficiency virus infection, Castleman disease, and amyloidosis.[38,43] LIP is rarely idiopathic. Lung cysts, seen in up to 80% of patients, are thought to result from airway obstruction due to peribronchiolar cellular infiltration.[38,43,44]

Clinically, patients with LIP commonly present with cough and dyspnea, although fever, night sweats, and weight loss may be seen.[45] A restrictive pattern and reduced decreased carbon monoxide diffusion capacity is usually seen at pulmonary function testing.[38,46] The clinical course of LIP is highly variable. Some patients improve or stabilize, whereas more than one-third undergo progressive disease despite therapy.[43]

Radiographic findings of LIP are nonspecific. Chest radiograph, if showing abnormal results, may show bilateral lower lung predominant reticular or reticulonodular opacities. Consolidation and ill-defined nodules may be seen.[46]

On HRCT, lung cysts are seen in 80% of patients, although the predominant finding described in the literature is that of diffuse ground-glass opacity, ill-defined centrilobular nodules, bronchovascular and interlobular septal thickening, and diffuse scattered cysts.[46,47] However, in the authors' clinical experience, LIP manifests most commonly as a predominantly cystic lung disease with middle and lower lung predominance, with perivascular location of the cysts (**Fig. 3**). Silva and colleagues[46] described a case with a similar pattern of middle and lower lung predominant cystic lung disease in a patient with no history of autoimmune disease or immunodeficiency. The cysts in that case ranged from 0.5 to 10 cm in diameter on HRCT, and there was minimal associated ground-glass opacity.

Some studies report that some imaging abnormalities, such as ground-glass opacity, may be

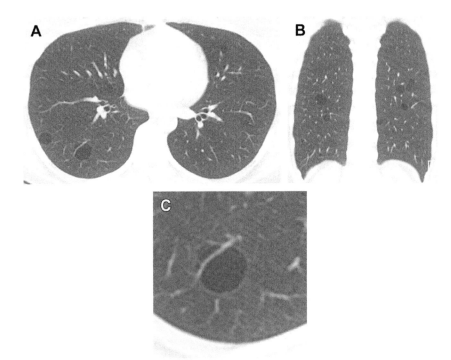

Fig. 3. Lymphocytic interstitial pneumonia. (*A*) Axial CT showing numerous thin-walled cysts, some of which are perivascular. (*B*) Note the slight lower lung predominance of cysts. (*C*) Cysts in LIP are characteristically perivascular, which can be a helpful clue.

reversible, whereas cystic changes are irreversible.[43,44] The role of HRCT in the follow-up of reversible findings is not yet determined.[44] Although lung biopsy definitively establishes the diagnosis, the presence of typical imaging findings with an appropriate clinical history is usually sufficient to establish a diagnosis.

Birt-Hogg-Dube Syndrome

Birt-Hogg-Dube (BHD) syndrome is a rare, autosomal dominant disorder initially described in 1977 with a characteristic triad of skin lesions: fibrofolliculomas, trichodiscomas, and skin tags.[48] Over the years, an association of BHD syndrome with renal tumors, including oncocytoma and renal cell carcinoma, pulmonary cysts, and spontaneous pneumothorax, has been described and better understood (**Fig. 4**).[49–51] It is known that mutations in the FLCN gene on chromosome 17p11.2, encoding the tumor-suppressor protein folliculin, are responsible for this inherited condition.[52] As a wide variety of mutations can occur in the FLCN gene, the combination of organ systems involved and severity of disease varies in affected patients.[52,53] Histopathology is nonspecific; typical findings include air-filled spaces, which may have a thin fibrous wall, and normal intervening lung parenchyma.[50] Prognosis of BHD syndrome depends mainly on other comorbid factors, such as renal cell carcinoma.[54] Genetic counseling is advised given its autosomal dominant inheritance.[54]

Most patients with BHD syndrome demonstrate thoracic abnormality at imaging; Agarwal and colleagues[55] described lungs cysts present in 15 of 17 patients in one cohort. Cysts in BHD syndrome tend to vary in size and morphology and show bilateral and lower lung zone predominance (see **Fig. 4**).[50,51,55] In the study by Agarwal and colleagues,[55] cyst size ranged from 0.2 to 7.8 cm, and morphology varied from round to oval and lentiform, with some of the larger cysts appearing multiseptated and lobulated. In the axial plane, the cysts are characteristically subpleural, often paramediastinal, and may extend along the proximal portion of lower lobe pulmonary arteries and veins.[56] Spontaneous pneumothorax may be a presenting feature.[57]

Light Chain Deposition Disease

Light chain deposition disorder (LCDD) is a rare disease characterized by the deposition of nonfibrillary, amorphous material that does not have β-pleated configuration and does not bind Congo

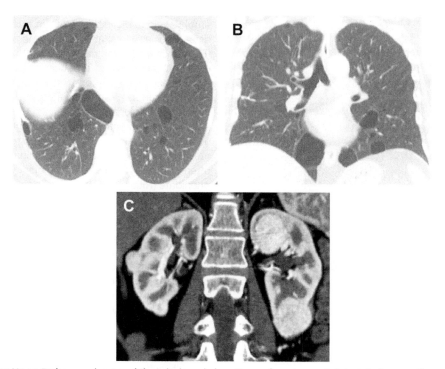

Fig. 4. Birt-Hogg-Dube syndrome. (*A*) Subpleural location of cysts and lobulated, sometimes septated morphology are a characteristic feature. (*B*) Coronal CT showing lower lung predominance. (*C*) Contrast-enhanced CT of the abdomen showing bilateral enhancing renal masses, which were oncocytomas, a benign lesion, in this patient.

red as in amyloidosis.[58] As initially described in 1976 by Randall and colleagues,[59] LCDD is a multiorgan disease with constant renal involvement. The heart and liver are the next most commonly affected organs.[58] Lung involvement is rare, usually asymptomatic, and most often diagnosed at the time of autopsy by systematic immunofluorescence study.[60]

Middle-aged men are the most commonly affected demographic, with 75% having an underlying plasma cell dyscrasia such as multiple myeloma or Waldenström macroglobulinemia.[59]

As described in the literature, LCDD manifests on imaging as pulmonary nodules of varying size and ranging from multiple and bilateral to solitary.[38,58] Nodule size varies from 2 to 5 cm. However, cystic lung disease is a known manifestation of LCDD (**Fig. 5**); Colombat and colleagues[58] reported 3 cases of LCDD presenting primarily as cystic lung disease associated with obstructive pulmonary chronic failure, eventually requiring lung transplant.[60] Cysts varied in size and were diffusely distributed, although lower lung zone predominance was present in one of the patients. In the other 2 patients, progression of cystic lung disease was noted on follow-up imaging, with development of nodules and consolidation.[58] Similar cysts may occur with amyloidosis, often associated with calcified nodules.

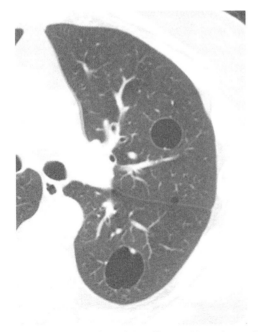

Fig. 5. Light chain deposition disease. Note the perivascular cysts in the left lung, a characteristic feature of light chain deposition disease in this patient with multiple myeloma.

Other Causes of Cysts

Solitary lung cysts are common in otherwise normal individuals. Some of these may be the residue of previous infection or barotrauma. Congenital lung cysts or cystic malformations are usually solitary. Cysts may also occur in other diffuse lung conditions, including *Pneumocystis jirovecii* pneumonia, hypersensitivity pneumonitis (HP), lung adenocarcinoma, and desquamative interstitial pneumonia (DIP). In all these conditions there are associated clinical and imaging features that should lead to the correct diagnosis.

MIMICS OF CYSTS
Emphysema

Emphysema represents destruction of lung parenchyma and is categorized relative to the pulmonary anatomy as centrilobular, paraseptal, and panlobular.[61] Centrilobular emphysema is the most common, usually associated with smoking, and can mimic cystic lung disease.[62]

On radiography, centrilobular emphysema is often not apparent given radiography's poor contrast resolution. However, there is often associated hyperinflation of the lungs, which presents as flattening of the diaphragms, barrel-shaped chest, small or tubular configuration of the heart, and diminished vascular markings.[38] Centrilobular emphysema is distinguished from true cystic lung disease on CT in that it lacks a perceptible wall (**Fig. 6**). These lucent, air-filled spaces can be multiple and bilateral and irregular in shape and are most often upper lung zone predominant. Paraseptal emphysema is also most often smoking related; given its upper lung and subpleural location, differentiation of this entity from cystic lung disease is usually not an issue. Panlobular emphysema is most often lower lung zone predominant and most often due to α-1 antitrypsin deficiency or methylphenidate (Ritalin) injection; the imaging presentation shares little overlap with cystic lung disease.

Honeycombing

From a pathologic standpoint, honeycombing represents destruction and fibrosis of the lung parenchyma with formation of cystic spaces, representing dilated respiratory bronchioles.[63] The Fleischner Society describes honeycombing as clustered cystic air spaces, typically of comparable diameters of the order of 3 to 10 mm but occasionally as large as 2.5 cm.[64] Honeycombing is typically subpleural in distribution.[65]

Although honeycombing is sometimes difficult to identify on chest radiographs, it may manifest as ring shadows with thin, perceptible walls.[38]

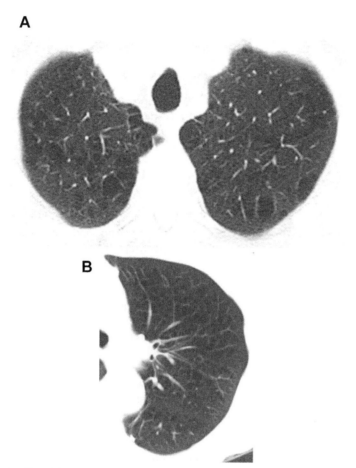

Fig. 6. Emphysema. (*A*, *B*) Axial CT in 2 separate patients showing several rounded, lucent areas in the upper lungs representing centrilobular emphysema in these patients with long smoking history. Note the lack of a thin, perceptible wall, which is a discriminative feature separating emphysema from a true lung cyst.

On HRCT, honeycombing is easier to identify and is characterized by rows and/or stacks of cystic spaces, which are similar in size and share walls (**Fig. 7**). Other signs of fibrosis are usually present, including traction bronchiectasis, architectural distortion, volume loss, and reticulation. As honeycombing typically implies end-stage fibrosis, the term should be used carefully, as it may directly affect patient care.

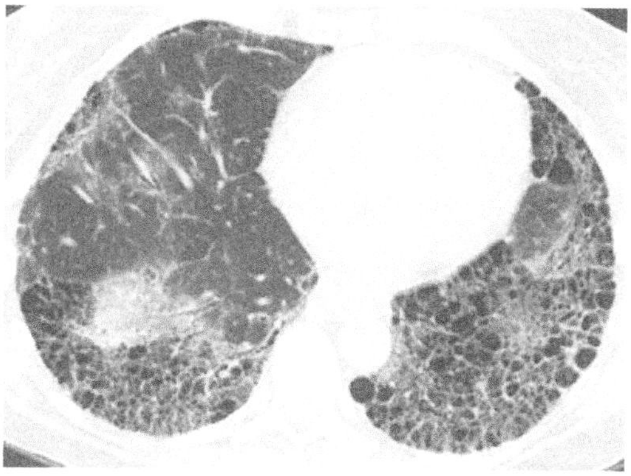

Cavities

A cavity is distinguished from a lung cyst primarily based on wall thickness, with greater than 4 mm being the cutoff (**Fig. 8**).[66] There are numerous causes, including neoplastic, infectious, autoimmune, and congenital causes. Evaluating for neoplastic cause is particularly important and may be aided by the wall thickness. Woodring and colleagues[67] evaluated 65 solitary cavities of the lung while measuring the thickest part of the cavity. They found 92% benignity with thickness less than 4 mm, 51% benignity and 49% malignancy with thickness between 5 and 15 mm, and more than 95% malignancy with thickness greater than 15 mm.

Fig. 7. Honeycombing. The cysts in honeycombing are subpleural in location and line up in rows or stacked on each other.

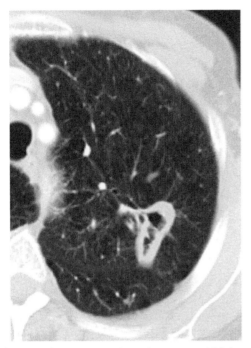

Fig. 8. Cavity. As opposed to a lung cyst, which has a thin wall, the wall in this lesion is thick. The lesion was resected as it caused concern for malignancy but was shown to represent a focus of granulomatous infection.

Bronchiectasis

Bronchiectasis refers to irreversible dilatation of the airways, which can be due to numerous causes. Three main forms are recognized (in order of increasing severity): cylindrical, varicoid, and cystic. Cystic bronchiectasis is the most common form to resemble a lung cyst but can be readily identified by tracing its contiguous relationship to an airway, which may be better appreciated on multiplanar reformations **(Fig. 9)**.[38]

NODULAR LUNG DISEASE

Nodular lung disease is characterized by numerous nodules ranging from 2 to 10 mm in diameter.[68] Approaching nodular lung disease often requires a multimodal approach, with close cooperation among clinicians, pathologists, and radiologists to reach an accurate, focused differential diagnosis. HRCT is a particularly useful modality in characterizing nodular lung disease, with the most useful clue being the distribution pattern relative to the SPL.[69] Distribution of nodules relative to the SPL can be segregated into 3 main patterns: centrilobular, perilymphatic, and random. The centrilobular pattern is the only pattern to spare subpleural lung and interlobular septa. Both the perilymphatic and random patterns involve the subpleural lung and interlobular septa, although the random pattern is much more uniformly distributed. An algorithm-based approach can guide the radiologist to the appropriate pattern. Features of these 3 patterns and some of their more common differential diagnoses are discussed.

Centrilobular Pattern

Knowledge of the anatomy of the SPL is key to understanding the imaging appearance of centrilobular nodules. The SPL measures 1 to 2.5 cm and is better defined at the lung periphery. Lymphatics and veins within the interlobular septa comprise the peripheral structure of the SPL, whereas lobular arteries/arterioles and their accompanying bronchi/bronchioles comprise the centrilobular structures. Each of these measures less than 1 mm in diameter and, aside from the artery/arteriole, is less than the resolution of HRCT, unless diseased. Thus, any disease process affecting the centrilobular structures manifests on imaging with sparing of the subpleural lung or interlobular septal surface.[70,71]

A

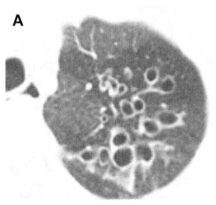

B

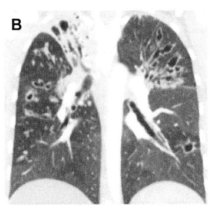

Fig. 9. Bronchiectasis. (*A*) Axial CT shows rounded lucent areas within the lung with thin wall. (*B*) However, coronal reformation shows these lucent areas to be contiguous with airways, consistent with bronchiectasis.

A

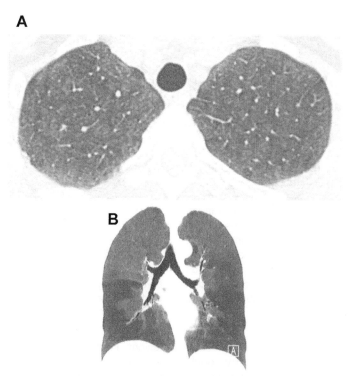

B

Fig. 10. Hypersensitivity pneumonitis. (*A*) HRCT image shows diffuse centrilobular ground-glass nodular lesions in this patient with HP. (*B*) Coronal minimum intensity projection shows mosaic attenuation in the mid and lower lung zones consistent with air trapping and upper lung zone ground-glass opacity with centrilobular preponderance.

Centrilobular nodules are commonly seen in subacute HP, although the differential diagnosis includes RB, pneumoconiosis, and, less commonly, vascular causes such as vasculitis, hemorrhage, or edema.[71,72] HP is a diffuse granulomatous interstitial lung disease caused by inhalation of antigenic organic particles.[73] Centrilobular nodules of ground-glass attenuation may be the predominant or only abnormal finding in subacute HP at HRCT.[74] Associated air trapping is quite common (**Fig. 10**). The nodules are typically small, ranging up to 10 mm in size; are usually innumerable; and can coalesce into more diffuse ground-glass attenuation in the lungs.[75]

RB is a smoking-related lung disease, histopathologically characterized by the accumulation of cytoplasmic golden brown–pigmented macrophages within respiratory bronchioles.[76] Most cases of RB are histologically too mild to produce visible abnormality on HRCT. However, when present, upper lung centrilobular ground-glass nodules are the main finding (**Fig. 11**).[77] Respiratory bronchiolitis–associated interstitial lung disease (RB-ILD) and DIP are also in the spectrum of smoking-related lung disease. HRCT findings in RB-ILD vary in regards to the major abnormality and zonal distribution, although imaging findings usually mirror those of RB; patients with RB-ILD

have abnormal clinical or physiologic abnormality, differentiating RB-ILD from RB.[77] DIP, a condition predominantly but not exclusively found in smokers,

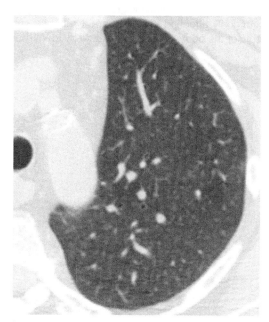

Fig. 11. Respiratory bronchiolitis. Coned-down axial CT in a long-time smoker shows diffuse centrilobular nodularity.

tends to show lower lung–predominant ground-glass abnormality and, rarely, pulmonary fibrosis; nodular disease from DIP would be highly unusual.[77,78]

The tree-in-bud pattern is a special subset of centrilobular nodules initially described in CT scans of patients with endobronchial spread of *Mycobacterium tuberculosis* infection.[79] Infection and aspiration are by far the most common causes of the tree-in-bud sign. Uncommonly this pattern can be seen in other entities that cause luminal impaction, bronchiolar dilatation, or wall thickening, including cystic fibrosis, immune deficiency, inflammatory bowel disease, and diffuse panbronchiolitis.[80,81] On CT, the tree-in-bud pattern manifests as small (2–4 mm), centrilobular, well-defined nodules connected to linear, branching opacities that have more than 1 contiguous branching site (**Fig. 12**).[81] As with centrilobular nodularity, there is sparing of the subpleural lung and interlobular septal surface.[81,82]

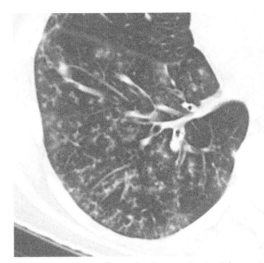

Fig. 12. Tree-in-bud opacity in a patient with nontuberculous mycobacterial infection. Note the sparing of the pleural surface, a characteristic feature of centrilobular and tree-in-bud nodules.

Perilymphatic Pattern

Perilymphatic pattern is characterized by nodule distribution preferentially involving the interlobular septa, peribronchovascular interstitium, and subpleural lung, including the fissures.[69,71] Although the perilymphatic pattern is characteristically described in sarcoidosis, it can also be seen in occupational lung disease, such as silicosis and coal workers pneumoconiosis, and in lymphangitic carcinomatosis.[71]

Sarcoidosis is a systemic granulomatous disease commonly affecting the lungs and lymphatic systems of the body. Diagnosis is made by identifying lesions in more than one organ system, while excluding other known causes of granulomatous disease.[83] Lung involvement is present in more than 90% of cases. Symptoms are seen in one-third to half of patients with lung involvement and include dyspnea, dry cough, and chest tightness. Most patients demonstrate pulmonary abnormalities by imaging at some stage of the disease. CT has proved superior to radiography in detection and characterization of this condition. The most predominant pattern is micronodules located along the peribronchovascular interstitium (**Fig. 13**). Associated findings include upper lung zone

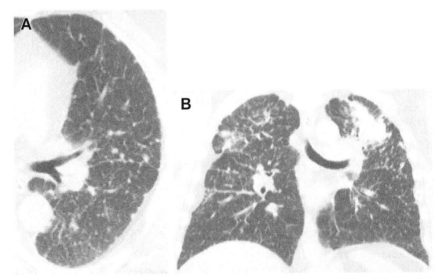

Fig. 13. Sarcoidosis. (*A, B*) Axial and coronal CT show a perilymphatic pattern with nodularity of the subpleural lung, fissures, and interlobular septa. Masslike fibrosis is present in the left upper lobe.

predominance, focal air trapping from bronchiolar obstruction, and diffuse hilar and mediastinal adenopathy, often calcified.[71] Although most cases of sarcoidosis are idiopathic, a sarcoidlike reaction has been described in the setting of malignancy, inflammatory bowel disease, and immunomodulatory therapy. Imaging features overlap with primary sarcoidosis with mediastinal and hilar adenopathy, middle and upper lung preponderant perilymphatic nodules, and ground-glass opacity.[84]

Silicosis is an occupational lung disease resulting from chronic inhalation of dust containing crystalline silica. Commonly reported occupations resulting in silicosis include construction, mining, sandblasting, and stone cutting. Symptoms typically develop 20 years after exposure and include cough, dyspnea, and increased sputum, although some individuals are asymptomatic.[85] The perilymphatic pattern of simple silicosis closely resembles sarcoidosis, with nodularity predominantly within the upper lung zones. However, in simple silicosis, nodules are usually concentrated in the centrilobular and subpleural portions of the lungs; significant degree of peribronchovascular disease would be unusual. Progressive massive fibrosis indicates complicated disease and is characterized by large opacities within the mid and upper lung zones, which tend to migrate toward the hila.[71,86] Eggshell calcification in mediastinal and hilar lymph nodes may be present.[86] Although imaging features of silicosis overlap with sarcoidosis, the 2 are usually easily diagnosed when correlated with clinical history.

Lymphangitic carcinomatosis results from metastasis to the lymphatic system. On CT, this manifests as smooth or nodular thickening of the interlobular septa and peribronchovascular interstitium, whereas lung architecture at the lobular level is preserved (**Fig. 14**).[85] The lungs are commonly asymmetrically involved, and there is usually accompanying adenopathy and effusions.[71]

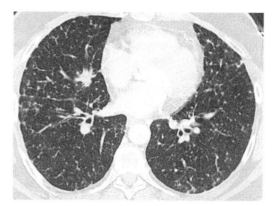

Fig. 14. Lymphangitic carcinomatosis. Axial CT showing nodularity of the fissures, pleura, and interlobular septa. Note the spiculated right middle lobe nodule, shown to represent adenocarcinoma.

Random Pattern

Random nodules are defined by the lack of a distinct relationship to the SPL or perilymphatic structures (**Fig. 15**). Entities that spread hematogenously, most commonly metastases and infection, give rise to a random pattern, with greatest profusion at the lung bases.[71]

Pulmonary metastases occur in 20% to 30% of malignancies, most commonly from hematogenous spread.[85] Nodules are usually well defined and lower lung predominant, although variable in size. The most common primary sites with pulmonary metastases, according to autopsy series, are the breast, colon, kidney, uterus, and head and neck.[87,88] Choriocarcinoma, osteosarcoma, testicular tumor, melanoma, Ewing tumor, and thyroid carcinoma have propensity to metastasize to the lung, although these primary tumors are low in frequency.[89]

Miliary infection is an important differential diagnosis for the random pattern. Miliary nodules are

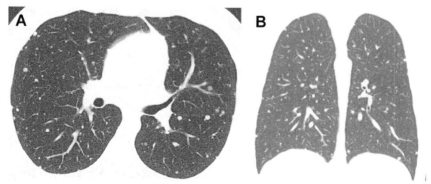

Fig. 15. Thyroid carcinoma metastases. (*A*, *B*) Axial and coronal CT images show a random distribution of small, well-defined pulmonary nodules. Although nodules involve the subpleural lung and fissural surfaces, most appear randomly distributed through the lung.

small, measuring 1 to 3 mm in diameter, and can be caused by at least 80 different entities.[90] Both primary and postprimary tuberculosis can produce a miliary pattern, most commonly in immunocompromised subjects. No correlation has been found between the size and number of nodules on imaging and the patient's clinical course.[91]

SUMMARY

For cystic lung disease, a pattern-based approach incorporating zonal distribution, cyst morphology, and associated clinical findings can often lead to an accurate diagnosis, obviating surgical lung biopsy. The most important step in evaluating nodular lung disease is establishing the nodular pattern relative to the SPL and lymphatic structures. Combining the nodular pattern with associated imaging findings, clinical history, and pertinent physical examination and laboratory findings can lead to a concise, appropriate differential diagnosis.

REFERENCES

1. Hansell DM, Bankier AA, MacMahon H, et al. Fleischner Society: glossary of terms for thoracic imaging. Radiology 2008;246(3):697–722.

2. McCormack FX. Lymphangioleiomyomatosis: a clinical update. Chest 2008;133(2):507–16.

3. Sullivan EJ. Lymphangioleiomyomatosis: a review. Chest 1998;114(6):1689–703.

4. Seaman DM, Meyer CA, Gilman MD, et al. Diffuse cystic lung disease at high-resolution CT. AJR Am J Roentgenol 2011;196(6):1305–11.

5. Grant LA, Babar J, Griffin N. Cysts, cavities, and honeycombing in multisystem disorders: differential diagnosis and findings on thin-section CT. Clin Radiol 2009;64(4):439–48.

6. Taylor JR, Ryu J, Colby TV, et al. Lymphangioleiomyomatosis. Clinical course in 32 patients. N Engl J Med 1990;323(18):1254–60.

7. Corrin B, Liebow AA, Friedman PJ. Pulmonary lymphangiomyomatosis. A review. Am J Pathol 1975; 79(2):348–82.

8. Berkman N, Bloom A, Cohen P, et al. Bilateral spontaneous pneumothorax as the presenting feature in lymphangioleiomyomatosis. Respir Med 1995; 89(5):381–3.

9. Muller NL, Chiles C, Kullnig P. Pulmonary lymphangiomyomatosis: correlation of CT with radiographic and functional findings. Radiology 1990;175(2):335–9.

10. Lenoir S, Grenier P, Brauner MW, et al. Pulmonary lymphangiomyomatosis and tuberous sclerosis: comparison of radiographic and thin-section CT findings. Radiology 1990;175(2):329–34.

11. Sherrier RH, Chiles C, Roggli V. Pulmonary lymphangioleiomyomatosis: CT findings. AJR Am J Roentgenol 1989;153(5):937–40.

12. Cudzilo CJ, Szczesniak RD, Brody AS, et al. Lymphangioleiomyomatosis screening in women with tuberous sclerosis. Chest 2013;144(2):578–85.

13. Ristagno RL, Biddinger PW, Pina EM, et al. Multifocal micronodular pneumocyte hyperplasia in tuberous sclerosis. AJR Am J Roentgenol 2005; 184(3 Suppl):S37–9.

14. Muir TE, Leslie KO, Popper H, et al. Micronodular pneumocyte hyperplasia. Am J Surg Pathol 1998; 22(4):465–72.

15. Avila NA, Kelly JA, Chu SC, et al. Lymphangioleiomyomatosis: abdominopelvic CT and US findings. Radiology 2000;216(1):147–53.

16. Bosniak MA. Angiomyolipoma (hamartoma) of the kidney: a preoperative diagnosis is possible in virtually every case. Urol Radiol 1981;3(3):135–42.

17. Wright T, Sooriakumaran P. Renal angiomyolipoma presenting with massive retroperitoneal haemorrhage due to deranged clotting factors: a case report. Cases J 2008;1(1):213.

18. Yoshida S, Hayashi T, Ishii N, et al. Bilateral renal angiomyolipoma coexistent with pulmonary lymphangioleiomyomatosis and tuberous sclerosis. Int Urol Nephrol 2006;38(3–4):413–5.

19. Oesterling JE, Fishman EK, Goldman SM, et al. The management of renal angiomyolipoma. J Urol 1986; 135(6):1121–4.

20. Johnson SR, Tattersfield AE. Lymphangioleiomyomatosis. Semin Respir Crit Care Med 2002;23(2): 85–92.

21. Johnson SR, Tattersfield AE. Clinical experience of lymphangioleiomyomatosis in the UK. Thorax 2000; 55(12):1052–7.

22. Abbott GF, Rosado-de-Christenson ML, Franks TJ, et al. From the archives of the AFIP: pulmonary Langerhans cell histiocytosis. Radiographics 2004; 24(3):821–41.

23. Rowden G. The Langerhans cell. Crit Rev Immunol 1981;3(2):95–180.

24. Friedman PJ, Liebow AA, Sokoloff J. Eosinophilic granuloma of lung. Clinical aspects of primary histiocytosis in the adult. Medicine (Baltimore) 1981; 60(6):385–96.

25. Favara BE, Feller AC, Pauli M, et al. Contemporary classification of histiocytic disorders. The WHO Committee on Histiocytic/Reticulum Cell Proliferations. Reclassification Working Group of the Histiocyte Society. Med Pediatr Oncol 1997; 29(3):157–66.

26. Kambouchner M, Basset F, Marchal J, et al. Three-dimensional characterization of pathologic lesions in pulmonary Langerhans cell histiocytosis. Am J Respir Crit Care Med 2002;166(11): 1483–90.

27. Myers JL, Aubry MC. Pulmonary Langerhans cell histiocytosis: what was the question? Am J Respir Crit Care Med 2002;166(11):1419–21.

28. Vassallo R, Ryu JH, Colby TV, et al. Pulmonary Langerhans' cell histiocytosis. N Engl J Med 2000; 342(26):1969–78.

29. Travis WD, Borok Z, Roum JH, et al. Pulmonary Langerhans cell granulomatosis (histiocytosis X). A clinicopathologic study of 48 cases. Am J Surg Pathol 1993;17(10):971–86.

30. Mendez JL, Nadrous HF, Vassallo R, et al. Pneumothorax in pulmonary Langerhans cell histiocytosis. Chest 2004;125(3):1028–32.

31. Lacronique J, Roth C, Battesti JP, et al. Chest radiological features of pulmonary histiocytosis X: a report based on 50 adult cases. Thorax 1982;37(2):104–9.

32. Moore AD, Godwin JD, Müller NL, et al. Pulmonary histiocytosis X: comparison of radiographic and CT findings. Radiology 1989;172(1):249–54.

33. Greiwe AC, Miller K, Farver C, et al. AIRP best cases in radiologic-pathologic correlation: pulmonary Langerhans cell histiocytosis. Radiographics 2012; 32(4):987–90.

34. Fraser RS. Fraser and Paré's diagnosis of diseases of the chest. 4th edition. Philadelphia: W.B. Saunders; 1999.

35. Grenier P, Valeyre D, Cluzel P, et al. Chronic diffuse interstitial lung disease: diagnostic value of chest radiography and high-resolution CT. Radiology 1991;179(1):123–32.

36. Bonelli FS, Hartman TE, Swensen SJ, et al. Accuracy of high-resolution CT in diagnosing lung diseases. AJR Am J Roentgenol 1998;170(6):1507–12.

37. Castoldi MC, Verrioli A, De Juli E, et al. Pulmonary Langerhans cell histiocytosis: the many faces of presentation at initial CT scan. Insights Imaging 2014; 5(4):483–92.

38. Jawad H, Walker CM, Wu CC, et al. Cystic interstitial lung diseases: recognizing the common and uncommon entities. Curr Probl Diagn Radiol 2014; 43(3):115–27.

39. Brauner MW, Grenier P, Mouelhi MM, et al. Pulmonary histiocytosis X: evaluation with high-resolution CT. Radiology 1989;172(1):255–8.

40. Soler P, Bergeron A, Kambouchner M, et al. Is high-resolution computed tomography a reliable tool to predict the histopathological activity of pulmonary Langerhans cell histiocytosis? Am J Respir Crit Care Med 2000;162(1):264–70.

41. Liebow AA, Carrington CB. Diffuse pulmonary lymphoreticular infiltrations associated with dysproteinemia. Med Clin North Am 1973;57(3):809–43.

42. Deheinzelin D, Capelozzi VL, Kairalla RA, et al. Interstitial lung disease in primary Sjogren's syndrome. Clinical-pathological evaluation and response to treatment. Am J Respir Crit Care Med 1996;154(3 Pt 1):794–9.

43. Johkoh T, Müller NL, Pickford HA, et al. Lymphocytic interstitial pneumonia: thin-section CT findings in 22 patients. Radiology 1999;212(2):567–72.

44. Johkoh T, Ichikado K, Akira M, et al. Lymphocytic interstitial pneumonia: follow-up CT findings in 14 patients. J Thorac Imaging 2000;15(3):162–7.

45. Koss MN, Hochholzer L, Langloss JM, et al. Lymphoid interstitial pneumonia: clinicopathological and immunopathological findings in 18 cases. Pathology 1987;19(2):178–85.

46. Silva CI, Flint JD, Levy RD, et al. Diffuse lung cysts in lymphoid interstitial pneumonia: high-resolution CT and pathologic findings. J Thorac Imaging 2006; 21(3):241–4.

47. Kanne JP. Idiopathic interstitial pneumonias. Semin Roentgenol 2010;45(1):8–21.

48. Birt AR, Hogg GR, Dube WJ. Hereditary multiple fibrofolliculomas with trichodiscomas and acrochordons. Arch Dermatol 1977;113(12):1674–7.

49. Pavlovich CP, Grubb RL 3rd, Hurley K, et al. Evaluation and management of renal tumors in the Birt-Hogg-Dube syndrome. J Urol 2005;173(5):1482–6.

50. Ayo DS, Aughenbaugh GL, Yi ES, et al. Cystic lung disease in Birt-Hogg-Dube syndrome. Chest 2007; 132(2):679–84.

51. Ardilouze P, Jacquin J, Ait Ali T, et al. Birt-Hogg-Dube syndrome: a little known cause of pulmonary cysts. Diagn Interv Imaging 2015;96:99–101.

52. Painter JN, Tapanainen H, Somer M, et al. A 4-bp deletion in the Birt-Hogg-Dube gene (FLCN) causes dominantly inherited spontaneous pneumothorax. Am J Hum Genet 2005;76(3):522–7.

53. Kluijt I, de Jong D, Teertstra HJ, et al. Early onset of renal cancer in a family with Birt-Hogg-Dube syndrome. Clin Genet 2009;75(6):537–43.

54. Souza CA, Finley R, Muller NL. Birt-Hogg-Dube syndrome: a rare cause of pulmonary cysts. AJR Am J Roentgenol 2005;185(5):1237–9.

55. Agarwal PP, Gross BH, Holloway BJ, et al. Thoracic CT findings in Birt-Hogg-Dube syndrome. AJR Am J Roentgenol 2011;196(2):349–52.

56. Tobino K, Gunji Y, Kurihara M, et al. Characteristics of pulmonary cysts in Birt-Hogg-Dube syndrome: thin-section CT findings of the chest in 12 patients. Eur J Radiol 2011;77(3):403–9.

57. Beddy P, Babar J, Devaraj A. A practical approach to cystic lung disease on HRCT. Insights Imaging 2011;2(1):1–7.

58. Colombat M, Stern M, Groussard O, et al. Pulmonary cystic disorder related to light chain deposition disease. Am J Respir Crit Care Med 2006;173(7): 777–80.

59. Randall RE, Williamson WC Jr, Mullinax F, et al. Manifestations of systemic light chain deposition. Am J Med 1976;60(2):293–9.

60. Colombat M, Mal H, Copie-Bergman C, et al. Primary cystic lung light chain deposition disease: a

clinicopathologic entity derived from unmutated B cells with a stereotyped IGHV4-34/IGKV1 receptor. Blood 2008;112(5):2004–12.

61. Cosio Piqueras MG, Cosio MG. Disease of the airways in chronic obstructive pulmonary disease. Eur Respir J Suppl 2001;34:41s–9s.

62. Takahashi M, Yamada G, Koba H, et al. Classification of centrilobular emphysema based on CT-pathologic correlations. Open Respir Med J 2012;6:155–9.

63. Echeveste J, Fernández-Velilla M, Torres MI, et al. Cystic diseases of the lung: high-resolution computed tomography findings. Arch Bronconeumol 2005;41(1):42–9 [in Spanish].

64. Johkoh T, Sakai F, Noma S, et al. Honeycombing on CT; its definition, pathologic correlation, and future direction of its diagnosis. Eur J Radiol 2014;83(1):27–31.

65. Muller NL, Miller RR, Webb WR, et al. Fibrosing alveolitis: CT-pathologic correlation. Radiology 1986; 160(3):585–8.

66. Cosgrove GP, Frankel SK, Brown KK. Challenges in pulmonary fibrosis. 3: cystic lung disease. Thorax 2007;62(9):820–9.

67. Woodring JH, Fried AM, Chuang VP. Solitary cavities of the lung: diagnostic implications of cavity wall thickness. AJR Am J Roentgenol 1980;135(6):1269–71.

68. Oikonomou A, Prassopoulos P. Mimics in chest disease: interstitial opacities. Insights Imaging 2013; 4(1):9–27.

69. Elicker B, Pereira CA, Webb R, et al. High-resolution computed tomography patterns of diffuse interstitial lung disease with clinical and pathological correlation. J Bras Pneumol 2008;34(9):715–44.

70. Abbott GF, Rosado-de-Christenson ML, Rossi SE, et al. Imaging of small airways disease. J Thorac Imaging 2009;24(4):285–98.

71. Raoof S, Amchentsev A, Vlahos I, et al. Pictorial essay: multinodular disease: a high-resolution CT scan diagnostic algorithm. Chest 2006;129(3):805–15.

72. Hansell DM, Wells AU, Padley SP, et al. Hypersensitivity pneumonitis: correlation of individual CT patterns with functional abnormalities. Radiology 1996;199(1):123–8.

73. Mohr LC. Hypersensitivity pneumonitis. Curr Opin Pulm Med 2004;10(5):401–11.

74. Lacasse Y, Selman M, Costabel U, et al. Clinical diagnosis of hypersensitivity pneumonitis. Am J Respir Crit Care Med 2003;168(8):952–8.

75. Silva CI, Churg A, Muller NL. Hypersensitivity pneumonitis: spectrum of high-resolution CT and pathologic findings. AJR Am J Roentgenol 2007;188(2):334–44.

76. Caminati A, Harari S. Smoking-related interstitial pneumonias and pulmonary Langerhans cell histiocytosis. Proc Am Thorac Soc 2006;3(4):299–306.

77. Heyneman LE, Ward S, Lynch DA, et al. Respiratory bronchiolitis, respiratory bronchiolitis-associated interstitial lung disease, and desquamative interstitial pneumonia: different entities or part of the spectrum of the same disease process? AJR Am J Roentgenol 1999;173(6): 1617–22.

78. Carrington CB, Gaensler EA, Coutu RE, et al. Natural history and treated course of usual and desquamative interstitial pneumonia. N Engl J Med 1978; 298(15):801–9.

79. Im JG, Itoh H, Shim YS, et al. Pulmonary tuberculosis: CT findings–early active disease and sequential change with antituberculous therapy. Radiology 1993;186(3):653–60.

80. Aquino SL, Gamsu G, Webb WR, et al. Tree-in-bud pattern: frequency and significance on thin section CT. J Comput Assist Tomogr 1996;20(4):594–9.

81. Eisenhuber E. The tree-in-bud sign. Radiology 2002; 222(3):771–2.

82. Collins J, Blankenbaker D, Stern EJ. CT patterns of bronchiolar disease: what is "tree-in-bud"? AJR Am J Roentgenol 1998;171(2):365–70.

83. Statement on sarcoidosis. Joint Statement of the American Thoracic Society (ATS), the European Respiratory Society (ERS) and the World Association of Sarcoidosis and Other Granulomatous Disorders (WASOG) adopted by the ATS Board of Directors and by the ERS Executive Committee, February 1999. Am J Respir Crit Care Med 1999; 160(2):736–55.

84. Lau RK, Takasugi JE, David Godwin J, et al. Sarcoid-like reaction - computed tomography features in 12 patients. J Comput Assist Tomogr 2015; 39(2):143–8.

85. Boitsios G, Bankier AA, Eisenberg RL. Diffuse pulmonary nodules. AJR Am J Roentgenol 2010; 194(5):W354–66.

86. Kim KI, Kim CW, Lee MK, et al. Imaging of occupational lung disease. Radiographics 2001;21(6): 1371–91.

87. Crow J, Slavin G, Kreel L. Pulmonary metastasis: a pathologic and radiologic study. Cancer 1981; 47(11):2595–602.

88. Coppage L, Shaw C, Curtis AM. Metastatic disease to the chest in patients with extrathoracic malignancy. J Thorac Imaging 1987;2(4):24–37.

89. Seo JB, Im JG, Goo JM, et al. Atypical pulmonary metastases: spectrum of radiologic findings. Radiographics 2001;21(2):403–17.

90. Andreu J, Mauleón S, Pallisa E, et al. Miliary lung disease revisited. Curr Probl Diagn Radiol 2002; 31(5):189–97.

91. Jamieson DH, Cremin BJ. High resolution CT of the lungs in acute disseminated tuberculosis and a pediatric radiology perspective of the term "miliary". Pediatr Radiol 1993;23(5):380–3.

Imaging of the Central Airways with Bronchoscopic Correlation
Pictorial Essay

Maria Shiau, MD[a],*, Timothy J. Harkin, MD[b],
David P. Naidich, MD[a]

KEYWORDS

- Central airways • Bronchoscopy • Computed tomography • Imaging

KEY POINTS

- Meticulous imaging technique is key to assessment of the central airways.
- Computed tomography assessment is complementary to bronchoscopy.
- Tracheal lesions can be classified into anatomic variants, focal tracheal narrowing, diffuse tracheal narrowing, and diffuse nodular disease.

INTRODUCTION

Despite the introduction of a wide range of imaging technologies over the past decade, including MRI and 18F-fluorodeoxyglucose (FDG) PET, computed tomography (CT) remains the most accurate noninvasive means for evaluating the central airways. There is a wide range of pathologic entities, both malignant and benign, for which CT imaging represents an essential component of both diagnosis and management. Indications for CT are generally in one of 2 broad categories: (1) symptomatic patients presenting with chronic cough, localized wheezing dyspnea, or hemoptysis, especially those with normal or nonlocalizing radiographs; and (2) cases in which there is endobronchial obstruction with or without associated atelectasis for which interventional bronchoscopic procedures are indicated, including for preprocedural planning as well as for postprocedural monitoring.[1,2]

This article will first review optimal CT techniques for imaging the central airways. Following

this, a classification of central airway disorders is presented with select illustrative examples. The central airways are defined as those airways that may be directly visualized by flexible bronchoscopy: the trachea, mainstem and lobar airways, as well as proximal segmental bronchi. A detailed description of central airway anatomy is not presented because this topic has previously been extensively reviewed.[3] In addition, emphasis is placed on CT-bronchoscopic correlations, in particular as pertains to both diagnostic and therapeutic interventional bronchoscopy.

TECHNIQUE

Following the introduction of multidetector CT scanners capable of imaging the entire thorax in a single breath hold, it is now standard to acquire both routine 5-mm sections spaced every 5 mm throughout the thorax reconstructed in the axial, coronal, and sagittal planes, as well as high-resolution 1-mm to 1.5-mm sections

a Department of Radiology, Center for Biological Imaging, NYU-Langone Medical Center, 660 1st Avenue, New York, NY 10016, USA; b Division of Pulmonary, Critical Care and Sleep Medicine, Department of Medicine, Icahn School of Medicine at Mount Sinai, One Gustave L. Levy Place, Box 1232, New York, NY 10029, USA
* Corresponding author.
E-mail address: maria.shiau@nyumc.org

Clin Chest Med 36 (2015) 313–334
http://dx.doi.org/10.1016/j.ccm.2015.02.012
0272-5231/15/$ – see front matter © 2015 Elsevier Inc. All rights reserved.

typically spaced at 10-mm intervals.[4] Although controversial, routine acquisition of contiguous high-resolution images throughout the thorax is recommended as well.[2] Contiguous high-resolution images with corresponding contiguous high-resolution coronal and sagittal images often prove essential for optimal imaging of the central airways both to enhance visualizing relationships between airways and adjacent mediastinal and hilar structures, as well as optimally visualizing select regions of interest, especially through lobar and proximal segmental airways. Additional advanced reconstruction techniques include curved multiplanar reconstructions, maximum intensity projection and minimum intensity projection (MINip) images (**Fig. 1**), external rendering with either three-dimensional (3D) shaded surface displays or volumetric rendering, and internal virtual bronchoscopic rendering. Although not routinely acquired, as discussed later, these techniques may be of value in select cases.[5,6]

We routinely use a low-dose technique (typically between 40 and 80 mAs) without loss of diagnostic accuracy. Scans are routinely performed in deep inspiration with the patient supine. Expiratory images may prove useful to either detect or confirm a suspicion of abnormal airway motility as occurs in patients with suspected tracheobronchomalacia (**Fig. 2**).[7,8] Expiratory high-resolution CT scans may be obtained either during suspended respiration after forced exhalation (static expiratory CT) or during forced exhalation (dynamic expiratory CT).[7,8] Accurate assessment of the central airways requires using a wide range of window settings with optimal evaluation of peripheral bronchial walls obtained with window centers between −250 and −700 HU, with corresponding window widths between 1000 and 1400 HU, respectively.[9] Administration of intravenous contrast material may be of value to enhance visualization of airways in relation to mediastinal or hilar structures, especially in cases in which atelectasis is radiographically identified, to facilitate differentiation between central tumor and peripheral consolidation, atelectasis, and pleural fluid (**Fig. 3**).

DISEASES AFFECTING THE CENTRAL AIRWAYS: COMPUTED TOMOGRAPHY CLASSIFICATION

Abnormalities affecting the central airways can be classified into one of 4 distinct patterns: anatomic variants (**Box 1**), focal versus diffuse airway narrowing (**Boxes 2** and **3**), and diffuse nodular disease (**Box 4**). Because there is considerable

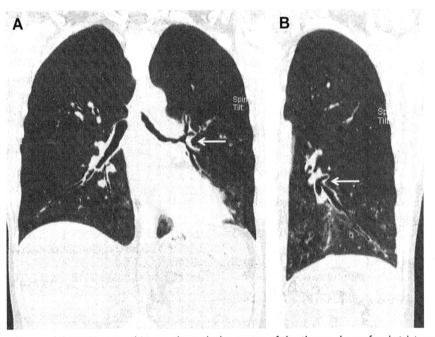

Fig. 1. Crohn disease. (*A*) MINiP coronal image through the center of the thorax shows focal strictures involving the distal left mainstem and proximal left lower lobe bronchus (*arrow* in *A*). (*B*) Enlargement of a MINiP coronal image through the left lower lobe basilar segmental airway shows a tight stenosis at the origin of the lateral basilar segmental bronchus associated with peripheral bronchiectasis (*arrow* in *B*). In this case airway disorder is secondary to inflammatory bowel disease. MINip images are particularly useful for enhancing visualization of airway lumens.

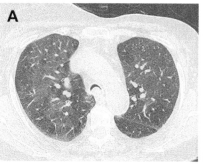
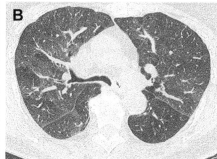

Fig. 2. Tracheomalacia. (*A, B*) Axial images through the distal trachea and carina, respectively, obtained in end-expiration show marked narrowing of the airway lumens caused by tracheomalacia. Note that there is also evidence of marked heterogeneous/mosaic lung density, consistent with associated obstructive small airway disease.

overlap in the appearance of diseases within each of these categories, only select entities are discussed here as sufficient to illustrate key distinguishing features. Although this approach emphasizes pattern recognition it should be emphasized that several entities may be placed in more than 1 category, reflecting variations in the extent and stage of disease.

ANATOMIC VARIANTS

In adults, the most commonly encountered anatomic variants are lung bud anomalies, either anomalous or supernumerary.[10] As proposed by Wu and colleagues,[11] there are 3 broad categories of anatomic variants (see **Box 1**).

Anomalies Arising from Normal Higher Order Bronchial Divisions

This category includes accessory superior segmental bronchi supplying the superior segment of the right lower lobe, and axillary bronchi, identifiable as a supernumerary segmental bronchus supplying the lateral aspect of the right upper lobe.

Anomalies Arising from Sites Typically Lacking Branches

This category includes tracheal bronchi (**Fig. 4**), which arise exclusively on the right side and must be differentiated from tracheoceles that occur because of weakness within the trachealis muscle. Accessory cardiac bronchi represent a true supernumerary anomalous bronchus of variable length arising from the medial wall of the bronchus intermedius proximal to the origin of the superior segmental bronchus (see **Fig. 4**). This bronchus is often associated with a rudimentary accessory lobe, and, depending on its length, may serve as a nidus for retained secretions resulting in subsequent recurrent pneumonia.[12]

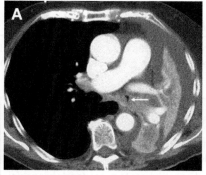
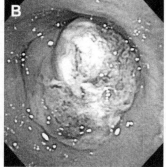
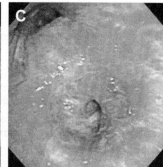

Fig. 3. Central airways obstruction: role of intravenous contrast administration. (*A*) Contrast-enhanced image through the distal left mainstem bronchus shows irregular narrowing of the airway associated with adjacent soft tissue density caused by central obstructing tumor (*white arrow*). Note that following contrast there is clear differentiation between central tumor and collapsed lung and surrounding effusion. The presence of patent mucus-filled airways suggests that there may be residual functional lung if the central airway obstruction can be relieved. (*B*) Bronchoscopic image showing tumor totally obstructing the left main bronchus. (*C*) Bronchoscopic image of the left main bronchus patent after removal of tumor with combination of electrocautery snare and argon plasma coagulation. Pathology revealed metastatic melanoma.

Box 1
Classification: anatomic variants

- Anomalies arising from normal airways
  - For example, supernumerary right upper lobe bronchus
- Anomalies arising from sites typically lacking branches
  - For example, tracheocele, cardiac bronchus, bridging bronchus
- Anomalies arising from abnormalities of situs
  - Simple left to right reversal
  - Bronchial isomerism
    - Bilateral left-sided airways (isolated, venolobar syndrome, polysplenia)
    - Bilateral right-sided airways (asplenia, congenital heart disease)

Anomalies Associated with Abnormalities of Situs

In this category, simple reversal of the right-sided and left-sided airways is the most commonly encountered anomaly. Less frequent are anomalies caused by bronchial isomerism, in which the pattern of airway branching and pulmonary lobation is identical in the 2 lungs. These anomalies include bilateral left-sided airway anatomy, either as an isolated finding or associated either with the venolobar syndrome or less commonly

---

Box 2
Focal tracheobronchial narrowing

- Posttraumatic strictures
- Postinfectious stenoses (eg, tuberculosis, rhinoscleroma)
- Tracheobronchial neoplasms
  - Primary: squamous cell carcinoma; adenoid cystic, carcinoid, mucoepidermoid tumors
  - Secondary: metastatic disease/direct invasion (eg, esophageal tumors)
- Inflammatory disease
  - Granulomatosis with polyangiitis (Wegener granulomatosis), sarcoidosis, inflammatory bowel disease (ulcerative colitis/Crohn disease)
- Extrinsic compression
  - Substernal thyroid tissue, mediastinal adenopathy

Box 3
Diffuse wall thickening/luminal narrowing

- Luminal narrowing
  - Infectious tracheobronchitis (eg, tuberculosis, aspergillosis)[a]
  - Relapsing polychondritis[b,c]
  - Tracheobronchial amyloidosis[b,a]
  - Tracheobronchopathia osteochondroplastica[b,c]
  - Tracheobronchitis associated with inflammatory bowel disease[a]
  - Saber sheath trachea
  - Tracheobronchomalacia[a]
  - Granulomatosis with polyangiitis[a]
  - Sarcoidosis[a]

[a]Circumferential involvement.
[b]Calcific deposits.
[c]Spares posterior/membranous portion of the trachea.

---

polysplenia; and bilateral right-sided airway anatomy. Right-sided airway isomerism is usually associated with asplenia and severe congenital heart disease and is only rarely seen in adults.

FOCAL CENTRAL AIRWAY NARROWING

Within this category are a wide range of entities, both benign and malignant, that have in common focal airway narrowing (see **Box 2**). Most important are benign strictures, as may result from prolonged intubation or prior trauma, and malignancy. Less commonly encountered is focal stenosis resulting from prior infection; in particular, prior tuberculosis.

Nonneoplastic Central Airway Stenosis

Benign airway strictures may be either congenital or acquired. In either case, accurate evaluation

---

Box 4
Diffuse nodular disease

- Granulomatosis with polyangiitis (Wegener granulomatosis)
- Tracheobronchial metastases (endobronchial and/or hematogenous spread)
- Laryngotracheobronchial papillomatosis
- Adenoid cystic carcinoma (multicentric)
- Tracheobronchial amyloidosis
- Tracheobronchopathia osteochondroplastica

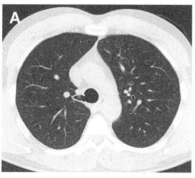
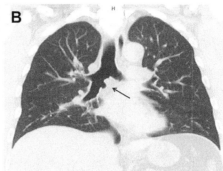

Fig. 4. Congenital airway abnormalities. (*A*) Axial image through the midtrachea shows characteristic appearance of an accessory tracheal bronchus leading to the right upper lobe. (*B*) Coronal image shows characteristic appearance of an accessory cardiac bronchus identifiable as an anomalous branch arising from the medial wall of the bronchus intermedius (*arrow*). (*From* [*B*] Naidich DP, Webb, WR, Grenier, AG, et al. Imaging of the airways. Philadelphia: Lippincott, Williams, and Wilkins; 2005. p. 25. Chapter 1, Figs. 1–23B; with permission.)

requires that the precise length and degree of stenosis be assessed along with associated peritracheal or bronchial abnormalities.[3]

Tracheal trauma: postintubation tracheal stenosis

Among acquired tracheal strictures, the most common cause is iatrogenic injury resulting from intubation, most often the result of overdistension of balloons of endotracheal or tracheostomy tubes (**Figs. 5** and **6**).[13] The 2 principal sites of postintubation stenosis are at the tracheostomy stoma site or at the level of the balloon of the endotracheal tube or tracheostomy tube. In both cases, strictures result from pressure necrosis, which causes ischemia and subsequent scarring, findings that are becoming less common because of improved tube management techniques. A similar mechanism also accounts for fibrous airway stenosis occurring following lung transplantation with narrowing resulting from necrosis, prominent granulation tissue, and malacia. Despite advanced imaging techniques, definitive diagnosis and therapy nearly always require bronchoscopy with primary tracheal and/or laryngotracheal resection and reconstruction remaining the optimal method for treating nonneoplastic stenosis.

Focal tracheal narrowing and obstruction may also follow blunt trauma, especially from automobile accidents: so-called steering-wheel injuries. This type of injury may lead to acute tracheal rupture, appearing as wall defects and/or a deformed lumen, almost invariably accompanied by pneumomediastinum. In contrast, pneumomediastinum may only occur in approximately 50% of patients with postintubation tracheobronchial lacerations (see **Fig. 6**).[14] In this setting, nonsurgical management may be appropriate for small

tears of less than 2 cm if these do not extend into the mainstem bronchi.

Postinfectious airway stenosis

In addition to postintubation stenoses, tracheobronchial strictures also occur as a result of infection, in particular caused by tuberculosis and histoplasmosis. Tuberculosis typically involves the distal trachea and proximal mainstem bronchi: isolated tracheal disease is rare.[15] Active inflammation typically results from extension of inflammation from peribronchial nodal disease and may be associated with endoluminal disease, with or without fistulization (**Fig. 7**). In some cases, smooth bronchial stenosis or occlusion persists or develops after resolution of active peribronchial inflammation (**Fig. 8**). Posttuberculous stenosis usually involves the left main bronchus, because this bronchus is longer than the right, with a larger number of contiguous mediastinal and hilar nodes (**Figs. 9** and **10**). Although CT findings of tuberculous airway stenosis are suggestive, definitive diagnosis typically requires endoscopic biopsy.

Tracheobronchial Neoplasia

Primary tracheobronchial neoplasia is rare.[16–19] The CT appearances of tracheobronchial neoplasms overlap, typically presenting as an endobronchial soft tissue mass or asymmetric tracheal or bronchial wall thickening causing eccentric airway narrowing; in nearly all cases, definitive diagnosis requires histologic evaluation. Squamous cell carcinoma and adenoid cystic carcinoma together account for 86% of primary tracheal lesions.[17]

Squamous cell carcinoma

Squamous cell carcinoma typically occurs in middle-aged male smokers. Characteristically

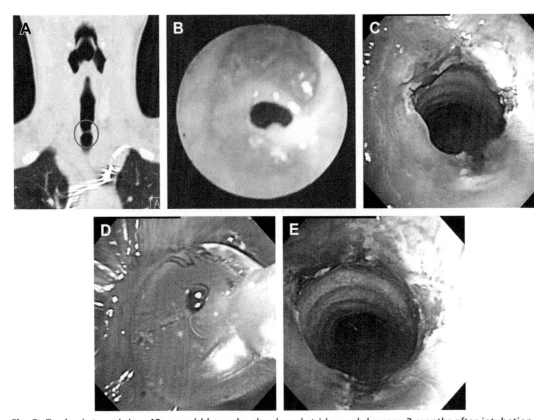

Fig. 5. Tracheal stenosis in a 12-year-old boy who developed stridor and dyspnea 3 months after intubation for sudden cardiac arrest. (*A*) Coronal images show weblike tracheal stenosis (*circle*). This type of tracheal stenosis is the most likely to permanently respond to bronchoscopic intervention. (*B*) Bronchoscopic image showing area of stenosis before therapeutic endoscopic intervention. (*C*) Bronchoscopic imaging showing 4 radial slits made with electrocautery needle knife. (*D*) Bronchoscopic image showing a dilating balloon catheter inflated in the trachea at the site of stenosis. (*E*) Bronchoscopic image showing tracheal patency following dilatation. Subsequent follow-up documented that stridor and dyspnea resolved with the development of a normal flow volume loop.

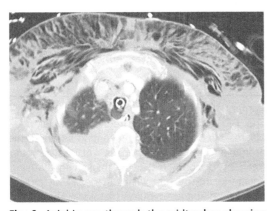

Fig. 6. Axial image through the midtrachea showing deformity of the posterior aspect of the trachea indicating tracheal disruption following traumatic intubation. Note the presence of subtle pneumomediastinum anteriorly and extensive subcutaneous emphysema. (*Courtesy of* Mark Bernstein, MD, NYU-Langone Medical center, NY.)

these tumors extend along a considerable length of the trachea. Direct mediastinal invasion, including esophageal invasion, is common, rendering surgical resection difficult, and local recurrence is common (see **Figs. 9** and **10**).[16–19] In approximately 10% of cases, squamous cell carcinoma proves to be multifocal. These cancers are frequently found to extend into the mainstem bronchi.

Tracheobronchial mucous gland tumors

These tumors primarily include adenoid cystic carcinomas and mucoepidermoid tumors, and are considered pulmonary analogs of the salivary glands. Adenoid cystic carcinomas are low-grade malignancies that typically appear as polypoid lesions, typically occurring in middle-aged patients without sex predilection, unrelated to cigarette smoking (**Fig. 11**).[20–22] Mucoepidermoid tumors arise from tracheobronchial mucous glands and may appear calcified and show enhancement following intravenous contrast

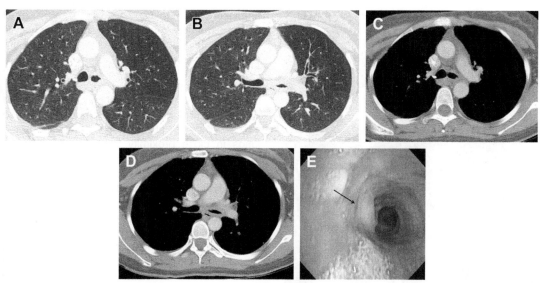

Fig. 7. Tuberculous tracheobronchitis. (*A, B*) Axial images though the carina and left mainstem bronchus, respectively, showing marked narrowing of the left main bronchus. (*C, D*) Identical images as shown in *A* and *B*, imaged with mediastinal windows showing to better advantage the extent of airway wall thickening. (*E*) Bronchoscopic image in a different patient than shown in *A* to *D* showing characteristic involvement of the airway mucosa and lumen with active infection (*arrow*).

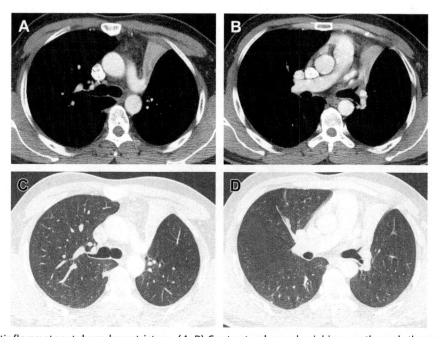

Fig. 8. Postinflammatory tuberculous stricture. (*A–D*) Contrast-enhanced axial images through the proximal left upper lobe bronchus imaged with narrow and wide windows show marked narrowing and obstruction of the proximal left upper lobe bronchus resulting in atelectasis of the left upper lobe. Note the similarity in appearance with active infection in **Fig. 7**. In this case bronchoscopic correlation confirmed the presence of a fibrous stricture consistent with a history of tuberculosis.

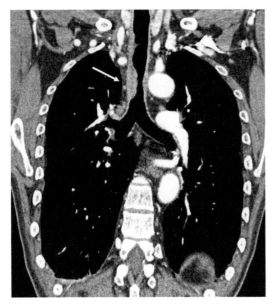

Fig. 9. Squamous cell carcinoma of the trachea. Coronal contrast-enhanced image through the trachea shows characteristic appearance of an eccentric soft tissue lesion extending along the right lateral wall of the trachea (*arrow*).

administration (**Fig. 12**). They comprise 5% of all primary tracheal neoplasms. More than half of the patients with mucoepidermoid tumors are younger than 30 years old.

Carcinoid tumors

Carcinoid tumors are the most frequently identified primary central airway neoplasms (**Figs. 13** and **14**).[18,19] They are also frequently identified in the lungs in close proximity to peripheral airways. These neuroendocrine neoplasms arise within bronchial or bronchiolar epithelium, and are classified as typical carcinoids, atypical carcinoids, and large cell neuroendocrine carcinomas, with the highest grades overlapping with small cell carcinoma. These tumors are hypervascular, which accounts for their marked enhancement following intravenous contrast administration (similar to mucoepidermoid tumors). Carcinoid tumors are also known to produce a variety of hormones and neuroamines, including adrenocorticotrophic hormone, serotonin, and somatostatin.[23,24] Characteristically, adenoid cystic carcinoma and carcinoid tumors extend extraluminally, resulting in so-called iceberg lesions (ie, only a small amount

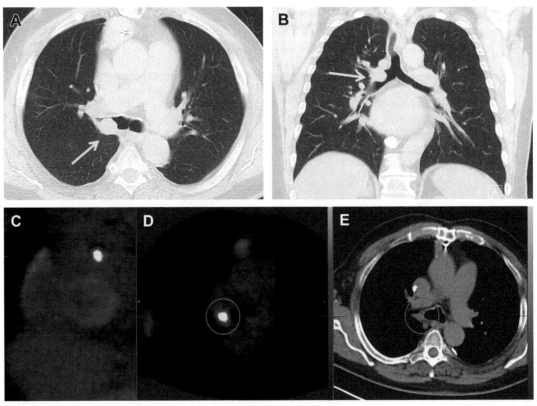

Fig. 10. Squamous cell carcinoma. (*A, B*) Axial and coronal images through the carina, respectively showing a well-defined endoluminal lesion (*arrows* in *A* and *B*). Although typically infiltrative, squamous cell carcinomas sometimes present as focal endoluminal lesions. (*C, D, E*) Images from a corresponding FDG-PET scan showing marked uptake of tracer in the primary lesion as well as in an anterior mediastinal node. FDG-PET images may play an indispensable role in accurately staging intrathoracic neoplasms.

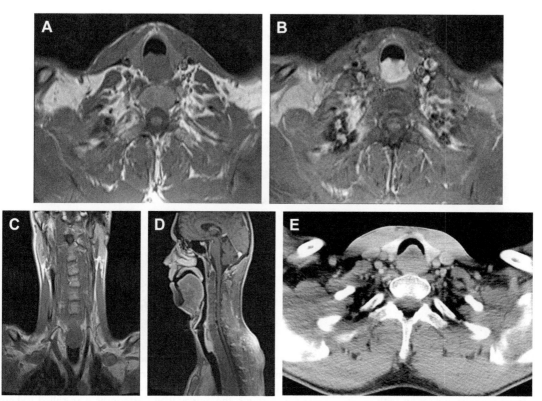

Fig. 11. Adenoid cystic carcinoma in a 45-year-old male nonsmoker presenting with shortness of breath and airflow obstruction. (*A–D*) Axial, coronal, and sagittal T1-weighted MRI, obtained before (*A* and *C*) and after (*B* and *D*) intravenous administration of gadolinium show a well-circumscribed enhancing tumor involving the cervical trachea and causing marked narrowing of the airway. (*E*) Corresponding contrast-enhanced CT image. Note that in this case the lesion is restricted to the airway lumen, making resection feasible.

of the tumor is visible endobronchially). With more peripheral lesions, airway obstruction may result in focal mucoid impaction.

Miscellaneous causes

In addition to primary lung tumors, the central airways may be secondarily involved either as a result of direct invasion (especially from lung, thyroid, and esophageal tumors) or by metastatic disease (see **Fig. 3**; **Figs. 15** and **16**).[18] Although distinct histologically, these entities as a group typically present with nonspecific symptoms of cough, wheezing, stridor, and hemoptysis.

Benign tracheobronchial lesions include hamartomas (**Fig. 17**) and papillomas (**Fig. 18**). The most common benign tracheal neoplasm is squamous

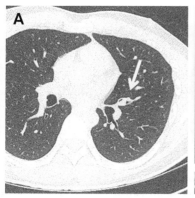
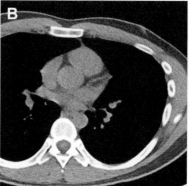
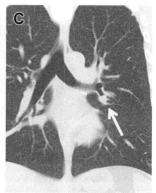

Fig. 12. Mucoepidermoid carcinoma. (*A, B*) Axial CT images through the proximal left inferior lingular bronchus with wide and narrow windows, respectively, show a subtle endoluminal lesion (*arrow* in *A*). (*C*) Coronal reconstruction also showing small well-circumscribed lesion (*arrow*). Biopsy proved mucoepidermoid carcinoma.

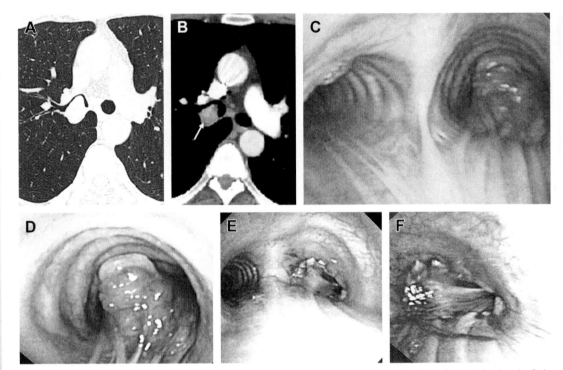

Fig. 13. Carcinoid tumor. (*A, B*) Contrast-enhanced image through the right main bronchus at the level of the origin of the right upper lobe bronchus, imaged with wide and narrow windows, respectively, show a well-defined endoluminal lesion with minimal extension through the airway wall posteriorly; a so-called iceberg lesion (*arrow* in *B*). (*C, D*) Bronchoscopic images confirm large intraluminal mass. (*E, F*) Bronchoscopic images following right upper lobe sleeve resection show patent right upper lobe bronchus. Precise depiction of the extent of this lesion is essential for presurgical planning.

cell papilloma. Squamous cell papillomas rarely involve the trachea, with extension limited to the tracheal wall.[18] Endobronchial hamartomas are rare mesenchymal lesions composed of a mixture of cartilage, fat, and fibrous tissue and are most often identified in segmental airways: tracheal involvement is unusual. On CT the presence of fat is considered diagnostic (see **Fig. 17**).[25]

DIFFUSE AIRWAY NARROWING

Diseases diffusely affecting the central airways are almost exclusively nonneoplastic and can be categorized based on whether they cause tracheal narrowing or dilatation, involve or spare the posterior tracheal membrane, or result in tracheal wall thickening (see **Box 3**).[3,26,27]

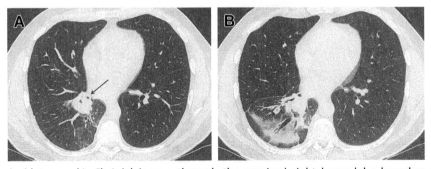

Fig. 14. Carcinoid tumor. (*A, B*) Axial images through the proximal right lower lobe bronchus and basilar segmental bronchi, respectively, show a well-circumscribed endoluminal lesion (*arrow* in *A*) associated with extensive consolidation with air bronchograms and volume loss in the right lower lobe. These findings are typical of long-standing airway obstruction by slow-growing benign endobronchial lesions, leading to chronic inflammation/infection.

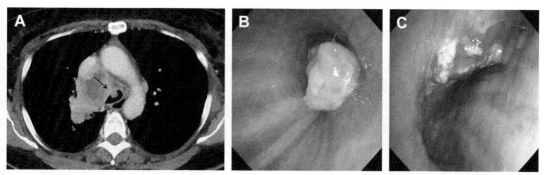

Fig. 15. Malignant tracheal invasion: renal cell carcinoma. (*A*) Contrast-enhanced axial image through the distal trachea shows a large necrotic right paratracheal mass (*arrow*) with direct extension into the tracheal lumen resulting in a polypoid mass. This appearance suggests that the lesions may be amenable to removal by electrocautery snare. (*B*) Bronchoscopic image showing tumor attached to the wall of the trachea. (*C*) Bronchoscopic image after complete removal of tumor by electrocautery snare.

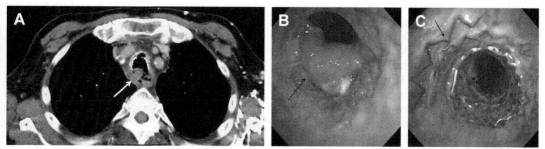

Fig. 16. Tracheoesophageal fistula from esophageal carcinoma. Following previous radiation and chemotherapy a tracheoesophageal fistula developed requiring placement of a tracheal stent. The patient subsequently presented with choking and coughing following meals. (*A*) Axial image through the midtrachea shows tumor infiltration into the posterior wall of the trachea (*arrow*). (*B*) Bronchoscopic image showing tumor invasion into the posterior trachea (*arrow*). (*C*) Bronchoscopic image showing placement of a second telescoping covered stent (*double arrows*) within the prior stent (*single arrow*) resulting in immediate resolution of symptoms.

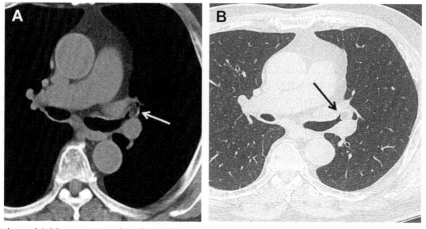

Fig. 17. Endobronchial hamartoma. (*A, B*) Axial images thought the left upper lobe bronchus imaged with narrow and wide windows, respectively, show a well-defined endoluminal lesion within which fat density can be identified (*arrows*). Surgically documented hamartoma.

A   **B**   **C**

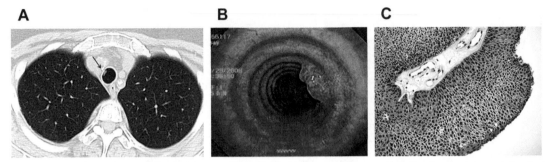

Fig. 18. Tracheal papilloma. (*A*) Axial image though the trachea shows a well-defined eccentric endoluminal lesion (*arrow*). (*B*) Corresponding bronchoscopic image showing good correlation with the CT finding. (*C*) Histologic specimen (H&E stain) documenting the lesions as papilloma. Air within airway lumens is a superb contrast agent allowing reliable identification of lesions as small as 2 mm. For lesions smaller than this, CT is of limited value compared with bronchoscopic evaluation.

Included in this group of patients are those with a variety of noninfectious disorders, including relapsing polychondritis, granulomatosis with polyangiitis, amyloidosis, sarcoidosis, and inflammatory bowel diseases including Crohn disease and ulcerative colitis.[28] Rarely, diffuse narrowing results from tracheobronchial infection, as may be seen flowing bacterial, viral, or fungal infections either primarily or secondarily resulting from adjacent mediastinitis. Although many of these have similar appearances in cross section, some are sufficiently distinctive to allow a definitive diagnosis with appropriate clinical correlation.[5]

Saber Sheath Trachea

Saber sheath trachea is a commonly encountered variant defined by an internal coronal diameter decreased to less than half the corresponding sagittal diameter. Further narrowing of the tracheal lumen is notable when expiratory images are obtained. Saber sheath trachea is invariably associated with chronic obstructive lung disease, and the severity of emphysema is related to the extent of trachea narrowing.[29]

Tracheobronchomalacia

Tracheobronchomalacia is an important cause of expiratory airway narrowing without airway thickening, and is best diagnosed with dynamic expiratory imaging.[30] Boiselle and Ernst[31] and Boiselle and colleagues[32] showed a wide range of collapsibility in normal individuals and therefore suggested that a threshold of greater than 75% decrease in cross-sectional diameter of the trachea on dynamic expiration provides optimal specificity for this diagnosis (see **Fig. 2**).[31,32] Tracheomalacia may be seen in association with most causes of diffuse tracheal inflammation, such as relapsing polychondritis, as well as

following trauma or in patients with chronic bronchitis. Symptoms are typically nonspecific and include chronic cough, dyspnea, and occasionally hemoptysis.

Tracheobronchomegaly

Tracheobronchomegaly refers to a heterogeneous group of entities defined by the presence of diffuse central airway dilatation. Although it may seem contradictory, tracheobronchomegaly is often associated with tracheomalacia in its more severe forms because of abnormalities of tracheal cartilage, tracheobronchial muscle fibers, and absence of the myenteric plexus (**Fig. 19**). It is often associated with recurrent lower respiratory tract infections and bronchiectasis and in association with a wide variety of additional diseases, including ankylosing spondylitis, Marfan syndrome, cystic fibrosis, Ehlers-Danlos syndrome, and cutis laxa in children.

Relapsing Polychondritis

Relapsing polychondritis is a multisystem disorder characterized by a combination of edema, granulation tissue, cartilage destruction, and ultimately fibrosis, variably affecting the trachea, pinna of the ear, nose, joints, and upper airways including the larynx and subglottic trachea.[33] Arteritis resulting in aortitis and aortic insufficiency, mitral insufficiency, and aneurysms involving medium-sized arteries has also been reported. It is most commonly diagnosed in the fourth and fifth decades. Fifty percent of patients develop respiratory tract involvement; a poor prognostic sign. On imaging there is smooth diffuse airway thickening, sparing of the posterior membrane, with progressive cartilage calcifications and frequently associated tracheomalacia (**Fig. 20**).[33]

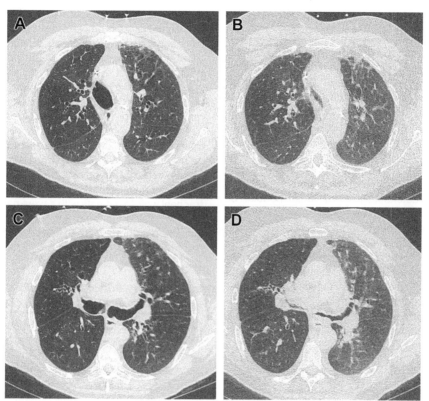

Fig. 19. Tracheobronchomegaly. (*A, C*) Axial images obtained in deep inspiration showing markedly dilated trachea and central bronchi. (*B, D*) Expiratory axial images at the same levels as *A* and *C*, respectively, showing marked collapse of these same airways, indicating tracheomalacia accompanying tracheobronchomegaly.

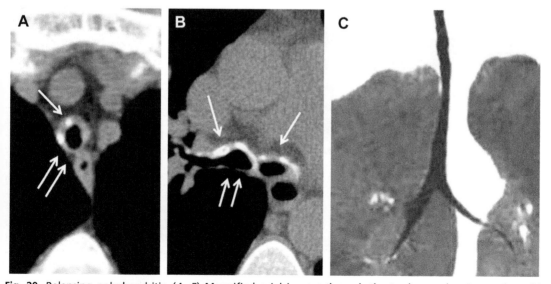

Fig. 20. Relapsing polychondritis. (*A, B*) Magnified axial images through the trachea and mainstem bronchi, showing marked airway narrowing associated with extensive calcification (*single arrows* in *A* and *B*). Note sparing of the posterior tracheal membrane (*double arrows* in *A* and *B*), which is characteristic of this lesion. (*C*) MINiP showing to good advantage diffuse trachea and bronchial narrowing. (*Courtesy of* Dr Jeffrey Kanne, University of Wisconsin Medical Center, WI.)

Granulomatosis and Polyangiitis (Formerly Known as Wegener Granulomatosis)

Granulomatosis and polyangiitis is a systemic necrotizing granulomatous vasculitis with a propensity for parenchymal and respiratory tract involvement.[34] In approximately 50% of patients, abnormalities involving the central airways may be identified by bronchoscopy, including inflammatory mucosal changes, ulcerations, and subglottic stenosis. Lesions may be either focal or diffuse and may involve any portion of the airways from the hypopharynx to the lobar bronchi. CT studies characteristically show focal nodular or diffuse tracheal and bronchial wall thickening, with luminal narrowing and calcification of the cartilaginous rings (**Fig. 21**).[34] In contrast with relapsing polychondritis, tracheal wall involvement is characteristically circumferential. Symptoms may include dyspnea, hoarseness, and stridor, which can be misdiagnosed as asthma. Associated renal and pulmonary involvement and a cytoplasmic pattern of antinuclear cytoplasmic antibodies may be helpful in supporting the diagnosis.

Amyloidosis

When it involves the central airways,[35,36] amyloidosis presents either as solitary or multinodular protrusions into the tracheal lumen, potentially mimicking tumor, or diffuse circumferential submucosal wall thickening with luminal narrowing caused by submucosal plaques or nodules (**Fig. 22**). Mural calcifications are prominent features, although calcifications are rarely identified bronchoscopically. Clinical manifestations reflect the portion of the tracheobronchial tree affected,[37] with proximal subglottic or laryngeal involvement leading to hoarseness or stridor, whereas distal tracheal, mainstem, or proximal bronchial involvement results in cough, wheezing, dyspnea, or hemoptysis. Involvement of the posterior tracheobronchial wall helps differentiate this entity from tracheobronchopathia osteochondroplastica (TO) and relapsing polychondritis, both of which spare the posterior tracheal wall. In patients with severe narrowing, debulking using forceps or neodymium:yttrium aluminum garnet (Nd:YAG) laser resection may be helpful. However, disease progression often necessitates repeated resections.[35,36]

Inflammatory Bowel Disease/Ulcerative Colitis and Crohn Disease

Chronic inflammatory bowel diseases are rare causes of large airways disease. Tracheobronchial involvement secondary to Crohn disease may result in wall thickening and luminal narrowing. Both Crohn disease and ulcerative colitis may result in airways mucosal ulceration with irregular tracheal and bronchial narrowing (see **Fig. 1**; **Fig. 23**). In both cases there is frequent association with peripheral airway involvement with proximal bronchiectasis caused by severe airway narrowing or obstruction and small airway

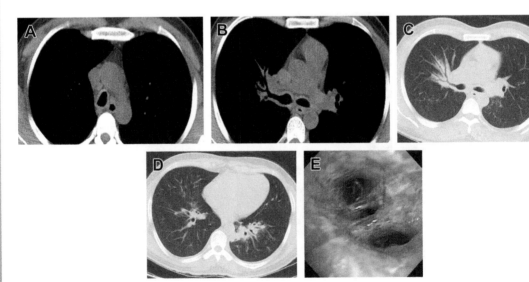

Fig. 21. Granulomatosis and polyangiitis. (*A, B*) Axial images though the distal trachea and carina, respectively, imaged with narrow windows, show circumferential airway wall thickening and narrowing. (*C, D*) Axial images though the right upper lobe bronchus and basilar segmental bronchi, respectively, imaged with a wide window, show to good advantage the extensive nature of airway involvement in patients with this disease. (*E*) Correlative bronchoscopic image showing diffuse airway inflammation and narrowing.

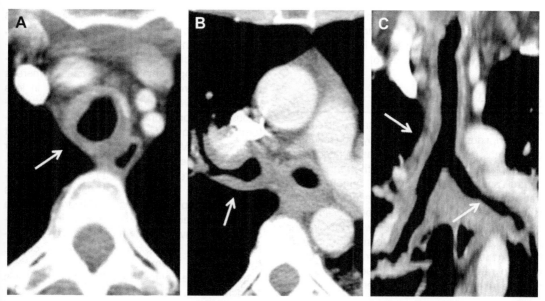

Fig. 22. Amyloidosis. (*A, B*) Axial images through the trachea and carina, respectively, show marked circumferential tracheal and bronchial wall thickening, similar in appearance to that seen in patients with granulomatosis and polyangiitis (*arrows*). (*C*) Coronal image documenting to good advantage the extent of disease (*arrow*). (*Courtesy of* Dr Jeffrey Kanne, University of Wisconsin Medical Center, WI.)

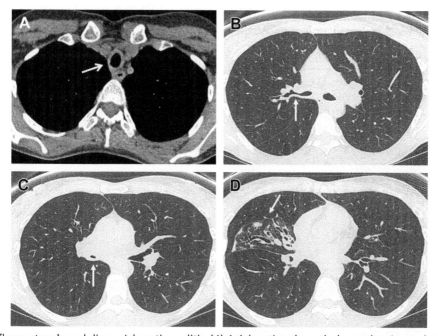

Fig. 23. Inflammatory bowel disease/ulcerative colitis. (*A*) Axial section through the trachea imaged with narrow windows (*A*) and mainstem, proximal lobar, and peripheral segmental airways imaged with wide windows (*B–D*) show typical appearance of diffuse circumferential airway narrowing (*arrows* in *A–C*). In this case there is focal middle lobe involvement with resulting severe bronchiectasis (*arrow* in *D*). Similar findings may also be seen in patients with Crohn disease.

involvement with constrictive bronchiolitis. On CT the tracheobronchial walls appear thickened, resulting in irregular narrowing that is indistinguishable from the other causes of diffuse airway narrowing.[38]

Sarcoidosis

Sarcoidosis is a systemic inflammatory disease of unknown cause characterized by noncaseating granulomas, characteristically associated with perilymphatic nodules involving the walls of the central and peripheral airways. Although rare, tracheal involvement may result either in nodular stenosis or, less commonly, smooth or irregular concentric tracheobronchial wall thickening (**Fig. 24**). Extrinsic bronchial compression from lymphadenopathy may also occur. On bronchoscopy, a raised cobblestone appearance of the mucosa when present is characteristic.[39]

MULTIFOCAL NODULAR CENTRAL AIRWAY DISEASE

Included in this category are a diverse group of diseases, both benign and malignant, that have in common a CT appearance of diffuse nodularity (see **Box 4**). As previously noted, many of the diseases already described may also present with diffuse airway nodularity. These diseases include, for example, central airway tumors, as well as diseases associated with diffuse airway narrowing, such as amyloidosis and relapsing polychondritis.

Laryngotracheobronchial Papillomatosis

Laryngotracheal papillomatosis is caused by human papilloma virus infection, and is often transmitted at birth. However, infection increasingly occurs in adults (including patients with acquired immunodeficiency syndrome), possibly secondary to oral-genital sexual transmission.[40] Tracheal and bronchial involvement occurs in only approximately 5% of cases, whereas pulmonary parenchymal disease occurs in less than 1%. However, unlike in childhood, spontaneous remission is unusual, with malignant transformation to squamous cell carcinoma a frequent complication. Malignant transformation may occur either within the central airways or the lung parenchyma, the latter most likely caused by endobronchial spread of disease.[41] Central lesions resemble skin papillary lesions, with large masslike protrusions causing airway obstruction. Parenchymal lung involvement may be cavitary. Symptoms include voice changes, stridor, cough, dyspnea, and recurrent pneumonia. Diagnosis initially may be confused with asthma or chronic bronchitis (**Fig. 25**).

Tracheobronchopathia Osteochondroplastica

TO is an uncommon incidental finding resulting in multiple submucosal nodules composed of bone, cartilage, and calcified acellular protein matrix.[27] TO classically affects the lower two-thirds of the trachea and proximal portions of the mainstem bronchi, resulting in diffuse airway nodularity; if sufficiently extensive, airway narrowing may also result. CT findings show thickened tracheal cartilage with wavy, irregular mucosal calcifications with characteristic sparing of the posterior wall.[38] Although usually asymptomatic, TO may cause hemoptysis in up to 25% of cases. Other symptoms include cough, dyspnea, hoarseness, stridor, and recurrent lower respiratory tract infections. Bronchoscopic findings include numerous firm

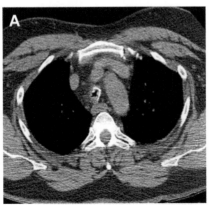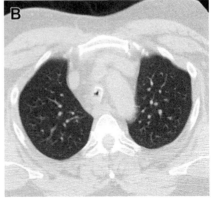

Fig. 24. Sarcoidosis. (*A, B*) Axial images through the midtrachea with narrow and wide windows, respectively, show irregular nodular circumferential tracheal wall thickening resulting in marked lumen narrowing. Note that disease is limited to the central airway without perilymphatic involvement of the lungs. (*Courtesy of* Dr Jane Ko, NYU-Langone Medical Center, NY)

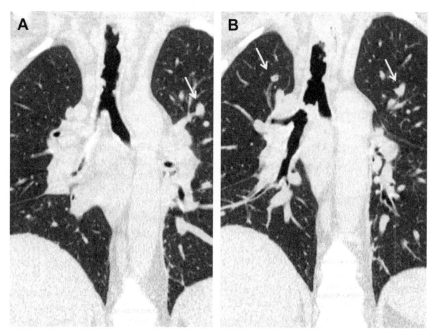

Fig. 25. Tracheobronchial papillomatosis. (*A, B*) Coronal images through the central airways show diffuse airway nodularity characteristic of this disease. There is also evidence of involvement of the lung parenchyma with well-defined lung nodules (*arrows*) caused by endogenous spread of tumor. Evidence of cavitation strongly suggests carcinomatous transformation.

white-yellow osteocartilaginous nodules around the cartilaginous rings (**Fig. 26**).

COMPUTED TOMOGRAPHY/ BRONCHOSCOPIC CORRELATIONS

Along with rapid advances in CT, PET, and MRI technology, the past decade has seen remarkable advances in diagnostic and therapeutic bronchoscopy (**Boxes 5** and **6**). Although CT may play a crucial role both in preinterventional and postinterventional assessment of airway disorders, optimal correlation between CT and diagnostic and therapeutic bronchoscopy requires meticulous attention to scan technique. As mentioned, a variety of CT imaging techniques are now available for

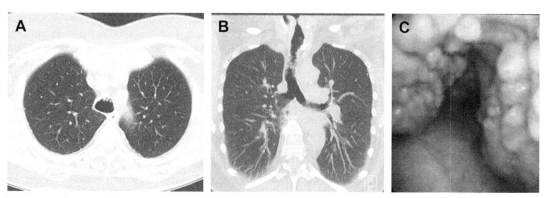

Fig. 26. Tracheobronchopathia osteochondroplastica. (*A, B*) Axial and coronal images through the midtrachea, respectively, show typical appearance of diffuse airway nodularity, sparing the posterior tracheal membrane, resulting in mild diffuse tracheal narrowing. This appearance is suggestive but nonspecific. (*C*) Endoscopic view in a different patient showing diffuse nodular appearance characteristic of TO. In cases in which the extent of nodularity is more limited, as shown in *A* and *B*, confirmation generally requires endoscopic evaluation. (*From* Naidich D, Richard Webb WR, Muller N, et al. Computed tomography and magnetic resonance of the thorax. 4th edition. Philadelphia: Lippincott Williams & Wilkins; 2007; with permission.)

(see **Box 5**)

Box 5
Techniques in diagnostic bronchoscopy

- EBUS
  - Radial probe (radial balloon EBUS)
  - Curvilinear probe EBUS-TBNA
  - Combined endoscopic ultrasonography/EUS
- Electromagnetic navigational bronchoscopy
- Autofluorescence bronchoscopy/narrow band imaging
- Optical coherence tomography
- Fibered confocal fluorescence microscopy

---

airway assessment, including routine two-dimensional axial and coronal, sagittal, and curved multiplanar reconstructions as well as a variety of 3D techniques, including volume-rendered surface images and virtual bronchoscopy (VB).[2]

It cannot be overemphasized that CT and bronchoscopy are complimentary techniques for assessing the central airways.[39] Advantages of CT include noninvasive visualization of the extent of

---

Box 6
Interventional/therapeutic bronchoscopy

- Indications
  - Palliation of both benign and malignant stenoses
  - Treatment of hemoptysis
  - Foreign body removal
  - Closure of persistent bronchopleural fistula
  - Treatment of severe asthma (bronchial thermoplasty)
  - Investigational: treatment of emphysema
- Techniques
  - Ablation
    - Immediate: balloon bronchoplasty, argon plasma coagulation, electrocautery, cryorecanalization, laser (Nd:YAG, CO_2), microdebrider
    - Delayed: brachytherapy, cryosurgery, photodynamic therapy
  - Stents: silicone versus self-expanding metal
    - Splinting extrinsic compression, maintenance of patency after ablation of endobronchial lesions, tracheoesophageal fistulas

---

lesions within and outside the airway lumen, visualization of airways distal to points of obstruction, and assessment of adjacent mediastinal and parenchymal abnormalities. In select cases, CT densitometry allows identification of calcification, as in broncholiths; intraluminal fat, as in endobronchial hamartomas; or increased vascularity following intravenous contrast administration, as occurs in carcinoid tumors. Limitations of CT include an inability to reliably differentiate mucosal from submucosal or extrinsic disease in the absence of a well-defined intraluminal abnormality, unreliable identification of lesions smaller than 2 to 3 mm, and inability to visualize flat mucosal lesions.

In contrast, bronchoscopic evaluation allows direct visualization of airway lumina to the fifth generation, enabling identification of and differentiation among subtle mucosal, submucosal, and endobronchial abnormalities. Bronchoscopy also allows acquisition of bacteriologic, cytologic, and histologic material from endobronchial, peribronchial, and parenchymal sites.[22] Of particular note is the marked increase in the sensitivity in diagnosing mediastinal and hilar adenopathy following the introduction of endobronchial ultrasonography (EBUS) guidance.[42–44]

Computed Tomography: Diagnostic Bronchoscopic Correlations

CT traditionally has proved essential for providing lymph node mapping to assist in the planning and performance of transbronchial needle aspiration (TBNA), especially in patients with known or suspected lung cancer (see **Box 5**).[5] Transbronchial needle aspiration allows access to mediastinal and hilar tissue through the bronchoscope, potentially obviating more invasive procedures such as mediastinoscopy or thoracotomy and in the process allowing precise staging of tumors. TBNA has an overall sensitivity of 78% (range, 14%–100%) and specificity of 99% (range, 96%–100%).[45] In select cases, TBNA may be performed under direct CT fluoroscopic guidance, which has the advantage of direct cine visualization of needle placement, although at the cost of greater radiation exposure. CT may also guide TBNA in patients with benign mediastinal or hilar disease.[46] Although CT remains an important method for localizing disease before TBNA, this approach has increasingly been replaced by the use of EBUS to perform transbronchial needle biopsy (**Fig. 27**). Compared with CT-directed TBNA, EBUS has the advantage of direct, real-time visualization and placement of biopsy needles, allowing diagnosis of malignant nodes as small as 3 to

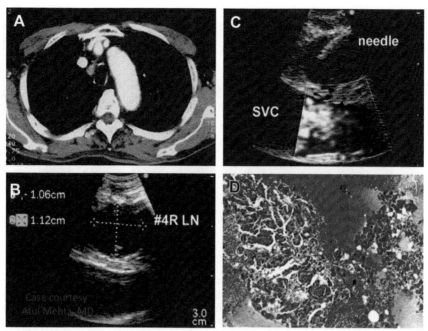

Fig. 27. EBUS. (*A*) Axial image shows a small right paratracheal node; a difficult location for routine TBNA/biopsy. (*B, C*) Endoscopic ultrasonography images showing the same node as in *A*, documenting in real time the placement of the transbronchial needle tip within the node. (*D*) Histologic confirmation of metastatic disease (H&E stain). Because of its ability to provide real-time guidance, EBUS has become a widely accepted standard for performing TBNA.

5 mm and establishing the diagnosis of benign causes of adenopathy such as sarcoidosis and tuberculosis.

Computed Tomography: Therapeutic Bronchoscopic Correlations

In addition to the use of CT for identifying and characterizing central airway disorder, CT plays a critical role in planning approaches for treating airway obstruction (see **Box 6**).[1] Current techniques for restoring airway patency from both benign and malignant causes include surgery (see **Fig. 13**), insertion of airway stents, as well as a wide variety of ablative techniques, either alone or in combination, including Nd:YAG laser phototherapy, photodynamic therapy, cryotherapy, electrocautery, brachytherapy, and argon plasma coagulation (see **Figs. 3** and **15**). Choices among these available treatment options reflect the type and extent of obstruction, as well as the overall medical status of individual patients.

Airway Stents

At present the common indication for the use of airway stents is palliation of malignant airway obstruction resulting from endoluminal disease,

extrinsic compression, or both (see **Fig. 16**; **Fig. 28**).[2,47] Stents are frequently used in conjunction with minimally invasive bronchoscopic tumor debulking procedures. Although treatment of benign tracheal strictures is generally surgical resection with primary reconstruction, in select cases stents may also be used to temporarily palliate patients with postintubation tracheal stenosis or patients with diffuse airway diseases, such as relapsing polychondritis, or fibrous tuberculous strictures. CT is of greatest utility in providing exact measurements of the size of the airway lumen and extent of airway obstruction. Although a detailed description of the various advantages and disadvantages of the various stents available is outside the scope of this article, a few comments are warranted. Stents most often used include silicone stents (easily inserted and removed, although requiring rigid bronchoscopy for insertion, providing smaller lumens and greater tendency to migrate); and metallic stents, both covered and uncovered. Uncovered stents allow epithelialization following placement, enabling mucociliary clearance, but are difficult to remove; uncovered stents also allow ventilation of the right upper lobe bronchus in cases in which a right main bronchial stent needs to extend into the bronchus intermedius. Covered stents prevent

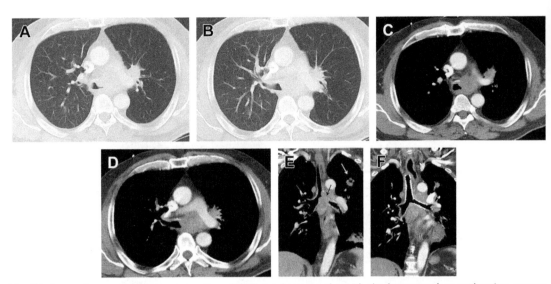

Fig. 28. Stent placement: airway obstruction. (*A, B*) Axial images through the lower trachea and carina, respectively, imaged with wide windows, show complete obstruction of the left mainstem bronchus by tumor –caused by metastatic non–small cell lung cancer. (*C, D*) Axial images corresponding with *A* and *B*, respectively, imaged with narrow windows, show to better advantage the extent of the soft tissue mass. (*E*) Coronal reconstruction before stent placement showing tumor obstructing the left main bronchus (*black arrow*). Note the cavitary lesion in the left upper lobe (*white arrow*). (*F*) Coronal reconstruction following insertion of stents in both the distal trachea and left mainstem bronchus.

ingrowth of tumor and granulation tissue and are easier to remove than uncovered stents, but are associated with greater incidence of infection.

In addition to providing preinsertion guidance, CT in conjunction with bronchoscopy plays an important role in identifying immediate and de-layed complications arising from stent placement. These complications include stent malposition, stent migration, stent fracture, and ingrowth of tu-mor or granulation tissue (**Fig. 29**).

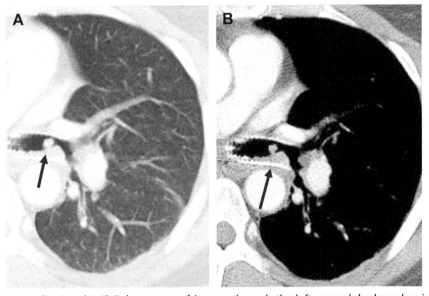

Fig. 29. Stent complication. (*A, B*) Enlargement of images through the left upper lobe bronchus imaged with wide and narrow windows, respectively, show the appearance of tumor growing through a left mainstem bron-chial stent (*arrows*).

SUMMARY

CT is an essential methodology for detecting, characterizing, and monitoring therapy for diseases affecting the central airways. CT provides a useful method of classifying the various causes of central airway disorder, allowing specific noninvasive diagnoses in select cases. In other cases, CT plays an essential role by determining optimal means for diagnosing lesions as needed by providing a plan for bronchoscopists. In this regard, the correlation of CT and bronchoscopic findings is of particular value in identifying optimal methods for interventional bronchoscopic procedures. Although not discussed in this article, the possibility of expanding the range of imaging modalities (in particular, the routine use of FDG-PET and MRI) holds considerable promise but still remains to be fully explored.

REFERENCES

1. Amdo T, Godoy MC, Ost DE, et al. Imaging-bronchoscopic correlations for interventional pulmonology. Radiol Clin North Am 2009;47:271–87.

2. Nair A, Godoy MC, Holden EL, et al. Multidetector CT and postprocessing in planning and assisting in minimally invasive bronchoscopic airway interventions. Radiographics 2012;32:E201–32.

3. Webb EM, Elicker BM, Webb WR. Using CT to diagnose nonneoplastic tracheal abnormalities: appearance of the tracheal wall. AJR Am J Roentgenol 2000;174(5):1315–21.

4. Beigelman-Aubrey C, Brillet PY, Grenier PA. MDCT of the airways: technique and normal results. Radiol Clin North Am 2009;4:185–201.

5. Naidich DP, Webb WR, Grenier PA, et al. Imaging of the airways. Philadelphia: Lippincott, Williams & Wilkins; 2005.

6. Naidich DP, Webb WR, Muller NL, et al. Computed tomography and magnetic resonance of the thorax. Philadelphia: Lippincott, Williams and Wilkins; 2007.

7. Bankier AA, Schaefer-Prokop C, De Maertelaer V, et al. Air trapping: comparison of standard-dose and simulated low-dose thin-section CT techniques. Radiology 2007;242(3):898–906.

8. Baroni RH, Feller-Kopman D, Nishino M. Tracheobronchomalacia: comparison between end-expiratory and dynamic expiratory CT for evaluation of central airway collapse. Radiology 2005;235:635–41.

9. Bankier AA, Fleischmann D, Mallek R, et al. Bronchial wall thickness: appropriate window settings for thin-section CT and radiologic-anatomic correlation. Radiology 1996;199(3):831–6.

10. Desir A, Ghaye B. Congenital abnormalities of the airways. Radiol Clin North Am 2009;47:203–25.

11. Wu JW, White CS, Meyer CA, et al. Variant bronchial anatomy: CT appearance and classification. AJR Am J Roentgenol 1999;72:741–4.

12. Zanetti G, Hochhegger B, Guimaraes MD, et al. Accessory cardiac bronchus causing recurrent pulmonary infection. J Bras Pneumol 2014;40:448–9.

13. Pulchalski J, Musani A. Traheobronchial stenosis: causes and advances in management. Clin Chest Med 2013;34:557–67.

14. Carbognani P, Baobbio A, Cattelani L, et al. Management of postintubation membranous tracheal rupture. Ann Thorac Surg 2004;77:406–9.

15. Choe KO, Jeong YJ, Sohn HY. Tuberculous bronchostenosis: CT findings in 28 cases. AJR Am J Roentgenol 1998;155:971–6.

16. Ferretti GR, Bithigoffer C, Righini CA, et al. Imaging of tumors of the trachea and central bronchi. Radiol Clin North Am 2009;47:227–41.

17. Macchiarini P. Primary tracheal tumors. Lancet Oncol 2006;7:83–91.

18. Ngo AV, Walker CM, Chung JH, et al. Tumors and tumorlike conditions of the large airways. AJR Am J Roentgenol 2013;201:301–13.

19. Park CM, Goo JM, Lee HJ, et al. Tumors in the tracheobronchial tree: CT and FDG PET features. Radiographics 2009;29:55–71.

20. Kim TS, Lee KS, Han J. Mucoepidermoid carcinoma of the tracheobronchial tree: radiographic and CT findings in 12 patients. Radiology 1999;121:643–8.

21. Song Z, Liu Z, Wang J, et al. Primary tracheobronchial mucoepidermoid carcinoma - a retrospective study of 32 patients. World J Surg Oncol 2013. http://dx.doi.org/10.1186/1477-2819-11-62.

22. Liu X, Zhang W, Wu X, et al. Mucoepidermoid carcinoma of the lung: common findings and unusual appearances on CT. Clin Imaging 2012;36:8–13.

23. Filosso PL, Oliaro A, Ruffini E, et al. Outcome and prognostic factors in bronchial carcinoids: a single-center experience. J Thorac Oncol 2013;10:1282–8.

24. Garcia-Yuste M, Matilla JM. The significance of histology: typical and atypical bronchial carcinoids. Thorac Surg Clin 2014;24:293–7.

25. Yilmaz S, Ekici A, Erdogan S, et al. Endobronchial lipomatous hamartoma. CT and MR imaging features. Eur Radiol 2004;14:1521–4.

26. Grenier P, Beigelman-Aubry C, Brillet PY. Nonneoplastic tracheal and bronchial stenosis. Radiol Clin North Am 2009;47:243–60.

27. Chung JH, Kanne JP, Gilman MD. CT of diffuse tracheal diseases. AJR Am J Roentgenol 2011;196:W240–6.

28. Javidan-Nejad C. MDCT of the trachea and main bronchi. Radiol Clin North Am 2010;48:157–76.

29. Ciccarese F, Poerio A, Stagni S, et al. Saber-sheath trachea as a marker of severe airflow obstruction in chronic obstructive pulmonary disease. Radiol Med 2014;119:90–6.

30. Lee EY, Litmanovich D, Boiselle PM. Multidetector CT evaluation of tracheobronchomalacia. Radiol Clin North Am 2009;47:261–9.

31. Boiselle PM, Ernst A. Tracheal morphology in patients with tracheomalacia: prevalence of inspiratory lunate and expiratory "frown" shapes. J Thorac Imaging 2006;21:190–6.

32. Boiselle PM, O'Donnell CR, Bankier AA, et al. Tracheal collapsibility in healthy volunteers during forced expiration: assessment with multidetector CT. Radiology 2009;252:255–62.

33. Sharma A, Gnanapandithan K, Sharma K, et al. Relapsing polychondritis: a review. Clin Rheumatol 2013;32:1575–83.

34. Lutalo PM, D'Cruz DP. Diagnosis and classification of granulomatosis with polyangiitis (aka Wegener's granulomatosis). J Autoimmun 2014. http://dx.doi.org/10.1016/j.jaut.2014.01.028.

35. Mares DC. Tracheobronchial amyloidosis: a review of clinical and radiographic characteristics, bronchoscopic diagnosis, and management. J Bronchol 1998;5:147–55.

36. Wang Q, Chen H, Wang S. Laryngo-tracheobronchial amyloidosis: a case report and review of literature. Int J Clin Exp Pathol 2014;15:7088–93.

37. O'Regan AS, Fenlon HM, Beamis JF Jr, et al. Tracheobronchial amyloidosis. The Boston University experience from 1984 to 1999. Medicine (Baltimore) 2000;79:69–79.

38. Marom EM, Goodman PC, McAdams HP. Focal abnormalities of the trachea and main bronchi. AJR Am J Roentgenol 2001;176:707–11.

39. Obusez EC, Jamjoom L, Kirsch J, et al. Computed tomography correlation of airway disease with bronchoscopy: part 1-nonneoplastic large airway diseases. Curr Probl Diagn Radiol 2014;43:268–77.

40. Harris K, Chalhoub M. Tracheal papillomatosis: what do we know so far? Chron Respir Dis 2011;8:233–5.

41. Rady PL, Schnadig VJ, Weiss RL, et al. Malignant transformation of recurrent respiratory papillomatosis associated with integrated human papillomavirus type 11 DNA and mutation of p53. Laryngoscope 1998;108:735–40.

42. Dincer HE. Linear EBUS in staging non-small cell lung cancer and diagnosing benign disease. J Bronchology Interv Pulmonol 2013;20:66–76.

43. Fielding DI, Kurimoto N. EBUS-TBNA/staging of lung cancer. Clin Chest Med 2013;34:385–94.

44. Kinsey CM, Arenberg DA. Endobronchial ultrasound-guided transbronchial needle aspiration for non-small cell lung cancer staging. Am J Respir Crit Care Med 2014;189:640–9.

45. Detterbeck FC, DeCamp MM Jr, Kohman LH, et al. Lung cancer. Invasive staging: the guidelines. Chest 2003;123(1 Suppl):167S–75S.

46. Harrow EM, Abi-Saleh W, Blum J, et al. The utility of transbronchial needle aspiration in the staging of bronchogenic carcinoma. Am J Respir Crit Care Med 2000;161:601–7.

47. Godoy MC, Saldana DA, Praveen PR, et al. Multidetector CT evaluation of airways stents: what the radiologist should know. Radiographics 2014;34:1793–806.

Imaging of Small Airways and Emphysema

Rachael M. Edwards, MD[a],*, Gregory Kicska, MD, PhD[a], Rodney Schmidt, MD, PhD[b],
Sudhakar N.J. Pipavath, MD[a]

KEYWORDS

- Bronchiolitis • Small airway disease • High-resolution computed tomography • Emphysema

KEY POINTS

- Diagnosing bronchiolitis with chest radiography is difficult.
- High-resolution computed tomography of the chest typically includes imaging during both inspiration and expiration. Images are acquired to allow for thin-section reconstruction (0.625 to 2 mm thickness).
- Expiratory imaging improves detection of air trapping.
- The 2 main categories of bronchiolitis are defined based on inflammatory/cellular or fibrotic/constrictive histopathologic features.
- Direct signs of bronchiolitis include centrilobular nodules, tree-in-bud pattern, and peribronchiolar ground-glass opacities.
- Indirect signs of bronchiolitis include air trapping and mosaic perfusion.
- Presence, absence, and distribution of direct and indirect signs can suggest a specific disease process.
- The 3 main subtypes of emphysema are centrilobular, paraseptal, and panlobular emphysema; each has a classic imaging appearance.

INTRODUCTION

Effectively using imaging to diagnose bronchiolitis or emphysema requires a basic knowledge of the imaging modalities used, exam protocols performed and the imaging findings that represent the hallmark of disease. With respect to bronchiolitis, high-resolution chest computed tomography (CT) is one of the most useful techniques available because it shows highly specific direct and indirect imaging signs. The direct signs of bronchiolitis include centrilobular nodules, tree-in-bud pattern, and centrilobular/peribronchial ground-glass opacities. The indirect signs of bronchiolitis include air trapping and mosaic perfusion. The distribution and combination of these various signs can further classify bronchiolitis as either cellular/inflammatory or fibrotic/constrictive. Emphysema is characterized by destruction of the airspaces, and a brief discussion of imaging findings of this class of disease is also included. Typical CT findings include destruction of airspace, attenuated vasculatures, and hyperlucent as well as hyperinflated lungs.

BRONCHIOLITIS

Tools for Imaging

Chest radiography

Chest radiography (CXR) is of low utility when evaluating bronchiolitis. The main value of CXR, which

Disclosures: none (R. Edwards, G. Kicska, R. Schmidt); consultant, Boehringer Ingelheim, Ridgefield, CT (S.N.J. Pipavath).
[a] Department of Radiology, University of Washington Medical Center, 1959 Northeast Pacific Street, Seattle, WA 98195, USA; [b] Department of Pathology, University of Washington Medical Center, 1959 Northeast Pacific Street, Seattle, WA 98195, USA
* Corresponding author.
E-mail address: edwards5@uw.edu

Clin Chest Med 36 (2015) 335–347
http://dx.doi.org/10.1016/j.ccm.2015.02.013
0272-5231/15/$ – see front matter © 2015 Elsevier Inc. All rights reserved.

has lower radiation and a quicker examination compared with CT, is in the exclusion of other diagnoses, such as pneumonia or pneumothorax.[1–3] The CXR often appears normal in cases of bronchiolitis until late in the disease course.[1,2]

Computed tomography

High-resolution CT (HRCT) is commonly used in adults when evaluating bronchiolitis. This technique uses more radiation compared with a routine chest CT so that thin-slice reconstructions of 0.625 mm can be created with an acceptable signal-to-noise ratio. HRCT examinations can vary based on the clinical indication and can contain a combination of prone or supine and inspiration or expiration images. Imaging patients in the prone position during inspiration is used to differentiate dependent atelectasis from early interstitial lung disease and can usually be omitted in the work-up of potential bronchiolitis.

The standard HRCT protocol at the authors' institution is described in **Table 1**. Inspiration and expiration images are important in diagnosing bronchiolitis because they can detect air trapping. A mosaic attenuation pattern that appears on expiratory images but not inspiratory images suggests the presence of air trapping, which has been suggested as one of the earliest imaging findings of small airway disease, specifically in obliterative bronchiolitis.[4] Additionally, the presence of air trapping on expiratory imaging has been shown to correlate well with obstructive findings on pulmonary function tests.[5,6] Although mosaic attenuation can be seen on the inspiratory images, a diagnosis of air trapping cannot be confidently made, as small vessel disease may also present with mosaic attenuation (**Fig. 1**). Expiratory imaging is usually performed using an axial acquisition, obtaining representative slices in the upper, mid, and lower lungs.[4] This axial acquisition technique is used instead of the helical acquisition because it decreases radiation but maintains diagnostic quality.

Several other methods of imaging the small airways have been described but are not commonly seen in clinical practice. One of these methods is dynamic imaging (4-dimensional CT) during inspiration and expiration. This method is currently used mainly as a research tool and not yet widely clinically accepted because of concerns over radiation dose, but studies have shown that results correlate with obstructive findings measured with pulmonary function tests.[7,8]

IMAGING FINDINGS

A thorough understanding of the anatomy of the secondary pulmonary lobule assists in understanding the direct and indirect imaging findings of bronchiolitis commonly seen on HRCT. The secondary pulmonary lobule is the smallest unit of the lung that can be imaged and has a polyhedral shape approximately 2 cm in diameter that is bordered by connective tissue planes of the interlobular septa (**Fig. 2**).[9] The secondary lobules are further subdivided into 6 to 8 polyhedral primary lobules (with central terminal bronchioles) and subsequently into pyramidal acini, with respiratory bronchioles at their apices. Importantly, the apices of the acini (the centers of the primary lobules) are located approximately halfway between the center of the secondary lobule and the interlobular septa; disease processes that affect them are commonly regarded as centrilobular even though they are not strictly located at the center of the secondary lobule.

Branches of the pulmonary artery accompany the bronchioles to the level of the respiratory bronchioles and are, thus, found at the apices of the acini. The pulmonary arterial system further branches into capillaries, which traverse the alveolar septa before coalescing in larger venules that run in the secondary lobular septa. One set of lymphatics originates near the respiratory bronchioles and tracks back to the hilum in the bronchovascular bundles. A second set tracks to the

		Patient			Slice Thickness	Reconstruction
Scan Type	Respiration	Position	Extent	Interval (mm)	(mm)	Algorithms
Helical	Inspiration	Supine	Lung apex to mid kidney	0.625	2.5 / 1.25	Standard / Bone
Axial	Expiration	Supine	Lung apex to diaphragm	20.0	1.25	Bone
Axial	Inspiration	Prone	Lung apex to diaphragm	20.0	1.25	Bone

Table 1
Computed tomography protocols

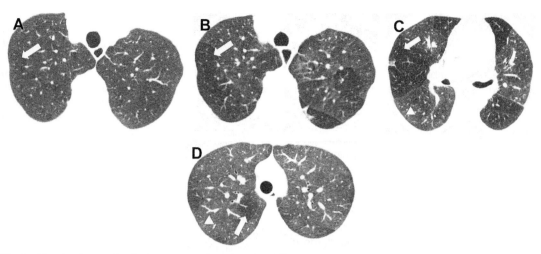

Fig. 1. *Mosaic attenuation* is the term used to describe differing attenuation of the lung parenchyma. Air trapping appears as areas of low attenuation conforming to the shape of pulmonary lobules (*white arrows*), which is accentuated on the expiratory images. (*A, B*) Images from an HRCT: (*A*) (inspiration) demonstrates subtle regions of low attenuation (mosaic attenuation); (*B*) (expiration) demonstrates accentuated segmental regions of low attenuation indicating air trapping. Mosaic perfusion (*C, D*) secondary to chronic thromboembolic disease presents as patchy regions of low attenuation (*white arrow*) compared with adjacent normal lung parenchyma (*arrowhead*) caused by combination of hypoperfusion secondary to vessel occlusion and hypoxic vasoconstriction.

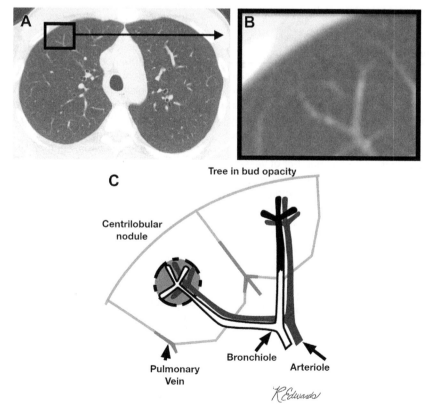

Fig. 2. Normal CT image of the chest (*A, B*) with correlative illustration (*C*) of the secondary pulmonary lobule depicting a representative centrilobular nodule and tree-in-bud opacity.

hilum along veins from secondary lobular septa. The secondary lobule can be identified on CT, unlike the primary lobule or pulmonary acinus, so common use of lobular in imaging generally refers to the secondary lobule. The apices of the acini and the lymphatics are generally not visible except in disease states.

Direct Signs of Bronchiolitis

Direct signs include centrilobular nodules, tree-in-bud pattern, and centrilobular/peribronchiolar ground-glass opacities. Normally, bronchioles in the pulmonary lobule are not visible on HRCT.[10] Centrilobular nodules, as the name implies, appear at or near the center of the secondary pulmonary lobule and, unless large, typically do not contact the pleural surface.[10] In the setting of bronchiolitis, centrilobular nodules result when the bronchiolar wall becomes inflamed or filled with debris (see **Fig. 2**C).

Tree-in-bud opacities are caused by impacted debris or fluid within the centrilobular bronchiole, which is often accompanied by centrilobular nodules caused by peribronchiolar inflammation. The combination of the bronchiolar branching pattern with the centrilobular nodules results in an appearance reminiscent of a tree branch with small buds on it, hence the name *tree-in-bud pattern* (see **Fig. 2**C).[10–12]

Indirect Signs of Bronchiolitis

Indirect signs include air trapping and mosaic attenuation. On inspiratory CT images, mosaic attenuation appears as lobular heterogeneous density of the lung parenchyma; this finding may represent air trapping or mosaic perfusion. The density of the lung parenchyma on CT predominantly depends on the size and number of vessels with comparatively less contribution from the interstitial tissue.[10,13] When describing variations in lung density (attenuation), it is important not to confuse the terms of mosaic attenuation, mosaic perfusion, and air trapping.

Air trapping results from partial outflow obstruction of the small airways that may be caused by premature collapse of the small airways during expiration, severe luminal narrowing that may be present in all phases of the respiratory cycle, or a combination of these findings.[4,14,15] Air trapping appears as areas of low attenuation conforming to the shape of a pulmonary lobule or groups of pulmonary lobules. The finding of air trapping can be appreciated at any phase of the respiratory cycle, although it is exaggerated on expiratory imaging. When normal lung decreases in volume at expiration, it results in an increase in attenuation. Lobules associated with abnormal small airways fail to decrease in volume resulting in a lower attenuation compared with adjacent normal lung (see **Fig. 1**).

Additionally, the presence of air trapping does not always indicate pulmonary disease as has been reported as a finding in normal asymptomatic individuals.[16–19] The radiologist and referring physician should be vigilant in assessing if any underlying disease is present before indicating that air trapping is only a normal incidental finding. Air trapping, a primary imaging finding in asthma and obliterative bronchiolitis, may be imperceptible on inspiratory CT images.[18]

In most cases, mosaic perfusion can be distinguished from air trapping on expiratory imaging; mosaic perfusion attributed to pulmonary vascular disease often does not demonstrate air trapping, although these findings can be seen together.[13] In areas of mosaic perfusion, the pulmonary vessels are often smaller than the adjacent blood vessels of the normally perfused lung parenchyma.[10] This finding is an important clue when distinguishing hypovascularity, with smaller vessels, from ground-glass opacity in which the blood vessels are similar in size when compared between the higher- and lower-density areas of the lung (see **Fig. 1**).[10]

Mosaic perfusion, often caused by hypoperfusion, is classically associated with pulmonary vascular disease, such as pulmonary hypertension or chronic pulmonary thromboembolism.[13] In chronic pulmonary thromboembolism, the vessels appear diminished because of distal vasculopathy in combination with hypoperfusion caused by vessel occlusion.[20] Albeit, it is important to note that decreased perfusion can occur in the setting of small airway diseases, such as bronchiolitis, as a compensatory physiologic reaction of hypoxic vasoconstriction in areas of abnormal airways.[10,21]

Major Categories of Bronchiolitis

Many classification systems of bronchiolitis exist with no current global agreement on which classification system should be used in practice.[11,21,22] This article uses a classification system based on a combination of radiologic and pathologic findings describing 2 major types of bronchiolitis: (1) inflammatory/cellular or (2) fibrotic.[22] The common findings on CT are discussed later and summarized in **Table 2**.

Inflammatory/Cellular Bronchiolitis

Inflammatory or cellular bronchiolitis includes infectious bronchiolitis, hypersensitivity pneumonitis, respiratory bronchiolitis, follicular bronchiolitis,

Table 2
Bronchiolitis characteristics

Type of Bronchiolitis	Causes or Associations	CT Features	Characteristic Distribution
Inflammatory bronchiolitis			
Infectious bronchiolitis	Acute or chronic infections	Centrilobular nodules Tree-in-bud opacities Ground-glass opacities	Variable
Hypersensitivity pneumonitis (subacute)	Inorganic and organic antigens	Ill-defined centrilobular nodules Ground-glass opacities Air trapping	Diffuse with basal sparing or upper-lung predominance
Respiratory bronchiolitis	Cigarette smoking	Centrilobular nodules Ground-glass opacities	Bilateral Upper-lobe predominant
Follicular bronchiolitis	Immunodeficiency syndromes, collagen vascular disorders	Centrilobular nodules Ground-glass opacities	Bilateral Lower-lung predominant
Panbronchiolitis	Unknown pathogenesis	Centrilobular nodules Tree-in-bud pattern Bronchiolectasis/bronchiectasis	Bilateral Basal predominant
Fibrotic/constrictive/obliterative bronchiolitis	Collagen vascular disorders, inflammatory bowel disease, transplant, inhalational injury, postinfectious	Mosaic attenuation Air trapping Bronchiolectasis/bronchiectasis	Variable

panbronchiolitis, and bronchiolitis related to bronchiectasis. In these disease processes, centrilobular nodules and tree-in-bud opacities predominate as findings on HRCT.[21,22]

Infectious Bronchiolitis

Centrilobular nodules and the tree-in-bud pattern, the dominant findings in infectious bronchiolitis, are caused by acute or chronic inflammation resulting in thickening of the bronchiolar walls with mucus and cellular exudates impacted within the small airways.[21,22] Most commonly, the centrilobular nodules and tree-in-bud opacities are well defined and can vary in distribution from unilateral to bilateral and patchy to diffuse.[11] Sometimes the centrilobular nodules can be ill defined if inflammation extends into the peribronchiolar tissue.[11] Additionally, classic findings of nodules and tree-in-bud opacities can be accompanied by airspace consolidation, ground-glass opacities, and air trapping (**Fig. 3**A).[11]

Acute or chronic viral, bacterial, *Mycoplasma*, or mycobacterial infections are associated with bronchiolitis.[21,22] In the pediatric population, acute infectious bronchiolitis is a common diagnosis, responsible for approximately 20% of pediatric

hospitalizations in the United States.[23] Rhinovirus and respiratory syncytial virus (RSV) are especially common causes of bronchiolitis that require hospitalization.[24] CXR and CT examinations are helpful in diagnosis but are performed less often than in adults because of the classic clinical presentation and a concern for the radiation dose in pediatric patients.[1,3] However, in severe cases, diagnostic imaging is sometimes performed to exclude an alternative diagnosis, such as pneumonia.[1]

Nontuberculous mycobacterial infection, such as Mycobacterium avium complex or *Mycobacterium intracellulare*, can present as bronchiolitis, though upper lobe cavitary disease mimicking tuberculosis may also occur.[25] The bronchiolitis pattern is most often present in postmenopausal women and usually involves the lingula and right middle lobe. Bronchiectasis, tree-in-bud nodularity, and centrilobular nodules on CT are typical of this condition.[25]

Hypersensitivity Pneumonitis

Hypersensitivity pneumonitis (HP) is caused by exposure to inorganic and organic antigens resulting in an immune-mediated inflammatory response within the lung.[26] Numerous antigens

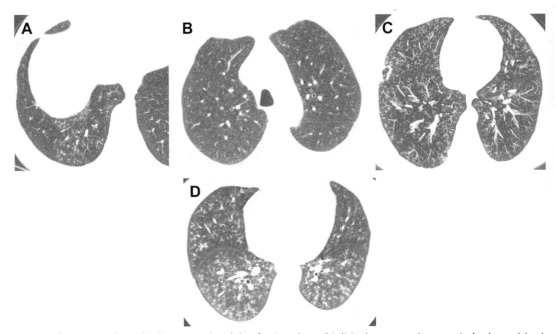

Fig. 3. Inflammatory bronchiolitis examples: (*A*) Infectious bronchiolitis demonstrating tree-in-bud opacities in the right lower lobe. (*B*) Respiratory bronchiolitis with subtle centrilobular nodules in the upper lungs. (*C*) Follicular bronchiolitis with diffuse bilateral tree-in-bud pattern on axial CT maximum intensity projection image. (*D*) Panbronchiolitis with diffuse bilateral tree-in-bud pattern.

have been described to incite HP, including protein from avian feces, bird plume, moldy hay, cork, and fluid used in metal cutting, to name only a few.[27]

The classic appearance of HP on HRCT is ill-defined centrilobular nodules with mosaic attenuation caused by air trapping, often diffusely distributed with sparing of the lung bases. Tree-in-bud opacities are less common in HP than other forms of bronchiolitis.[22,27] This HRCT appearance correlates with the histopathology in which interstitial lymphocytic infiltrates and poorly formed granulomas are smaller than the voxels of HRCT and typically involve alveolar lung tissue more than airway mucosa (**Fig. 4**).[28]

There are 3 stages of HP: (1) acute, (2) subacute, and (3) chronic. The subacute phase is characterized by symptomatic bronchiolitis and alveolitis with the acute phase rarely imaged caused by resolution of initial symptoms. Further medical evaluation is often only sought if symptoms persist; by this time point, the disease has progressed to the subacute or chronic stage. Chronic HP is different from subacute and acute HP in that patients have radiologic evidence of pulmonary fibrosis.[26]

Respiratory Bronchiolitis

Respiratory bronchiolitis (RB) is seen most commonly in cigarette smokers. RB demonstrates

ill-defined centrilobular nodules and ground-glass opacities on HRCT, with relative upper lung predominance **Fig. 3**B.[22,29] These findings at CT result from pigment-laden macrophages accumulating within the bronchioles and alveolar ducts resulting in ill-defined centrilobular nodules. Macrophages within the alveolar spaces result in the centrilobular ground-glass opacities often seen in RB.[29] Sometimes RB is associated with mild fibrosis of the respiratory bronchioles.[22,29]

Although both RB and RB-ILD (Respiratory bronchiolitis-Interstitial Lung Disease) share many features, RB-ILD is classified as an idiopathic interstitial pneumonia and patients present with impairment of lung function and gas exchange; RB is asymptomatic.[11,22] When patients with RB or RB-ILD stop smoking, findings on CT may regress or stabilize. Continued exposure to cigarette smoke may result in emphysema, another disease with centrilobular predominance.[22]

Follicular Bronchiolitis

Follicular bronchiolitis (FB) is most often seen in the setting of immunodeficiency syndromes, both congenital and acquired; collagen vascular diseases, such as rheumatoid arthritis and Sjögren syndrome; hypersensitivity reactions; and lymphoproliferative disorders.[11,22] Histology reveals polyclonal hyperplasia of the bronchial mucosa–associated

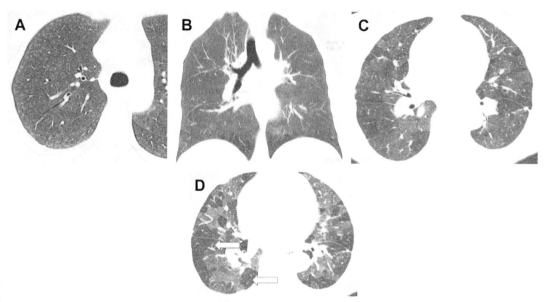

Fig. 4. Inflammatory bronchiolitis-HP. (*A, B*) Different patient with subacute HP demonstrating diffuse ill-defined centrilobular nodules on axial and coronal CT images with relative sparing of the bases. (*C*) Inspiratory axial CT image demonstrating mosaic attenuation in setting of subacute hypersensitivity pneumonitis. (*D*) Same patient as in (*C*), expiratory axial CT image demonstrating multifocal lobular air trapping (*white arrows*) in HP.

lymphoid tissue and the formation of lymphoid follicles in the walls of bronchioles.[30] FB is most common in adults, with a more progressive form seen in patients younger than 30 years.[30]

The most commonly encountered appearance on CT is bilateral, diffuse, or lower lung–predominant, well-defined centrilobular nodules with a tree-in-bud pattern and peribronchial nodules (see **Fig. 3**C). Ground-glass opacities are variably present.[31–33]

Panbronchiolitis

Panbronchiolitis is most often seen in patients of East Asian descent.[32,34] Although certain human leukocyte antigens have shown a predisposition toward panbronchiolitis, the cause and pathogenesis remains unknown.[11,34] Additionally, many patients with panbronchiolitis also have chronic sinusitis.[11]

Typically, panbronchiolitis demonstrates both centrilobular nodules and a tree-in-bud pattern on CT with progressive bronchiolectasis and bronchiectasis (see **Fig. 3**D).[11,22,34] Often, the abnormalities show lower lung predominance.[22] This appearance on CT is the result of chronic inflammation with accumulation of foamy macrophages in the walls of the bronchioles; most of the infiltration by inflammatory cells is in the respiratory bronchioles.[34,35]

Bronchiectasis

Although bronchiectasis is not a subtype of bronchiolitis, it warrants a mention in this discussion

as bronchiolitis is commonly seen in the setting of bronchiectasis. Bronchiectasis is often associated with impaired mucociliary clearance, either focally or globally, which may predispose to bronchiolitis.[36] The causes of bronchiectasis are numerous: chronic infection, ciliary motility disorders, and disease affecting mucociliary clearance, such as cystic fibrosis.

Fibrotic and Constrictive Bronchiolitis

Fibrotic bronchiolitis is a category of disorders characterized by narrowing of the bronchiolar lumen, which can be progressive, caused by fibrosis that can be a primary process or secondary to prior infection, inhalational injury, or other insult to the airway.[22,37–39] Fibrotic bronchiolitis includes constrictive/obliterative bronchiolitis (CB) and nonspecific scarring. These diseases share submucosal fibrosis in the membranous and respiratory bronchioles resulting in fixed luminal narrowing. Importantly, this fibrosis is irreversible.[11,22] CB is a disease of submillimeter diameter conducting bronchioles characterized by concentric fibrosis localized to the inner part of the bronchiolar wall. Nonspecific scarring results in full-thickness scarring of the bronchioles. Numerous underlying diseases and exposures have been associated with fibrotic bronchiolitis, including previous severe pneumonia, collagen vascular disorders, inflammatory bowel disease, stem cell and lung transplant, toxic fume exposure, and medications, to name a few; rarely is the disease idiopathic.[11,21,22,37,38]

CT imaging typically demonstrates air trapping and variable occurrence of bronchiolectasis/bronchiectasis. The direct signs of bronchiolar inflammation, such as centrilobular nodules, are much less common.[39] Some of the more commonly discussed causes and associations of fibrotic bronchiolitis are discussed later.

Postinfectious Constrictive Bronchiolitis

Postinfectious constrictive (obliterative) bronchiolitis is a diagnosis based on several diagnostic characteristics, including prior severe lower respiratory tract infection and abnormal lung function with obstructive symptoms.[40] Some of the more common infectious causes associated with postinfectious CB (PICB) are adenovirus, RSV, and *Mycoplasma*. PICB is more common in the pediatric population and relatively rare in adults.[41] In young adults, viral infection and *Mycoplasma* infection is the most common cause of PICB.[41]

PICB demonstrates mosaic attenuation with air trapping on CT; centrilobular nodules or tree-in-bud opacities are rare. The findings can be unilateral or bilateral following a distribution similar to the inciting infectious bronchiolitis.

Swyer-James or Macleod Syndrome

It is important for the clinician and radiologist to distinguish Swyer-James/Macleod (SJM) syndrome from PICB. SJM is a variant of PICB and

appears most often on CXR as a hyperlucent unilateral lung.[42] CT imaging often demonstrates segmental or lobar air trapping with both a compensatory decrease in perfusion and pulmonary artery hypoplasia of the affected segments of the lung (**Fig. 5**A, B).[42,43] Bilateral involvement on CT is the rule, though usually one lung is more severely affected. Because the original infectious insult in SJM syndrome occurs before the lung is mature, the affected segment/lobe or sometimes the entire lung may have a decreased number of alveoli or dilated airspaces caused by alveolar destruction.[43,44] The most common cause of SJM syndrome is prior adenovirus infection.[41]

Constrictive Bronchiolitis Resulting from Inhalational Injury

CB has been documented following a multitude of inhalational injuries. There is usually an acute inhalational injury, which may or may not be symptomatic depending on the characteristics of the inhaled substance. In some cases, the initial inhalational injury may be followed by the development of CB. The acute injury can range from mild pneumonitis to diffuse alveolar hemorrhage or alveolar damage.[45] Flavor worker's lung is a specific pattern of inhalation injury seen in patients who have been exposed to diacetyl, a ketone formerly used as butter flavoring in microwave popcorn.[46] CT findings most often include mosaic attenuation with air trapping. Bronchiectasis and bronchial wall thickening are more variable in appearance.[46]

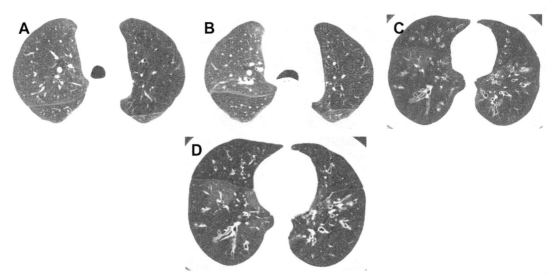

Fig. 5. Fibrotic bronchiolitis examples: (*A, B*) Patient with Swyer-James syndrome with hyperlucent left upper lobe on inspiratory examination (*A*) and air trapping on expiratory examination (*B*). (*C, D*) Patient with obliterative bronchiolitis following stem cell transplant. Axial inspiratory examination (*C*) demonstrates bronchiectasis with bronchial wall thickening and mosaic attenuation. Expiratory axial image (*D*) demonstrate diffuse air trapping.

Obliterative Bronchiolitis Following Transplantation

CB has been documented in both patients who have received lung transplants and those who have received allogeneic stem cell transplants.[47] CB following lung transplantation and allogeneic hematopoietic stem cell transplant (HSCT) are different disease processes, although they share some characteristics.[47]

Following lung transplantation, there is microvascular insufficiency in the small airways of the transplanted lung, which is thought to predispose to developing CB as cellular repair may be limited in this setting.[39] CB has been shown to be present in 70% of long-term lung transplant survivors at 10 years following transplant in the International Heart and Lung Transplant Registry.[39,47] Additionally, CB also affects those patients who recently received lung transplants and is a well-known cause of death in the first few years following the transplant.[47]

Importantly, the diagnosis of CB requires histologic confirmation with demonstration of fibrous tissue in the wall of the membranous bronchioles with specific localization internal to the airway elastica.[32] As biopsy is not always possible, the term bronchiolitis obliterans syndrome (BOS) has been developed to describe patients with the clinical manifestations of obliterative bronchiolitis without histologic documentation of disease.[47]

Patients with BOS or CB following lung transplant typically demonstrate mosaic perfusion and air trapping with bronchiolectasis and bronchial wall thickening in the transplanted lung.[22] The presence of air trapping on HRCT has been demonstrated to be fairly sensitive for CB/BOS but not specific. Correlation of imaging findings with clinical presentation and pulmonary functions is often required in the absence of histologic confirmation.[48]

CB following allogeneic HSCT occurs as a manifestation of chronic graft-versus-host disease and is the most common noninfectious pulmonary complication following allogeneic HSCT.[22,39,47,49] The term BOS is also used in the setting of HSCT-related pulmonary complications, as invasive biopsy is usually not pursued.[47] The incidence of CB or BOS in patients with allogeneic HSCT has been estimated to be between 2% and 10% and is most commonly identified 15 to 18 months following transplantation.[50] CT findings of CB/BOS following HSCT are similar to those following lung transplantation with mosaic attenuation, air trapping, bronchiolectasis, and bronchiolar wall thickening being the most common.[32] CT in patients with HSCT may also demonstrate findings suggesting graft-versus-host disease in additional organ systems (see **Fig. 5**C, D).[47,51]

EMPHYSEMA

Emphysema is a disease characterized by destruction of alveolar and respiratory bronchiolar walls with permanently enlarged airspaces distal to the terminal bronchiole.[14,52] There are 3 main subtypes of emphysema: centrilobular, paraseptal, and panlobular (**Fig. 6**A–F). These subtypes can occur in combination. Centrilobular and paraseptal emphysema were the most common subtypes in the MESA COPD (Multiethnic study of atherosclerosis chronic obstructive pulmonary disease) study population.[52] A fourth subtype is paracicatricial emphysema that is associated with preexisting pulmonary scarring disease (see **Fig. 6**H).[53]

Imaging findings on CT are unique to each subtype of emphysema, although the appearance of the CXR in each of the 3 emphysema subtypes can appear similar. On CXR, the lungs are hyperinflated because of the airspace destruction and dilation resulting in flattening of the normal curvature of the diaphragm.[53] Additionally, there can be widening of the retrosternal clear space caused by lung hyperinflation.[53] The regions of airspace dilation and destruction appear as increasingly radiolucent as the disease worsens, and the distribution of the airspace destruction can suggest a subtype of emphysema; but this distribution may not always be confidently appreciated on the CXR alone.[53]

Centrilobular Emphysema

Centrilobular emphysema demonstrates destruction of alveolar and respiratory bronchiolar walls centered in the pulmonary lobule. It is commonly associated with cigarette smoking, although is also seen in dust (specifically silica) inhalation.[52,54] CT demonstrates foci of low attenuation within the center of the pulmonary lobule, which can be of a variety of sizes in an upper lung–predominant distribution (see **Fig. 6**A, B).[52] The pulmonary artery branch within the pulmonary lobule can appear as a central dot surrounded by the low attenuation of the destroyed and dilated airspaces. These centrilobular low-attenuation regions can become confluent as the disease progresses resulting in the formation of bullae.[55]

Paraseptal Emphysema

Paraseptal emphysema results from alveolar and respiratory bronchiolar wall destruction adjacent to the pleura and the septa of the pulmonary lobule.[52] CT typically reveals rounded foci of low attenuation arranged in a linear pattern along the pleura and

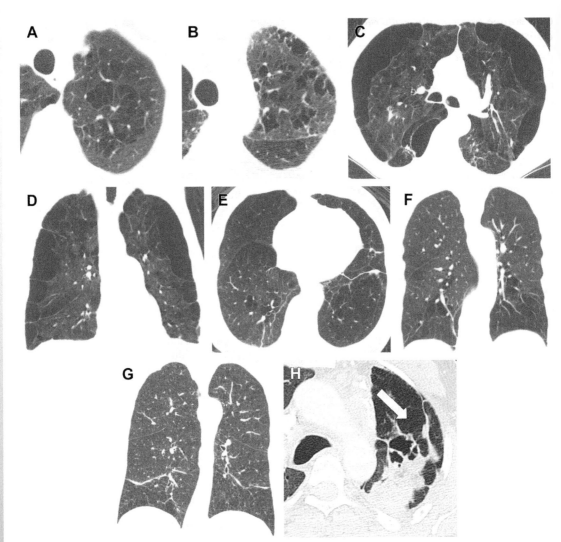

Fig. 6. Emphysema examples: (*A*) Axial CT in a patient with centrilobular emphysema demonstrating areas of lucency at the center of the pulmonary lobule. (*B*) Axial CT in a patient with areas of lucency at the center of the pulmonary lobule (centrilobular emphysema and arranged in a linear fashion at the periphery of the lung [paraseptal emphysema]). (*C, D*) Axial (*B*) and coronal (*D*) CT images in a patient with giant bullous emphysema. Multiple large bullae are seen displacing lung parenchyma. (*E, F*) Axial CT in a patient with panlobular emphysema secondary to alpha-1-antitrypsin deficiency with homogeneous low attenuation in the lower lobes corresponding to panlobular emphysema. (*G*) Coronal CT in a patient with panlobular emphysema, predominantly in the lower lobes, secondary to intravenous injection of methylphenidate tablets (Ritalin lung). (*H*) Axial CT in a patient with progressive massive fibrosis caused by silicosis. Abnormal airspace dilation (*white arrow*) seen adjacent to left upper lobe consolidation consistent with paracicatricial emphysema.

pulmonary lobule septa (see **Fig. 6**B).[52] Vanishing lung syndrome, a form of paraseptal emphysema, also known as giant bullous emphysema, occurs when the dilated airspaces in paraseptal emphysema coalesce to form giant bullae (see **Fig. 6**C, D). This disease has upper lung predilection.[56]

Panlobular Emphysema

Panlobular emphysema is classically described as diffuse uniform destruction of the alveolar and

respiratory bronchiolar walls resulting in global airspace expansion. This disease differs from paraseptal and centrilobular emphysema, as the destruction of the alveoli and respiratory bronchioles is homogeneous and not localized to the center of the pulmonary lobule (centrilobular emphysema) or the peripheral airspaces (paraseptal emphysema).[52] Panlobular emphysema is associated with alpha-1-antitrypsin deficiency, an autosomal recessive disease, which results in uniform destruction of lung parenchyma by proteolytic enzymes that are not inactivated in this disorder.[53] Panlobular emphysema on CT has lower-lobe predominance with characteristic homogenous decrease in attenuation of the entire secondary pulmonary lobule (see **Fig. 6**E, F).

Although panlobular emphysema is most often associated with alpha-1-antitrypsin deficiency, it has also been demonstrated in a rare condition called the Ritalin lung. Ritalin lung is caused by intravenous injection of crushed methylphenidate (RitalinTM) tablets intended for oral use (see **Fig. 6**G).[57] In addition to panlobular emphysema, high attenuation consolidations caused by local excipient deposition may act as a clue to the cause when present.[57,58]

Paracicatricial Emphysema

Paracicatricial emphysema, also known as irregular or scar emphysema, is characterized by airspace dilation that occurs adjacent to pulmonary parenchymal scar from disease, such as sarcoidosis or silicosis, or granulomatous infections, such as tuberculosis (see **Fig. 6**H).[53,59] Paracicatricial emphysema can also be associated with fibrosis.[60] This subtype of emphysema is usually asymptomatic, although patients may have symptoms from the primary pulmonary disease.[61]

SUMMARY

Bronchiolitis may be classified based on histopathologic appearance into either inflammatory/cellular or fibrotic/constrictive groups. Imaging, specifically HRCT, can be used to help differentiate between these subtypes of bronchiolitis based on the presence of direct or indirect signs of disease. Direct signs of bronchiolitis include centrilobular nodules, tree-in-bud pattern, and centrilobular/peribronchiolar ground-glass opacity. Indirect signs include air trapping, mosaic attenuation, and hypovascularity. Emphysema is characterized by destruction and permanent enlargement of airspaces distal to the terminal bronchiole and is subcategorized into centrilobular, paraseptal, and panlobular subtypes with characteristic imaging appearances.[14]

REFERENCES

1. Schuh S, Lalani A, Allen U, et al. Evaluation of the utility of radiography in acute bronchiolitis. J Pediatr 2007;150(4):429–33.
2. Carsin A, Gorincour G, Bresson V, et al. Chest radiographs in infants hospitalized for acute bronchiolitis: real information or just irradiation? Arch Pediatr 2012;19(12):1308–15.
3. Swingler GH, Hussey GD, Zwarenstein M. Randomised controlled trial of clinical outcome after chest radiograph in ambulatory acute lower-respiratory infection in children. Lancet 1998;351(9100):404–8.
4. Arakawa H, Webb WR. Air trapping on expiratory high-resolution CT scans in the absence of inspiratory scan abnormalities: correlation with pulmonary function tests and differential diagnosis. Am J Roentgenol 1998;170(5):1349–53.
5. Zaporozhan J, Ley S, Eberhardt R, et al. Paired inspiratory/expiratory volumetric thin-slice CT scan for emphysema analysis: comparison of different quantitative evaluations and pulmonary function test. Chest 2005;128(5):3212–20.
6. Arakawa H, Fujimoto K, Fukushima Y, et al. Thin-section CT imaging that correlates with pulmonary function tests in obstructive airway disease. Eur J Radiol 2011;80(2):e157–63.
7. Mistry NN, Diwanji T, Shi X, et al. Evaluation of fractional regional ventilation using 4D-CT and effects of breathing maneuvers on ventilation. Int J Radiat Oncol Biol Phys 2013;87(4):825–31.
8. Liu Z, Araki T, Okajima Y, et al. Pulmonary hyperpolarized noble gas MRI: recent advances and perspectives in clinical application. Eur J Radiol 2014; 83(7):1282–91.
9. Webb WR. High resolution lung computed tomography. Normal anatomic and pathologic findings. Radiol Clin North Am 1991;29(5):1051–63.
10. Webb WR. Thin-section CT of the secondary pulmonary lobule: anatomy and the image–the 2004 Fleischner lecture. Radiology 2006;239:322–38.
11. Kang EY, Woo OH, Shin BK, et al. Bronchiolitis: classification, computed tomographic and histopathologic features, and radiologic approach. J Comput Assist Tomogr 2009;33(1):32–41.
12. Abbott GF, Rosado-de-Christenson ML, Rossi SE, et al. Imaging of small airways disease. J Thorac Imaging 2009;24(4):285–98.
13. Ridge CA, Bankier AA, Eisenberg RL. Mosaic attenuation. AJR Am J Roentgenol 2011;197(6):W970–7.
14. Austin JH, Müller NL, Friedman PJ, et al. Glossary of terms for CT of the lungs: recommendations of the Nomenclature Committee of the Fleischner Society. Radiology 1996;200:327–31.
15. Chen D, Webb WR, Storto ML, et al. Assessment of air trapping using postexpiratory high-resolution computed tomography. J Thorac Imaging 1998; 13(2):135–43.
16. Mastora I, Remy-Jardin M, Sobaszek A, et al. Thin-section CT finding in 250 volunteers: assessment of the relationship of CT findings with smoking history and pulmonary function test results. Radiology 2001;218(3):695–702.
17. Mets OM, van Hulst RA, Jacobs C, et al. Normal range of emphysema and air trapping on CT in young men. Am J Roentgenol 2012;199(2):336–40.

18. Tanaka N, Matsumoto T, Miura G, et al. Air trapping at CT: high prevalence in asymptomatic subjects with normal pulmonary function1. Radiology 2003; 227(3):776–85.

19. Lee KW, Chung SY, Yang I, et al. Correlation of aging and smoking with air trapping at thin-section CT of the lung in asymptomatic subjects. Radiology 2000;214(3):831–6.

20. Castañer E, Gallardo X, Ballesteros E, et al. Diagnosis of chronic pulmonary thromboembolism. Radiographics 2009;29(1):31–50.

21. Devakonda A, Raoof S, Sung A, et al. Bronchiolar disorders: a clinical-radiological diagnostic algorithm. Chest 2010;137(4):938–51.

22. Pipavath SJ, Lynch DA, Cool C, et al. Radiologic and pathologic features of bronchiolitis. Am J Roentgenol 2005;185(2):354–63.

23. Ralston S, Comick A, Nichols E, et al. Effectiveness of quality improvement in hospitalization for bronchiolitis: a systematic review. Pediatrics 2014; 134(3):571–81.

24. Hasegawa K, Mansbach JM, Teach SJ, et al. Multicenter study of viral etiology and relapse in hospitalized children with bronchiolitis. Pediatr Infect Dis J 2014;33(8):809–13.

25. Lee G, Kim HS, Lee KS, et al. Serial CT findings of nodular bronchiectatic Mycobacterium avium complex pulmonary disease with antibiotic treatment. Am J Roentgenol 2013;201(4):764–72.

26. Walsh SL, Sverzellati N, Devaraj A, et al. Chronic hypersensitivity pneumonitis: high resolution computed tomography patterns and pulmonary function indices as prognostic determinants. Eur Radiol 2012;22(8):1672–9.

27. Hirschmann JV, Pipavath SN, Godwin JD. Hypersensitivity pneumonitis: a historical, clinical, and radiologic review. Radiographics 2009;29(7): 1921–38.

28. Barrios RJ. Hypersensitivity pneumonitis: histopathology. Arch Pathol Lab Med 2008;132(2):199–203.

29. Churg A, Hall R, Bilawich A. Respiratory bronchiolitis with fibrosis-interstitial lung disease: a new form of smoking-induced interstitial lung disease. Arch Pathol Lab Med 2014;46(Suppl 2):S38.

30. Hare SS, Souza CA, Bain G, et al. The radiological spectrum of pulmonary lymphoproliferative disease. Br J Radiol 2012;85(1015):848–64.

31. Do KH, Lee JS, Seo JB, et al. Pulmonary parenchymal involvement of low-grade lymphoproliferative disorders. J Comput Assist Tomogr 2005; 29(6):825–30.

32. Pipavath SN, Stern EJ. Imaging of small airway disease (SAD). Radiol Clin North Am 2009;47(2): 307–16.

33. Howling SJ, Hansell DM, Wells AU, et al. Follicular bronchiolitis: thin-section CT and histologic findings. Radiology 1999;212(3):637–42.

34. Kudoh S, Keicho N. Diffuse panbronchiolitis. Clin Chest Med 2012;33(2):297–305.

35. Allen TC. Pathology of small airways disease. Arch Pathol Lab Med 2010;134(5):702–18.

36. Miller WT, Panosian JS. Causes and imaging patterns of tree-in-bud opacities. Chest 2013;144(6): 1883–92.

37. King MS, Eisenberg R, Newman JH, et al. Constrictive bronchiolitis in soldiers returning from Iraq and Afghanistan. N Engl J Med 2011; 365(3):222–30.

38. Bergeron A, Godet C, Chevret S, et al. Bronchiolitis obliterans syndrome after allogeneic hematopoietic SCT: phenotypes and prognosis. Bone Marrow Transpl 2013;48(6):819–24.

39. Barker AF, Bergeron A, Rom WN, et al. Obliterative bronchiolitis. N Engl J Med 2014;370(19):1820–8.

40. Mattiello R, Sarria EE, Mallol J, et al. Post-infectious bronchiolitis obliterans: can CT scan findings at early age anticipate lung function? Pediatr Pulmonol 2010;45(4):315–9.

41. McLoud TC, Epler GR, Colby TV, et al. Bronchiolitis obliterans. Radiology 1986;159(1):1–8.

42. Wasilewska E, Lee EY, Eisenberg RL. Unilateral hyperlucent lung in children. Am J Roentgenol 2012;198(5):W400–14.

43. Gottlieb LS, Turner AF. Swyer-James (Macleod's) syndrome. Variations in pulmonary-bronchial arterial blood flow. Chest 1976;69(1):62–6.

44. Cumming GR, Macpherson RI, Chernick V. Unilateral hyperlucent lung syndrome in children. J Pediatr 1971;78(2):250–60.

45. Akira M, Suganuma N. Acute and subacute chemical-induced lung injuries: HRCT findings. Eur J Radiol 2014;83(8):1461–9.

46. Sirajuddin A, Kanne JP. Occupational lung disease. J Thorac Imaging 2009;24(4):310–20.

47. Burgel PR, Bergeron A, de Blic J, et al. Small airways diseases, excluding asthma and COPD: an overview. Eur Respir Rev 2013;22:131–47.

48. Lee ES, Gotway MB, Reddy GP, et al. Early bronchiolitis obliterans following lung transplantation: accuracy of expiratory thin-section CT for diagnosis. Radiology 2000;216(2):472–7.

49. Gazourian L, Rogers AJ, Ibanga R, et al. Factors associated with bronchiolitis obliterans syndrome and chronic graft-versus-host disease after allogeneic hematopoietic cell transplantation. Am J Hematol 2014;89(4):404–9.

50. Gunn ML, Godwin JD, Kanne JP, et al. High-resolution CT findings of bronchiolitis obliterans syndrome after hematopoietic stem cell transplantation. J Thorac Imaging 2008;23(4):244–50.

51. Ditschkowski M, Elmaagacli AH, Koldehoff M, et al. Bronchiolitis obliterans after allogeneic hematopoietic SCT: further insight–new perspectives? Bone Marrow Transpl 2013;48(9):1224–9.

52. Smith BM, Austin JH, Newell JD, et al. Pulmonary emphysema subtypes on computed tomography: the MESA COPD study. Am J Med 2014;127(1):94. e7–23.

53. Foster WL, Gimenez EI, Roubidoux MA, et al. The emphysemas: radiologic-pathologic correlations. Radiographics 1993;13(2):311–28.

54. Takahashi M, Fukuoka J, Nitta N, et al. Imaging of pulmonary emphysema: a pictorial review. Int J Chron Obstruct Pulmon Dis 2008;3(2):193–204. Dove Press.

55. Webb WR. Radiology of obstructive pulmonary disease. AJR Am J Roentgenol 1997;169(3):637–47.

56. Sharma N, Justaniah AM, Kanne JP, et al. Vanishing lung syndrome (giant bullous emphysema): CT findings in 7 patients and a literature review. J Thorac Imaging 2009;24(3):227–30.

57. Stern EJ, Frank MS, Schmutz JF, et al. Panlobular pulmonary emphysema caused by i.v. injection of methylphenidate (Ritalin): findings on chest radiographs and CT scans. AJR Am J Roentgenol 1994; 162(3):555–60.

58. Chong S, Lee KS, Chung MJ, et al. Pneumoconiosis: comparison of imaging and pathologic findings. Radiographics 2006;26(1):59–77.

59. Bégin R, Filion R, Ostiguy G. Emphysema in silica- and asbestos-exposed workers seeking compensation. A CT scan study. Chest 1995;108(3):647–55.

60. Bergin CJ, Müller NL, Miller RR. CT in the qualitative assessment of emphysema. J Thorac Imaging 1986; 1(2):94–103.

61. Thurlbeck WM. The pathobiology and epidemiology of human emphysema. J Toxicol Environ Health 1984;13(2–3):323–43.

Functional Imaging
Computed Tomography and MRI

Saeed Mirsadraee, MD, PhD, Edwin J.R. van Beek, MD, PhD*

KEYWORDS

- CT • Airways • Parenchyma • Ventilation • Perfusion • Computer-aided detection • Lung function
- MRI

KEY POINTS

- Standard imaging for the lungs has limited specificity, does not always diagnose pathology at a treatable stage, and does not provide physiologic information.
- In the past decade, advances in imaging technology and analytical methods allowed more physiologic approach in lung imaging, functional imaging.
- Novel CT and MRI techniques, such as ventilation and perfusion, have been developed in imaging of the lungs.

INTRODUCTION

Since the previous review on this topic of functional computed tomography (CT) and MRI of the lung, significant advances have been made into the development of imaging based biomarkers for evaluation of lung diseases.[1] The increased utility of multidetector row CT (MDCT) has incorporated traditional high-resolution lung imaging, allowing multiplanar reconstructions at hitherto unimaginable spatial resolution. The incorporation of contrast-enhanced CT methodologies is still expanding, thereby not just yielding us the capacity to study vascular pathology in great detail, but, in combination with greater speed and coverage of the chest, also bringing us closer to true lung perfusion in clinical practice. Techniques like spirometry-controlled MDCT have paved the way for introduction of routinely applicable protocols where patients are monitored more closely and coached to obtain better quantifiable CT imaging data. In addition to these parenchymal and vascular imaging improvements, inhaled contrast has also continued further development and xenon gas is now being piloted in patients with a range of lung pathologies. Last, but not least,

software has continued to develop, enabling quantification of parenchymal disease, quantification of ventilation–perfusion ratios and giving us insights into airway disease like never before.

In the meantime, MRI is beginning to overcome its problems related to lung imaging (mainly field inhomogeneity and lack of protons in the lung), both with applications of proton MRI sequences as well as by using injected (gadolinium-based) and inhaled (oxygen, hyperpolarized gases such as ^{3}He, ^{129}Xe, and ^{19}F) contrast methods. These advances are starting to make an impact on the management of particularly radiation-sensitive patients (children, pregnancy, those with chronic conditions requiring repeated investigations) and in areas where CT is disadvantaged in providing soft tissue detail (eg, lung cancer staging in the lung apex, mediastinal involvement, and chest wall assessment). The faster imaging speed also allows MRI to give a comprehensive assessment of the effects of heart and lung pathologies on each organ system. Although some of these techniques were limited initially to a few centers, there is now a gradual expansion of knowledge making these technologies more widely available.

Disclosure: None.

Clinical Research Imaging Centre, Queen's Medical Research Institute, University of Edinburgh, 47 Little France Crescent, Edinburgh EH16 4TJ, UK

* Corresponding author.

E-mail address: edwin-vanbeek@ed.ac.uk

Clin Chest Med 36 (2015) 349–363
http://dx.doi.org/10.1016/j.ccm.2015.02.014

chestmed.theclinics.com

This article describes the new applications of CT and MRI in relation to obtaining functional and quantifiable tools for the study of pulmonary parenchymal and vascular disorders. We hope that it will familiarize the community with the translation of techniques from research into clinical applied methodologies.

COMPUTED TOMOGRAPHY
Computed Tomography Hardware Systems Developments

As described, CT has developed rapidly into one of the most clinically requested investigations in medicine.[1] A recent review of the history and development of CT on the occasion of the centenary meeting of the Radiological Society of North America is worth reading in this context.[2] Clearly, much progress has been made as we have moved from the dynamic spatial reconstructor, the prototype of dynamic volumetric x-ray CT designed and installed at the Mayo Clinic in the mid 1970s.[3] From the initial beginnings of computed transverse axial scanning tomography,[4] via electron beam CT[5] to the current 16-cm coverage electrocardiography-gated imaging within a single heartbeat,[6] CT has been at the heart of changes in medical diagnosis and management. It is difficult to imagine that even Hounsfield in his visionary acceptance speech of the Nobel Prize could have quite foreseen the impact CT has made.[7]

Apart from the high temporal resolution now available on CT systems, the spatial resolution has also improved and 0.4-mm isotropic resolution is now achievable using the latest scanner technology.[8] Furthermore, the application of novel reconstruction methods has resulted in significant reductions in radiation dose, and all vendors now routinely include iterative reconstruction as part of their standard protocols with the latest techniques resulting in very low-dose CT with exposure for lung parenchymal disease in the order of 0.15 mSv[9] and for lung nodule detection with exposures less than traditional chest radiographs at 0.06 mSv.[10]

These developments have had both positive and negative impacts on the application of CT. The surge in use of CT has resulted in a significant increase in radiation burden in the overall population,[11,12] although it is important to realize that the use of CT has a greater benefit to patients, which justifies its risks.[13] Moreover, radiation exposure is now being addressed by stricter guidance on indications and monitoring of radiation dose.[14] Furthermore, novel reconstruction methods, such as iterative reconstruction, have allowed

introduction of dose limitation while maintaining signal-to-noise ratio and image quality. Another issue with different scanner manufacturers and different reconstruction techniques is that this has an effect on density measurements, and this may impact on interpretation of images and the use of different CT systems in cohort and clinical studies.[15,16]

The advanced technologies now enable structural imaging of the chest in great detail and with 0.4 to 0.6 mm isotropic resolution. This is all achieved with a z-axis coverage of 4 to 16 cm in a rotation time of 0.3 seconds or less. This speed makes the examination more robust and full coverage of the chest in a single breath-hold is easier to achieve. At the same time, it is crucial to coach patients to full inspiration as well as forced residual volume expiration where air trapping or airway collapse is being investigated.

The application of contrast has yielded anatomic images of the vasculature in the chest, including the coronary arteries, aorta, and pulmonary vessels. However, with dual-energy application, where 2 scans are performed using different keV settings, it is feasible separate out particular high-density compounds such as iodine or xenon. Thus, it is now feasible to obtain the distribution of vascular contrast (resulting in a measure of pulmonary blood volume),[17,18] as well as to evaluate the distribution of inhaled contrast like xenon gas.[19,20] Similarly, dynamic contrast-enhanced methods are able to track a tight contrast bolus of 5 to 9 mL/s during a 20-second period to yield true perfusion, mean transit times (MTT) and even assess pulmonary and systemic supply of the pulmonary vascular bed.

Clearly, the versatility of CT is expanding as the radiation dose, and temporal and spatial resolution are all optimized. This expansion will give impetus to the development of more individual approaches, with a combination of morphologic and functional information. However, radiation will always need to be a matter of concern and, despite these developments, we need to take into consideration that MRI may be preferred wherever the information gained can be on a similar setting compared with CT. For future studies, it is very likely that there will be an interleaved approach to ordering MRI and CT investigations in patients where longitudinal studies are required.

Quantitative Image Analysis and Distilling Functional Information

Quantification of disease using CT methods depends on a number of fundamental steps: protocol standardization, coaching of patients during the procedure and post processing using advanced software. Using the latest technology, it is now possible to reliably define the airway tree down to the sixth or seventh generation, obtain measurement of airway wall thickness and luminal cross-section and their relationship (wall area percentage), categorize these results (eg, using the Pi10 definition) and additionally allocate histogram analysis of airspace density during inspiration and expiration resulting in parametric response map (**Fig. 1**).[21]

These methods have resulted in large cohort classification, and highlighted different phenotypes in chronic obstructive pulmonary disease (COPD; **Fig. 2**)[22] and asthma.[23] In addition, using different threshold and computer-assisted diagnosis, it has become feasible to perform texture analysis and quantify this, for instance, in interstitial lung disease.[24,25]

Clearly, all these new opportunities will gradually make their way into clinical practice, as the quest for more quantitative analysis in relation to lung function continues to drive new therapeutic approaches. The traditional lung function tests are not able to give regional information, and using CT methods as biomarkers is very likely going to impact on how new treatments will be developed.

In addition to these noncontrast methods, application of ventilation and intravenous contrast agents has allowed the study of direct functional parameters of the lungs. In this respect, CT is of interest, even though there is a radiation exposure issue that requires close attention. At this interface, there is a trade-off with MRI methods described elsewhere in this review.

MRI

With its inherent image acquisition speed, lack of ionizing radiation, and the resolution and capability to resolve different tissues, MRI has significant potential in medical imaging. However, despite these advantages being exploited in other areas of the body, chest MRI has lagged behind owing to the problems with moving organs, lack of protons in the lungs, and field inhomogeneities causing artifacts. Over the past several years, several approaches have been taken to overcome these barriers, and as things are today, MRI can deliver on a number of morphologic and functional clinical parameters that rival CT, and in some cases supersede it.

MRI Systems Hardware and Software Developments

The optimal field strength for pulmonary MRI is debatable, but most 1.5 T systems can yield good quality proton images. Adaptations of MRI hardware include greater field gradients (allowing for faster image acquisition—ultrafast imaging), options to perform multinuclear imaging (given access to hyperpolarized noble gas inhaled contrast agent applications) and dedicated radio-frequency (RF) coils to improve signal-to-noise ratios as well as to improve patient tolerance.

The use of intravenous contrast based on gadolinium is commonplace, because it allows for better visualization of the main blood vessels, and dynamic contrast-enhanced MRI offers the capability to study the contrast bolus traveling through the entire cardiac cycle, giving rise to perfusion, blood volume, and transit time measurements. The technique is increasingly finding use in routine clinical practice, particularly in centers of excellence where patients are investigated for pulmonary hypertension.[26,27] Last, but not least, MRI offers an integrated assessment of the lung–heart axis, incorporating a dynamic assessment of the right ventricle as well as assessment of myocardial health.

Functional Imaging

Numerous methods have been developed to assess ventilation, perfusion, or their functional outcome—gas exchange. Subsequently, we provide examples of the use of MRI and MDCT imaging technology to probe normal and abnormal cardiopulmonary structure and function. We argue that these technologies offer a unique and comprehensive approach to evaluating the structural and functional complexity of the respiratory and cardiopulmonary systems.

ASSESSMENT OF REGIONAL PULMONARY VENTILATION AND GAS EXCHANGE
Oxygen-Enhanced MRI

Oxygen has paramagnetic properties that can be detected by subtraction of the signal obtained in the lung during normal respiration of room air (concentration 20%) from the signal obtained after sustained breathing of 100% oxygen.[28–30] Although there are some limitations, such as full saturation of all lung tissue over time, the technique has been shown to be able to delineate ventilation, whereas several studies have shown that this technique may be useful in prediction of outcome after lung resection for lung cancer (**Fig. 3**) and more recently for the assessment of treatment response in asthma.[29,30] Oxygen's paramagnetic properties lead to depolarization of hyperpolarized gas, and this effect is directly correlated with the partial oxygen tension. This effect is thus a direct measure of the presence

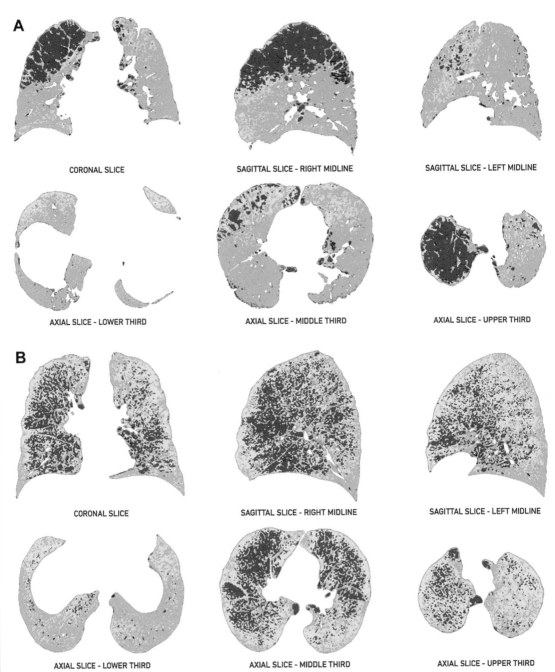

Fig. 1. Advanced analysis techniques in evaluation of emphysema. Patient with regional emphysema (*A*) and diffuse emphysema (*B*). The co-registered inspiration and expiration images demonstrate normal lung tissue (*green*), areas of air trapping (density between -950 and -856 HU; *yellow*) and fixed low attenuation areas where there is no longer any dynamic airflow (*red*). (*Courtesy of* Imbio, Minneapolis, USA; and *Adapted from* Galbán CJ, Han MK, Boes JL, et al. Computed tomography-based biomarker provides unique signature for diagnosis of COPD phenotypes and disease progression. Nat Med 2012;18(11):1711–5; with permission.)

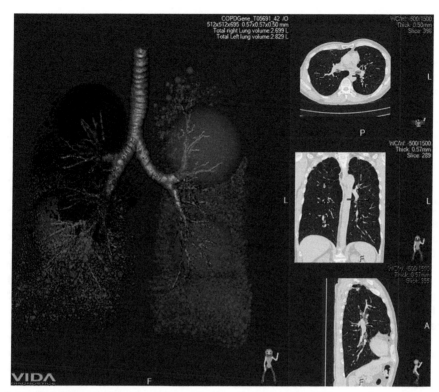

Fig. 2. Smoker with GOLD zero status based on pulmonary function tests, with extensive emphysema based on advanced CT quantification. The 3-dimensional image provides a schematic representation of the size of emphysematous "holes." (*Courtesy of* the NIH supported COPDGene study; and *Adapted from* Barr CC, Berkowitz EA, Bigazzi F, et al. A combined pulmonary-radiology workshop for visual evaluation of COPD: study design, chest CT findings and concordance with quantitative evaluation. COPD 2012;9:151–9; with permission.)

of oxygen, and the higher the oxygen concentration the sooner the hyperpolarized gas signal will be lost. This can be used to produce 3-dimensional oxygen maps, a measure of lung's oxygen exchange effectiveness[31] in patients with major perfusion–ventilation mismatch, such as those with (chronic) thromboembolic disease, and where patients are considered for radical surgery

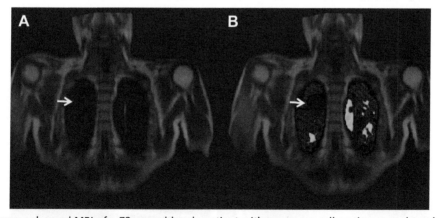

Fig. 3. Oxygen-enhanced MRI of a 73-year-old male patient with squamous cell carcinoma and emphysema. (*A*) Source image of O₂-enhanced MRI. (*B*) Relative enhancement map of O₂-enhanced MRI. On source and relative enhancement map, lung cancer with cavity (*arrow*) is clearly demonstrated. Relative enhancement map shows heterogeneous enhancement within lung owing to pulmonary emphysema. Relative enhancement map is color coded from dark blue to red. (*Courtesy of* Prof Y. Ohno, MD, PhD, University of Kobe, Kobe, Japan.)

or radiation therapy, but whose pulmonary function tests are borderline.

The technique is inexpensive (oxygen is normally available in every MRI suite), but technically the imaging remains challenging and requires image post-processing, which is not available uniformly. As a result, only a few centers use the technology in a research setting, although expectations are that the technology will grow with simplification and increased availability of regulators and automated image analysis software.

Hyperpolarized Gas MRI

MRI is based on tuning RF amplifiers to a particular transmission/receiving frequency, which is 64 MHz at 1.5 T for proton. By changing this frequency, it is possible to tune into other nuclear signals (referred to as multinuclear spectroscopy), and this has been successfully applied for lung imaging of inert noble gases, like [3]He,[32] and [129]X,[33] whereas other gases are also undergoing tests (^{19}F, for instance[34]). These gases have no signal in their normal resting state, but they can be excited by laser light, resulting in a hyperpolarized state. This state can then be used to visualize these nuclei during MRI, where the loss of polarization results in an RF signal that can be detected by appropriately tuned RF coils. **Figs. 4** and **5** demonstrate the advantage of hyperpolarized [3]He MRI in evaluation of lung ventilation, compared with proton MRI.

The technique was well advanced in the utility of hyperpolarized [3]He imaging, which has excellent signal-to-noise properties and a good safety profile, because it does not pass the alveolar–blood barrier, and has been applied in a multicenter trial in emphysema patients.[35] More recently, in response to a general lack of supply of [3]He,[36] which is also being used for nuclear detector systems, researchers have also begun to take another look at [129]X. Polarization systems have been developed that create higher polarization levels for this agent, and thus a better signal-to-noise ratio.[37] This gas is lipid soluble and can diffuse to the blood; the phenomenon is used for measurement of alveolar surface and alveolar–blood barrier thickness, which both offer new insights compared with [3]He MRI.[38,39]

Although the high signal introduced with hyperpolarized gas makes this technique relatively less dependent on field strength, most research has been performed on 1.5 T systems that are fairly routinely available in most hospitals. Nonstandard imaging sequences have been developed to allow maximal use of the hyperpolarization. Unfortunately, it takes a well-trained team and dedicated equipment to produce hyperpolarized gas, and therefore it has remained limited to advanced research centers, where it has elicited interesting insights into pathophysiologic relationships and its potential to serve as a quantifiable biomarker for disease and treatment response in a variety of clinical conditions.

Ventilation distribution is largely homogeneous in normal volunteers, whereas patients with airflow obstruction will develop nonventilated lung regions. It has been shown that the extent of these defects correlate with pulmonary function tests, but of course, this technique offers a direct spatial delineation, which may be important for therapy planning, for instance.[40] This method has been used to study asthma (**Fig. 6**),[41] COPD,[35] measuring response to treatment in cystic fibrosis and COPD,[42,43] and also recently in predicting risk of COPD exacerbations.[44]

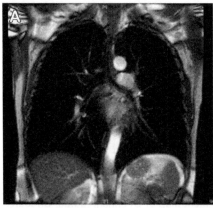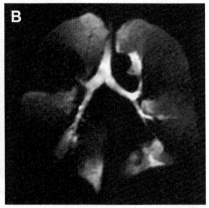

Fig. 4. Hyperpolarized [3]He MRI of lung ventilation. (A) Proton MRI shows lack of signal in the lungs, and the corresponding hyperpolarized [3]He MRI (B) demonstrates multiple hypoventilated lung segments in this patient with chronic obstructive pulmonary disease.

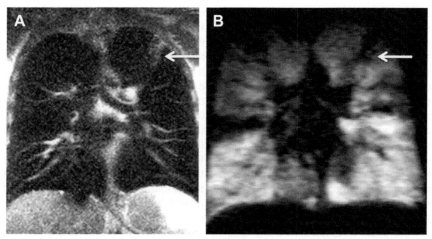

Fig. 5. Examples of hyperpolarized ³He MRI in cystic fibrosis. A 12-year-old with cystic fibrosis, demonstrating slightly increased signal in left apex and right upper lobe on proton sequence (*arrow; A*) and more extensive ventilation defects on the hyperpolarized ³He image (*arrow; B*).

Initial pilot studies have suggested the combined use of hyperpolarized ³He MRI with proton MRI and CT can improve radiation therapy planning.[45] Another pilot study suggested that this technique was more sensitive to detect early signs of lung transplant rejection compared with CT or spirometry.[46]

Xenon Computed Tomography

Xenon is denser than air and therefore acts as a contrast agent when inhaled. The greater the density of inhaled xenon in a particular area, the greater the ventilation in that region. Xenon has anesthetic effects that may limit its use at higher concentrations.[47] The gas diffuses through the lung into the circulation and although this can potentially provide information on local diffusion and perfusion, it can also complicate the analysis.

CT can be used for dynamic or static evaluation of regional ventilation. Dual energy CT (DECT) is used to enhance initiation of xenon from air and lung tissue by 3-material decomposition.[48] The technique is used for evaluation of ventilation in various conditions, such as COPD,[49] asthma,[50] bronchiolitis obliterans.[51]

ASSESSMENT OF PULMONARY PERFUSION BY COMPUTED TOMOGRAPHY AND MRI

Pulmonary perfusion can be assessed by CT and MRI after the administration of contrast material. Compared with the normal lung parenchyma, areas with altered perfusion demonstrate slower and less intense enhancement, or no perfusion (infarcted tissue). Delayed perfusion from arterial sources other than lobar pulmonary artery

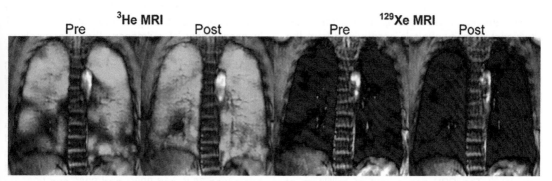

Fig. 6. Hyperpolarized ³He (*blue*) and ¹²⁹Xe (*purple*) MRI ventilation registered to the anatomic ¹H MRI of the thorax (*gray scale*) before and after salbutamol for a representative asthmatic patient (43-year-old man; presalbutamol FEV_1 = 82% pred; FEV_1/FVC = 69%; postsalbutamol FEV_1 = 93% predicted; FEV_1/FVC = 72%). Both images show multiple ventilation defects. FEV_1, forced expiratory volume in 1 second; FVC, forced vital capacity. (*Courtesy of* Svenningsen and Parraga, Robarts Research Institute, Western University, London, Canada.)

branches (eg, from systemic arteries or collaterals) is observed in benign and malignant pulmonary conditions. The physiologic perfusion values differ in lung lobes and segments of the lungs.

There are 2 approaches to image lung perfusion—static peak enhancement imaging and dynamic contrast-enhanced imaging. In the former approach, a single CT scan is performed at a particular time point, for example, at the peak of normal lung parenchymal enhancement. The differences in the density of the lung tissue imply changes in the perfusion. DECT can be used to produce iodine maps of the lungs by material decomposition based on attenuation differences at different energy levels.[52] The main advantage of the peak enhancement imaging is the relatively ease of the technique. Wrong timing of the scan may, however, result in falsification of the results. Moreover, single time point imaging would not take into account the physiologic differences in the regional perfusion of the lungs. Although the DECT has been extensively used in the evaluation of various benign and malignant pulmonary conditions, the technique suffers from limitations such as restriction of the field of view of the second tube in 1 scanner model, which resulted in the loss of peripheral lung coverage, especially in larger patients, increased radiation dose, and additional noise at lower tube voltage that is especially important in patients with a greater body mass index. Breathing artifact would result in misregistration artifact.[52,53]

Dynamic contrast-enhanced perfusion studies can be performed by CT or MR and involve serial CT/MRI at fixed or variable time intervals while the iodinated contrast is administrated. The method used to measure perfusion is derived from first-pass indicator dilution theory. The assumption is that the indicator (contrast agent) does not disturb flow, mixes uniformly with blood, and remains intravascular.[54]

After intravenous contrast injection, a time–density/signal intensity curve is constructed from the change in CT density or MR signal intensity of the imaged tissues as the agent passes through the vasculature from which several perfusion parameters are calculated. Time to peak is defined as the time from the start of the contrast injection to maximal tissue enhancement and is measured in seconds. The pulmonary blood volume (PBV) is a measure of the total volume of blood within an imaging voxel (tissues and blood vessels).[55] The PBV has a unit of milliliters of blood per 100 g of tissue (mL/100 g) and is determined by mathematic integration of the area under the tissue time-density/signal curve.[56] Pulmonary blood flow (PBF) is defined as the volume of blood moving through a given region per unit time (mL/100 mg/min), representing the capillary flow in the tissue. The MTT is the average transit time of all the contrast medium molecules through a given volume of tissue and is measured in seconds and can be approximated according to the central volume principle: MTT = central blood volume/central blood flow.[55] Various models are used to calculate perfusion values from the time–density curves, including the deconvolution techniques and maximum slope technique. In the latter model, the steepest slope of the lung tissue enhancement is divided by the peak of the arterial input function (pulmonary artery) to estimate PBF.[57] Absolute measurement of perfusion depends on the cardiac output at the time of measurement. To compare perfusion values of a patient, it has been proposed that the values are normalized to the cardiac output[58] that can be calculated from the input function time–density curve.[59]

In principal, signal–time curves are converted into concentration–time curves for quantitative perfusion evaluation. Therefore, a linear relationship between signal intensity and concentration is mandatory. This is especially important for the arterial input function, where all contrast media bolus passes during the first pass.[60] Compared with iodinated contrast agent, where there is a linear relationship between contrast dose and CT density, the relationship between the MR signal and gadolinium is nonlinear, which makes quantification more complex. Therefore, the MR contrast dose has to be kept to a minimum to avoid signal saturation.[61]

CLINICAL APPLICATIONS OF PULMONARY PERFUSION IMAGING

Pulmonary perfusion imaging has been used in many benign and malignant lung diseases. Many studies reported the application of perfusion CT in assessment of pulmonary thromboembolism. A small observational study comparing DECT perfusion with CT pulmonary angiogram (CTPA) demonstrated a sensitivity and specificity of 100% on a per-patient basis, and 60% to 66.7% and 99.5% to 99.8% on a per-segment basis the sensitivity and specificity ranged between 60% and 66.7% and 99.5% and 99.8%.[62] Compared with scintigraphy, the reported sensitivity and specificity of DECT perfusion on a per-patient basis was 75% and 80%, and 83% and 99% on a per-segment basis.[63] Other studies reported application of dynamic MR perfusion imaging to be superior to MR and CT angiography in extent assessment of disease severity assessment and outcome prediction for acute pulmonary thrombo-embolism.[64] **Fig. 7** shows the advantage of CT perfusion over CTPA in the detection of peripheral pulmonary arterial vascular obstruction that is often missed on CTPA, especially in the subacute cases of pulmonary embolism.

Both CT and MRI technologies are being used in the assessment of pulmonary arteries and right ventricular function in patients with chronic thromboembolic disorders.[65,66] A recently published study suggested that tortuosity as well as 3-dimensional fractal dimension of the pulmonary vessels that were segmented from pulmonary CT angiogram correlated with mean pulmonary arterial pressure ($r = 0.60$) and other relevant parameters, like pulmonary vascular resistance ($r = 0.59$), arteriovenous difference in oxygen ($r = 0.54$), arterial ($r = 20.54$) and venous oxygen saturation ($r = 20.68$), and may provide a tool to evaluate the severity of pulmonary hypertension.[67] Another study suggested that the vortex flow patterns (eg, period of existence) in the pulmonary artery on time-resolved 3-dimensional MR phase-contrast imaging correlated with pulmonary artery pressure.[68]

Perfusion studies demonstrate ventilation changes and localized/wedge-shaped perfusion defects in chronic thromboembolic diseases, whereas in pulmonary hypertension the perfusion is overall reduced and inhomogeneous.[69] **Fig. 8** shows an example of ventilation and perfusion assessment in a patient with chronic thromboembolic pulmonary hypertension.

A good correlation between the mosaic attenuation and the DECT perfusion changes is observed

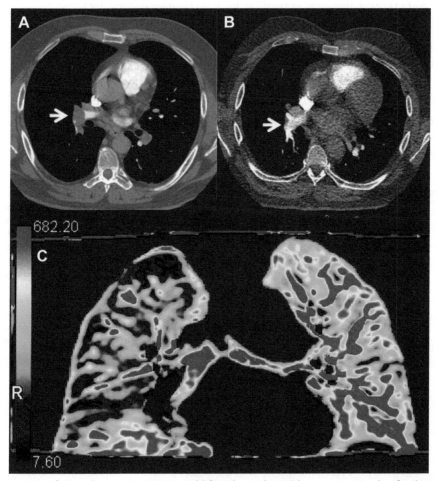

Fig. 7. Pulmonary perfusion changes in a 52-year-old female smoker with a recent episode of pulmonary embolism (PE). This patient presented with large volume bilateral PE (*arrow; A*). The patient remained symptomatic at 6 months despite treatment. (*B*) Resolution of PE in the lobar and segmental branches (*arrow*). (*C*) Dynamic CT perfusion, however, demonstrated significant residual perfusion reduction in the right lung accounting for patient's symptoms. Pixels are color coded in the parametric maps according to the degree of perfusion (from high to low perfusion values: *red, yellow, green, blue/black*).

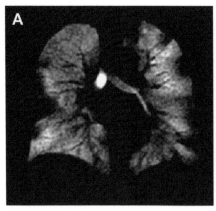
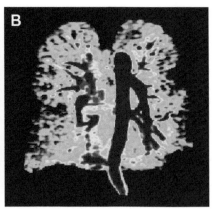

Fig. 8. MR ventilation and perfusion imaging in a patient with chronic thromboembolic pulmonary hypertension. Hyperpolarized ³He MRI (*A*) demonstrated multiple peripheral ventilation defects. The dynamic gadolinium-enhanced ¹H perfusion study (*B*) showed more extensive bilateral segmental perfusion abnormalities in segments with abnormal and normal ventilation (matched and mismatched VQ). (*B*) Pixels are color coded in the parametric maps according to the degree of perfusion (from high to low perfusion values: *red, yellow, green, blue/black*). (*Courtesy of* Prof J.M. Wild, University of Sheffield, Royal Hallamshire Hospital, UK.)

in chronic thromboembolic pulmonary hypertension.[70] Various studies reported delayed regional perfusion in chronic thromboembolic disease when compared with acute pulmonary embolism.[71] This phenomenon is explained by perfusion from systemic collateral formation.[71] **Fig. 9** shows an example of segmental delayed perfusion in a patient with previous pulmonary embolism and apparent perfusion defect in the pulmonary artery phase.

Ohno and colleagues[72] investigated perfusion parameters derived from 3-dimensional dynamic contrast-enhanced MRI, and pulmonary vascular resistance and mean pulmonary artery pressure in patients with primary pulmonary hypertension and healthy volunteers. The authors reported

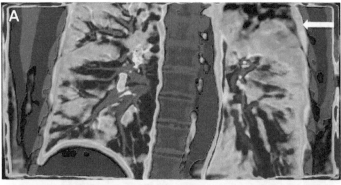
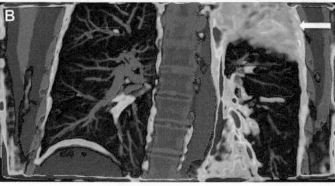

Fig. 9. Delayed perfusion after an episode of recent pulmonary embolism. Pixels are color coded in the parametric maps according to the degree of perfusion (from high to low perfusion values: *red, yellow, green, blue/black*). Dual phase perfusion analysis shows lack of perfusion from pulmonary artery in the left upper lobe (*arrow; A*), but perfusion from other sources (*arrow; B*). The time delay was approximately 4 seconds.

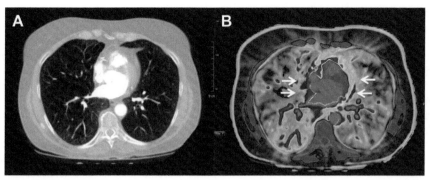

Fig. 10. Pulmonary perfusion changes in a 63-year-old female smoker with diffuse emphysema (*A*, lung window CT; *B*, parametric perfusion map). Perfusion map from dynamic contrast-enhanced CT shows diffusely abnormal perfusion throughout both lungs. Pixels are color coded in the parametric maps according to the degree of perfusion (from high to low perfusion values: *red, yellow, green, blue/black*). The perfusion is much better in the right lower lobe, compared with the other lobes (note homogenous higher perfusion as coded in *green/yellow* in the right posterior zone, compared with patchy darker pixels in the other regions indicating lower perfusion). Note artifactual increased perfusion around the heart (*arrows*) secondary to cardiac motion.

significantly different mean regional PBF in primary pulmonary hypertension, when compared with healthy volunteers. PBF was correlated negatively with pulmonary vascular resistance and mean pulmonary artery pressure, but the MTT had a moderate positive correlation.

Previous studies suggested that endothelial dysfunction and abnormal pulmonary vascular response play a role in pathogenesis COPD.[73–75] A study of dynamic CT perfusion in patients with minor emphysema versus control (healthy volunteers and smokers without emphysema) reported globally increased heterogeneity in the early emphysema group, but not in the control group. The authors suggested that the CT perfusion might be able to differentiate smokers at risk of emphysema.[76] When emphysema is established, alveolar surface reduction is associated with reduction in

capillary volume.[77,78] As a result, the reduction in perfusion on CT correlated with severity of emphysema.[79] **Fig. 10** shows diffuse perfusion changes in a patient with emphysema.

Microvascular thrombosis and injury is reported to play a role in the pathogenesis of pulmonary fibrosis.[80] CT and MRI examinations in these patients demonstrated lower MTT, time to peak, and PBF in areas with pulmonary fibrosis.[81,82] **Fig. 11** shows perfusion changes in areas with apparent fibrosis, but also areas without CT evidence of established fibrosis.

Dynamic perfusion CT is reported to be more specific and accurate than static positron emission tomography/CT for differentiating malignant from benign pulmonary nodules of less than 3 cm.[83] A study of solitary pulmonary nodules in 51 patients that was investigated with dynamic

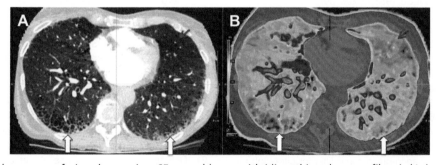

Fig. 11. Pulmonary perfusion changes in a 65-year-old man with idiopathic pulmonary fibrosis (*A*, lung window CT; *B*, parametric perfusion map). Pixels are color coded in the parametric maps according to the degree of perfusion (from high to low perfusion values: *red, yellow, green, blue/black*). Perfusion map from dynamic contrast-enhanced CT shows diffusely abnormal perfusion in the subpleural regions of both lungs. The maps demonstrated diffusely abnormal perfusion in areas without apparent pulmonary fibrosis on CT images (*red arrow*). White arrows show significantly reduced perfusion in areas with established honeycombing which is partly owing to the replacement of lung tissue by air spaces.

contrast-enhanced MRI demonstrated higher maximum peak, faster enhancement slope, and significant washout with malignant nodules, the sensitivity, specificity, and accuracy in diagnosis of malignant from benign nodules was 100%, 79%, and 90%, respectively.[84] The results can be explained by knowledge of increased vascularity in malignant tumors.[85-87] A strong relationship is also reported between thin peripheral enhancement and benign nodules, which is thought to be an inflammatory response.[84]

SUMMARY

This article shows the breadth of functional lung assessment that can now be achieved with excellent image quality in the chest. A combination of perfusion and ventilation assessment is feasible with great detail, and this may help study the effects of treatments. The technologies have clearly made significant strides over the past 5 to 10 years, and there is an increasing role for functional imaging for study of pathophysiologic processes in the lungs.

REFERENCES

1. van Beek EJ, Hoffman EA. Functional imaging: CT and MRI. Clin Chest Med 2008;29:195–216.
2. Rubin GD. Computed tomography: revolutionizing the practice of medicine for 40 years. Radiology 2014;273(2 Suppl):S45–74.
3. Ritman EL, Robb RA, Harris LD. Imaging physiological functions: experience with the DSR. Philadelphia: Praeger; 1985.
4. Hounsfield GN. Computerized transverse axial scanning (tomography). Description of system. Br J Radiol 1973;46:1016–22.
5. Boyd DP, Lipton MJ. Cardiac computed tomography. Proc IEEE 1983;71:298–307.
6. Kasai J, Sugiura T, Tanabe N, et al. Electrocardiogram-gated 320-slice multidetector computed tomography for the measurement of pulmonary arterial distensibility in chronic thromboembolic pulmonary hypertension. PLoS One 2014;9:e111563.
7. Hounsfield GN. Computed medical imaging. Nobel lecture, December 8, 1973. J Comput Assist Tomogr 1980;4:665–74.
8. Meyer M, Haubenreisser H, Raupach R, et al. Initial results of a new generation dual source CT system using only an in-plane comb filter for ultra-high resolution temporal bone imaging. Eur Radiol 2015; 25(1):178–85.
9. Newell JD Jr, Fuld MK, Allmendinger T, et al. Very low-dose (0.15 mGy) chest CT protocols using the COPDGene 2 test object and a third-generation dual source CT scanner with corresponding third-

10. Gordic S, Morsbach F, Schmidt B, et al. Ultralow-dose chest computed tomography for pulmonary nodule detection: first performance evaluation of single energy scanning with spectral shaping. Invest Radiol 2014;49:465–73.
11. National Council on Radiation Protection and Measurements. Ionizing radiation exposure of the population of the United States. NCRP Report No. 160. Bethesda (MD): National Council on Radiation Protection and Measurements; 2009.
12. Brenner DJ, Hall EJ. Computed tomography: an increasing source of radiation exposure. N Engl J Med 2007;357(22):2277–84.
13. Hendee ER, O'Connor MK. Radiation risk of medical imaging: separating fact from fantasy. Radiology 2012;264:312–21.
14. Boone JM, Hendee WR, McNitt-Gray F, et al. Radiation exposure from CT scans: how to close our knowledge gap and safeguard exposure – proceedings and recommendations of the radiation dose summit, sponsored by NIBIB, February 24-25, 2011. Radiology 2012;265:544–54.
15. Sieren JP, Newell JP, Judy PF, et al. Reference standard and statistical model for intersite and temporal comparison of CT attenuation in a multicenter quantitative lung study. Med Phys 2012;39:5757–67.
16. Sieren JP, Hoffman EA, Fuld MK, et al. Sinogram affirmed iterative reconstruction (SAFIRE) versus weighted filtered back projection (WFBP) effects on quantitative measure in the COPDgene 2 test object. Med Phys 2014;41:091910.
17. Ameli-Renani S, Rahman F, Nair A, et al. Dual-energy CT for imaging of pulmonary hypertension: challenges and opportunities. Radiographics 2014; 34:1769–90.
18. Sakamoto A, Sakamoto I, Nagayama H, et al. Quantification of lung perfusion blood volume with dual-energy CT: assessment of the severity of acute pulmonary thromboembolism. Am J Roentgenol 2014;203:287–91.
19. Zhang LJ, Zhou CS, Schoepf UJ, et al. Dual-energy CT lung ventilation/perfusion imaging for diagnosing pulmonary embolism. Eur Radiol 2013;23:2666–75.
20. Fuld MK, Halaweish AF, Newell JD Jr, et al. Optimization of dual-energy xenon-computed tomography for quantitative assessment of regional pulmonary ventilation. Invest Radiol 2013;48:629–37.
21. Galbán CJ, Han MK, Boes JL, et al. Computed tomography-based biomarker provides unique signature for diagnosis of COPD phenotypes and disease progression. Nat Med 2012;18(11):1711–5.
22. Barr CC, Berkowitz EA, Bigazzi F, et al. A combined pulmonary-radiology workshop for visual evaluation of COPD: study design, chest CT findings and

concordance with quantitative evaluation. COPD 2012;9:151–9.

23. Choi S, Hoffman EA, Wenzel SE, et al. Registration-based assessment of regional lung function via volumetric CT images of normal subjects vs. severe asthmatics. J Appl Physiol (1985) 2013;115: 730–42.

24. Xu Y, van Beek EJ, Hwanjo Y, et al. Computer-aided classification of interstitial lung diseases via MDCT: 3D adaptive multiple feature method (3D AMFM). Acad Radiol 2006;13(8):969–78.

25. Kim HG, Tashkin DP, Clements PJ, et al. A computer-aided diagnosis system for quantitative scoring of extent of lung fibrosis in scleroderma patients. Clin Exp Rheumatol 2010;28:S26–35.

26. Rajaram S, Swift AJ, Telfer A, et al. 3D contrast-enhanced lung perfusion MRI is an effective screening tool for thromboembolic pulmonary hypertension: results from the ASPIRE registry. Thorax 2013;68:677–8.

27. Swift AJ, Wild J, Nagle S, et al. Quantitative MR imaging of pulmonary hypertension: a practical approach to the current state of the art. J Thorac Imaging 2014;29:68–79.

28. Edelman RR, Hatabu H, Tadamura E, et al. Noninvasive assessment of regional ventilation in the human lung using oxygen-enhanced magnetic resonance imaging. Nat Med 1996;2:1236–9.

29. Ohno Y, Iwasawa T, Seo JB, et al. Oxygen-enhanced magnetic resonance imaging versus computed tomography: multicentre study for clinical stage classification of smoking-related chronic obstructive pulmonary disease. Am J Respir Crit Care Med 2008;177:1095–102.

30. Ohno Y, Nishio M, Koyama H, et al. Asthma: comparison of dynamic oxygen-enhanced MR imaging and quantitative thin-section CT for evaluation of clinical treatment. Radiology 2014;273:907–16.

31. Wild JM, Woodhouse N, Fichele S, et al. 3D volume-localized pO2 measurement in the human lung with 3He MRI. Magn Reson Med 2005;20:1055–64.

32. De Lange EE, Altes TA, Patrie JT, et al. Changes in regional airflow obstruction over time in the lungs of patients with asthma: evaluation with 3He MR imaging. Radiology 2009;250:567–75.

33. Mugler JP 3rd, Altes TA, Ruset IC, et al. Simultaneous magnetic resonance imaging of ventilation distribution and gas uptake in the human lung using hyperpolarized xenon-129. Proc Natl Acad Sci U S A 2010;107:21707–12.

34. Couch MJ, Ball IK, Li T, et al. Pulmonary ultrashort echo time 19F MR imaging with inhaled fluorinated gas mixtures in healthy volunteers: feasibility. Radiology 2013;269:903–9.

35. Van Beek EJ, Dahmen AM, Stavngaard T, et al. Comparison of hyperpolarised 3-He MRI and HRCT in normal volunteers, patients with COPD and patients with alpha-1-antitrypsin deficiency – PHIL trial. Eur Respir J 2009;34:1–11.

36. Cho A. Helium-3 shortage could put freeze on low-temperature research. Science 2009;326:778–9.

37. Hersman FW, Ruset IC, Ketel S, et al. Large production system for hyperpolarized 129Xe for human lung imaging studies. Acad Radiol 2008;15:683–92.

38. Patz S, Muradian I, Hrovat MI, et al. Human pulmonary imaging and spectroscopy with hyperpolarized 129-Xe at 0.2T. Radiology 2008;15:713–27.

39. Patz S, Muradyan I, Hrovat MI, et al. Diffusion of hyperpolarized 129Xe in the lung: simplified model of 129Xe septal uptake & experimental results. New J Phys 2011;13:015009.

40. Kirby M, Mathew L, Heydarian M, et al. Chronic obstructive pulmonary disease: quantification of bronchodilator effects using hyperpolarized 3He MR imaging. Radiology 2011;261:283–92.

41. Samee S, Altes T, Powers P, et al. Imaging the lungs in asthmatic patients by using hyperpolarized helium-3 magnetic resonance: assessment of response to methocholine and exercise challenge. J Allergy Clin Immunol 2003;111:1205–11.

42. Woodhouse N, Wild JM, van Beek EJ, et al. Hyperpolarized 3He-MRI for the evaluation of CF therapies. J Magn Reson Imaging 2009;30:981–8.

43. Kirby M, Heydarian M, Wheatley A, et al. Evaluating bronchodilator effects in chronic obstructive pulmonary disease using diffusion-weighted hyperpolarized helium-3 magnetic resonance imaging. J Appl Physiol (1985) 2012;112:651–7.

44. Kirby M, Pike D, Coxson HO, et al. Hyperpolarized 3He ventilation defects used to predict pulmonary exacerbations in mild to moderate chronic obstructive pulmonary disease. Radiology 2014;273:887–96.

45. Ireland RH, Din O, Swinscoe JA, et al. Detection of radiation-induced lung injury in non-small cell lung cancer patients using hyperpolarized helium-3 magnetic resonance imaging. Radiother Oncol 2010;97: 244–8.

46. Ley-Zaporozhan J, Ley S, Gast KK, et al. Functional analysis in single-lung transplant recipients. A comparative study of high-resolution Ct, 3He MRI and pulmonary function tests. Chest 2004;125: 173–81.

47. Cullen SC, Gross EG. The anesthetic properties of xenon in animals and human beings, with additional observations on krypton. Science 1951;113:580–2.

48. Kong X, Sheng HX, Lu GM, et al. Xenon-enhanced dual-energy CT lung ventilation imaging: techniques and clinical applications. AJR Am J Roentgenol 2014;202(2):309–17.

49. Park EA, Goo JM, Park SJ, et al. Chronic obstructive pulmonary disease: quantitative and visual ventilation pattern analysis at xenon ventilation CT performed by using a dual-energy technique. Radiology 2010;256:985–97.

50. Chae EJ, Seo JB, Lee J, et al. Xenon ventilation imaging using dual-energy computed tomography in asthmatics: initial experience. Invest Radiol 2010; 45:354–61.

51. Goo HW, Yang DH, Hong SJ, et al. Xenon ventilation CT using dual-source and dual-energy technique in children with bronchiolitis obliterans: correlation of xenon and CT density values with pulmonary function test results. Pediatr Radiol 2010;40:1490–7.

52. Kang MJ, Park CM, Lee CH, et al. Dual-energy CT: clinical applications in various pulmonary diseases. Radiographics 2010;30(3):685–98.

53. Karçaaltıncaba M, Aktaş A. Dual-energy CT revisited with multidetector CT: review of principles and clinical applications. Diagn Interv Radiol 2011;17(3): 181–94.

54. Gould RG. Perfusion quantitation by ultrafast computed tomography. Invest Radiol 1992;27: S18–21.

55. Allmendinger AM, Tang ER, Lui YW, et al. Imaging of stroke: part 1, Perfusion CT—overview of imaging technique, interpretation pearls, and common pitfalls. Am J Roentgenol 2012;198(1):52–62.

56. Aksoy FG, Lev MH. Dynamic contrast-enhanced brain perfusion imaging: technique and clinical applications. Semin Ultrasound CT MR 2000;21(6): 462–77.

57. Brix G, Zwick S, Griebel J, et al. Estimation of tissue perfusion by dynamic contrast-enhanced imaging: simulation-based evaluation of the steepest slope method. Eur Radiol 2010;20(9):2166–75.

58. Miles KA, Griffiths MR, Fuentes MA. Standardized perfusion value: universal CT contrast enhancement scale that correlates with FDG PET in lung nodules. Radiology 2001;220:548–53.

59. Miles KA, Griffiths MR. Perfusion CT: a worthwhile enhancement? Br J Radiol 2003;76(904):220–31.

60. Kostler H, Ritter C, Lipp M, et al. Prebolus quantitative MR heart perfusion imaging. Magn Reson Med 2004;52:296–9.

61. Puderbach M, Risse F, Biederer J, et al. In vivo Gd-DTPA concentration for MR lung perfusion measurements: assessment with computed tomography in a porcine model. Eur Radiol 2008;18(10):2102–7.

62. Fink C, Johnson TR, Michaely HJ, et al. Dual-energy CT angiography of the lung in patients with suspected pulmonary embolism: initial results. Rofo 2008;180(10):879–83.

63. Thieme SF, Becker CR, Hacker M, et al. Dual energy CT for the assessment of lung perfusion: correlation to scintigraphy. Eur J Radiol 2008;68(3):369–74.

64. Ohno Y, Koyama H, Matsumoto K, et al. Dynamic MR perfusion imaging: capability for quantitative assessment of disease extent and prediction of outcome for patients with acute pulmonary thromboembolism. J Magn Reson Imaging 2010;31(5): 1081–90.

65. Pena E, Dennie C, Veinot J, et al. Pulmonary hypertension: how the radiologist can help. Radiographics 2012;32:9–32.

66. Tsai IC, Tsai WL, Wang KY, et al. Comprehensive MDCT evaluation of patients with pulmonary hypertension: diagnosing underlying causes with the updated Dana Point 2008 classification. Am J Roentgenol 2011;197:W471–81.

67. Helmberger M, Pienn M, Urschler M, et al. Quantification of tortuosity and fractal dimension of the lung vessels in pulmonary hypertension patients. PLoS One 2014;9:e87515.

68. Reiter G, Reiter U, Kovacs G, et al. Magnetic resonance-derived 3-dimensional blood flow patterns in the main pulmonary artery as a marker of pulmonary hypertension and a measure of elevated mean pulmonary arterial pressure. Circ Cardiovasc Imaging 2008;1(1):23–30.

69. Ley S, Fink C, Ley-Zaporozhan J, et al. Value of high spatial and high temporal resolution magnetic resonance angiography for differentiation between idiopathic and thromboembolic pulmonary hypertension: initial results. Eur Radiol 2005;15:2256–63.

70. Hoey ET, Mirsadraee S, Pepke-Zaba J, et al. Dual-energy CT angiography for assessment of regional pulmonary perfusion in patients with chronic thromboembolic pulmonary hypertension: initial experience. AJR Am J Roentgenol 2011;196(3):524–32.

71. Hong YJ, Kim JY, Choe KO, et al. Different perfusion pattern between acute and chronic pulmonary thromboembolism: evaluation with two-phase dual-energy perfusion CT. AJR Am J Roentgenol 2013; 200(4):812–7.

72. Ohno Y, Hatabu H, Murase K, et al. Primary pulmonary hypertension: 3D dynamic perfusion MRI for quantitative analysis of regional pulmonary perfusion. AJR Am J Roentgenol 2007;188(1):48–56.

73. Barr RG, Mesia-Vela S, Austin JH, et al. Impaired flow-mediated dilation is associated with low pulmonary function and emphysema in ex-smokers: the Emphysema and Cancer Action Project (EMCAP) Study. Am J Respir Crit Care Med 2007; 176:1200–7.

74. Kanazawa H, Asai K, Hirata K, et al. Possible effects of vascular endothelial growth factor in the pathogenesis of chronic obstructive pulmonary disease. Am J Med 2003;114:354–8.

75. McAllister DA, Maclay JD, Mills NL, et al. Arterial stiffness is independently associated with emphysema severity in patients with chronic obstructive pulmonary disease. Am J Respir Crit Care Med 2007;176:1208–14.

76. Alford SK, van Beek EJ, McLennan G, et al. Heterogeneity of pulmonary perfusion as a mechanistic image-based phenotype in emphysema susceptible smokers. Proc Natl Acad Sci U S A 2010;107(16): 7485–90.

77. Morrison NJ, Abboud RT, Müller NL, et al. Pulmonary capillary blood volume in emphysema. Am Rev Respir Dis 1990;141(1):53–61.

78. Barberà JA, Riverola A, Roca J, et al. Pulmonary vascular abnormalities and ventilation-perfusion relationships in mild chronic obstructive pulmonary disease. Am J Respir Crit Care Med 1994;149(2 Pt 1):423–9.

79. Pansini V, Remy-Jardin M, Faivre JB, et al. Assessment of lobar perfusion in smokers according to the presence and severity of emphysema: preliminary experience with dual-energy CT angiography. Eur Radiol 2009;19(12):2834–43.

80. Magro CM, Allen J, Pope-Harman A, et al. The role of microvascular injury in the evolution of idiopathic pulmonary fibrosis. Am J Clin Pathol 2003;119(4): 556–67.

81. Kim BH, Seo JB, Chae EJ, et al. Analysis of perfusion defects by causes other than acute pulmonary thromboembolism on contrast-enhanced dual-energy CT in consecutive 537 patients. Eur J Radiol 2012;81(4):e647–52.

82. Sergiacomi G, Bolacchi F, Cadioli M, et al. Combined pulmonary fibrosis and emphysema: 3D time-resolved MR angiographic evaluation of pulmonary arterial mean transit time and time to peak enhancement. Radiology 2010;254(2):601–8.

83. Ohno Y, Koyama H, Matsumoto K, et al. Differentiation of malignant and benign pulmonary nodules with quantitative first-pass 320-detector row perfusion CT versus FDG PET/CT. Radiology 2011; 258(2):599–609.

84. Schaefer JF, Vollmar J, Schick F, et al. Solitary pulmonary nodules: dynamic contrast-enhanced MR imaging– differences in malignant and benign lesions. Radiology 2004;232:544–53.

85. Dean PB, Niemi P, Kivisaari L, et al. Comparative pharmacokinetics of gadolinium DTPA and gadolinium chloride. Invest Radiol 1988;23(Suppl 1): S258–60.

86. Milne EN, Noonan CD, Margulis AR, et al. Vascular supply of pulmonary metastases: experimental study in rats. Invest Radiol 1969;4:215–29.

87. Milne EN, Zerhouni EA. Blood supply of pulmonary metastases. J Thorac Imaging 1987;2:15–23.

Index

Clin Chest Med 36 (2015) 365–372
http://dx.doi.org/10.1016/S0272-5231(15)00046-5
0272-5231/15/$ – see front matter © 2015 Elsevier Inc. All rights reserved.

Printed and bound by CPI Group (UK) Ltd, Croydon, CR0 4YY

03/10/2024

01040378-0006